1993
YEAR BOOK OF
NEUROLOGY AND
NEUROSURGERY®

Statement of Purpose

The YEAR BOOK Service

The YEAR BOOK series was devised in 1901 by practicing health professionals who observed that the literature of medicine and related disciplines had become so voluminous that no one individual could read and place in perspective every potential advance in a major specialty. In the final decade of the 20th century, this recognition is more acutely true than it was in 1901.

More than merely a series of books, YEAR BOOK volumes are the tangible results of a unique service designed to accomplish the following:

- to *survey* a wide range of journals of proven value
- to *select* from those journals papers representing significant advances and statements of important clinical principles
- to provide *abstracts* of those articles that are readable, convenient summaries of their key points
- to provide *commentary* about those articles to place them in perspective.

These publications grow out of a unique process that calls on the talents of outstanding authorities in clinical and fundamental disciplines, trained literature specialists, and professional writers, all supported by the resources of Mosby, the world's preeminent publisher for the health professions.

The Literature Base

Mosby subscribes to nearly 1,000 journals published worldwide, covering the full range of the health professions. On an annual basis, the publisher examines usage patterns and polls its expert authorities to add new journals to the literature base and to delete journals that are no longer useful as potential Year Book sources.

The Literature Survey

The publisher's team of literature specialists, all of whom are trained and experienced health professionals, examines every original, peer-reviewed article in each journal issue. More than 250,000 articles per year are scanned systematically, including title, text, illustrations, tables, and references. Each scan is compared, article by article, to the search strategies that the publisher has developed in consultation with the 270 outside experts who form the pool of Year Book editors. A given article may be reviewed by any number of editors, from one to a dozen or more, regardless of the discipline for which the paper was originally published. In turn, each editor who receives the article reviews it to determine whether or not the article should be included in the Year Book . This decision is based on the article's inherent quality, its probable usefulness to readers of that Year Book , and the editor's goal to represent a balanced picture of a given field in each volume of the Year Book . In addition, the editor indicates when to include figures and tables from the article to help the Year Book reader better understand the information.

Of the quarter million articles scanned each year, only 5% are selected for detailed analysis within the Year Book series, thereby assuring readers of the high value of every selection.

The Abstract

The publisher's abstracting staff is headed by a physician-writer and includes individuals with training in the life sciences, medicine, and other areas, plus extensive experience in writing for the health professions and related industries. Each selected article is assigned to a specific writer on this abstracting staff. The abstracter, guided in many cases by notations supplied by the expert editor, writes a structured, condensed summary designed so that the reader can rapidly acquire the essential information contained in the article.

The Commentary

The Year Book editorial boards, sometimes assisted by guest commentators, write comments that place each article in perspective for the reader. This provides the reader with the equivalent of a personal consultation with a leading international authority—an opportunity to better understand the value of the article and to benefit from the authority's thought processes in assessing the article.

Additional Editorial Features

The editorial boards of each Year Book organize the abstracts and comments to provide a logical and satisfying sequence of information. To enhance the organization, editors also provide introductions to sections or individual chapters, comments linking a number of abstracts, citations to additional literature, and other features.

The published Year Book contains enhanced bibliographic citations for each selected article, including extended listings of multiple authors and identification of author affiliations. Each Year Book contains a Table of Contents specific to that year's volume. From year to year, the Table of Contents for a given Year Book will vary depending on developments within the field.

Every Year Book contains a list of the journals from which papers have been selected. This list represents a subset of the nearly 1,000 journals surveyed by the publisher, and occasionally reflects a particularly pertinent article from a journal that is not surveyed on a routine basis.

Finally, each volume contains a comprehensive subject index and an index to authors of each selected paper.

The 1993 Year Book® Series

Year Book of Anesthesia and Pain Management: Drs. Miller, Abram, Kirby, Ostheimer, Roizen, and Stoelting

Year Book of Cardiology®: Drs. Schlant, Collins, Engle, Gersh, Kaplan, and Waldo

Year Book of Chiropractic: Drs. Phillips and Adams

Year Book of Critical Care Medicine®: Drs. Rogers and Parrillo

Year Book of Dentistry®: Drs. Meskin, Currier, Kennedy, Leinfelder, Berry, Roser, and Zakariasen

Year Book of Dermatologic Surgery: Drs. Swanson, Salasche, and Glogau

Year Book of Dermatology®: Drs. Sober and Fitzpatrick

Year Book of Diagnostic Radiology®: Drs. Federle, Clark, Gross, Madewell, Maynard, Sackett, and Young

Year Book of Digestive Disease®: Drs. Greenberger and Moody

Year Book of Drug Therapy®: Drs. Lasagna and Weintraub

Year Book of Emergency Medicine®: Drs. Wagner, Burdick, Davidson, Roberts, and Spivey

Year Book of Endocrinology®: Drs. Bagdade, Braverman, Horton, Kannan, Landsberg, Molitch, Morley, Odell, Rogol, Ryan, and Sherwin

Year Book of Family Practice®: Drs. Berg, Bowman, Davidson, Dietrich, and Scherger

Year Book of Geriatrics and Gerontology®: Drs. Beck, Reuben, Burton, Small, Whitehouse, and Goldstein

Year Book of Hand Surgery®: Drs. Amadio and Hentz

Year Book of Health Care Management: Drs. Heyssel, Brock, Moses, and Steinberg, Ms. Avakian, and Messrs. Berman, Kues, and Rosenberg

Year Book of Hematology®: Drs. Spivak, Bell, Ness, Quesenberry, and Wiernik

Year Book of Infectious Diseases®: Drs. Wolff, Barza, Keusch, Klempner, and Snydman

Year Book of Infertility: Drs. Mishell, Paulsen, and Lobo

Year Book of Medicine®: Drs. Rogers, Bone, Cline, O'Rourke, Greenberger, Utiger, Epstein, and Malawista

Year Book of Neonatal and Perinatal Medicine®: Drs. Klaus and Fanaroff

Year Book of Nephrology: Drs. Coe, Favus, Henderson, Kashgarian, Luke, Myers, and Curtis

Year Book of Neurology and Neurosurgery®: Drs. Bradley and Crowell

Year Book of Neuroradiology: Drs. Osborn, Eskridge, Harnsberger, and Grossman

Year Book of Nuclear Medicine®: Drs. Hoffer, Gore, Gottschalk, Zaret, and Zubal

Year Book of Obstetrics and Gynecology®: Drs. Mishell, Kirschbaum, and Morrow

Year Book of Occupational and Environmental Medicine: Drs. Emmett, Brooks, Frank, and Hammad

Year Book of Oncology®: Drs. Young, Longo, Ozols, Simone, Steele, and Glatstein

Year Book of Ophthalmology®: Drs. Laibson, Adams, Augsburger, Benson, Cohen, Eagle, Flanagan, Nelson, Rapuano, Reinecke, Sergott, and Wilson

Year Book of Orthopedics®: Drs. Sledge, Poss, Cofield, Frymoyer, Griffin, Hansen, Johnson, Simmons, and Springfield

Year Book of Otolaryngology–Head and Neck Surgery®: Drs. Holt and Paparella

Year Book of Pathology and Clinical Pathology®: Drs. Gardner, Bennett, Cousar, Garvin, and Worsham

Year Book of Pediatrics®: Dr. Stockman

Year Book of Plastic, Reconstructive, and Aesthetic Surgery: Drs. Miller, Cohen, McKinney, Robson, Ruberg, and Whitaker

Year Book of Podiatric Medicine and Surgery®: Dr. Kominsky

Year Book of Psychiatry and Applied Mental Health®: Drs. Talbott, Frances, Freedman, Meltzer, Perry, Schowalter, and Yudofsky

Year Book of Pulmonary Disease®: Drs. Bone and Petty

Year Book of Sports Medicine®: Drs. Shephard, Eichner, Sutton, and Torg, Col. Anderson, and Mr. George

Year Book of Surgery®: Drs. Copeland, Deitch, Eberlein, Howard, Ritchie, Robson, Souba, and Sugarbaker

Year Book of Transplantation®: Drs. Ascher, Hansen, and Strom

Year Book of Ultrasound: Drs. Merritt, Mittelstaedt, Carroll, Babcock, and Goldstein

Year Book of Urology®: Drs. Gillenwater and Howards

Year Book of Vascular Surgery®: Dr. Porter

Roundsmanship® '93–'94: A Student's Survival Guide to Clinical Medicine Using Current Literature: Drs. Dan, Feigin, Quilligan, Schrock, Stein, and Talbott

1993

The Year Book of NEUROLOGY AND NEUROSURGERY®

"Published without interruption since 1902"

Neurology

Editor

Walter G. Bradley, D.M., F.R.C.P.

Professor and Chairman, Department of Neurology, University of Miami School of Medicine, Miami, Florida

Neurosurgery

Editor

Robert M. Crowell, M.D.

Director of Cerebrovascular Surgery, Massachusetts General Hospital and Harvard Medical School, Boston, Massachusetts

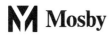 Mosby

St. Louis Baltimore Boston Chicago London Philadelphia Sydney Toronto

Editor-in-Chief, Year Book Publishing: Kenneth H. Killion
Associate Acquisitions Editor: Gretchen C. Templeton
Sponsoring Editor: Linda Steiner
Manager, Literature Services: Edith M. Podrazik
Senior Information Specialist: Terri Santo
Senior Medical Writer: David A. Cramer, M.D.
Assistant Director, Manuscript Services: Frances M. Perveiler
Associate Managing Editor, Year Book Editing Services: Connie Murray
Senior Production/Desktop Publishing Manager: Max F. Perez
Proofroom Manager: Barbara M. Kelly

Editorial Office:
Mosby
200 North LaSalle St.
Chicago, IL 60601

International Standard Serial Number: 0513-5117
International Standard Book Number: 0-8151-2142-3

Contributing Editors

Associate Editors

Joseph Berger, M.D.
Professor of Neurology, Department of Neurology, University of Miami School of Medicine, Miami, Florida

John Blass, M.D., Ph.D.
Professor of Neurology, The Burke Rehabilitation Center, White Plains, New York

Robert Davidoff, M.D.
Professor of Neurology, Department of Neurology, University of Miami School of Medicine, Miami, Florida

Gerald Fenichel, M.D.
Professor and Chairman of Neurology, Department of Neurology, Vanderbilt University School of Medicine, Nashville, Tennessee

Albert M. Galaburda, M.D.
Associate Professor of Neurology; Director, Dyslexia Neuroanatomical Laboratory, Beth Israel Hospital, Boston, Massachusetts

Myron D. Ginsberg, M.D.
Professor and Vice-Chairman of Neurology; Director of Cerebral Vascular Disease, Research Center and Neurotrauma Clinical Research Center, University of Miami School of Medicine, Miami, Florida

Jerome D. Posner, M.D.
Chairman and Professor of Neurology Department, Memorial Sloan-Kettering Cancer Center, New York, New York

Robert M. Quencer, M.D.
Professor of Radiology, Neurological Surgery, and Ophthalmology; Director, Division of Magnetic Resonance Imaging, University of Miami School of Medicine, Miami, Florida

Eugene R. Ramsay, M.D.
Professor of Neurology, Department of Neurology, University of Miami School of Medicine, Miami, Florida

Peter Spencer, M.D., Ph.D.
Professor of Neurology, Oregon Health Sciences University School of Medicine, Portland, Oregon

Subramaniam Sriram, M.D.
Associate Professor of Neurology, Department of Neurology, University Health Center, University of Vermont College of Medicine, Burlington, Vermont

David Stumpf, M.D., Ph.D.
Benjamin and Virginia T. Boshes Professor of Neurology; Chairman, Department of Neurology, Professor of Pediatrics, Northwestern University Medical School, Chicago, Illinois

William Weiner, M.D.
Professor of Neurology, Department of Neurology, University of Miami School of Medicine, Miami, Florida

Special Article Contributors

Dalia M. Araujo, Ph.D.
Department of Gerontology, University of Southern California, Ethel Percy Andrus Gerontology Center, Los Angeles, California
Phillip F. Chance, M.D.
Assistant Professor of Pediatrics, Division of Medical Genetics and the MDA Muscle Clinic, University of Utah Medical Center, Salt Lake City, Utah
Franz Hefti, Ph.D.
Department of Gerontology, University of Southern California, Ethel Percy Andrus Gerontology Center, Los Angeles, California
Donald R. Johns, M.D.
Assistant Professor of Neurology, Johns Hopkins University School of Medicine, Baltimore, Maryland
Paul A. Lapchak, Ph.D.
Department of Gerontology, University of Southern California, Ethel Percy Andrus Gerontology Center, Los Angeles, California

Table of Contents

Journals Represented

Mosby subscribes to and surveys nearly 900 U.S. and foreign medical and allied health journals. From these journals, the Editors select the articles to be abstracted. Journals represented in this YEAR BOOK are listed below.

Acta Neurochirurgica
Acta Neurologica Scandinavica
Acta Paediatrica Scandinavica
American Journal of Human Genetics
American Journal of Neuroradiology
American Journal of Roentgenology
American Journal of Surgery
Annals of Internal Medicine
Annals of Neurology
Annals of Otology, Rhinology and Laryngology
Annals of Vascular Surgery
Archives of General Psychiatry
Archives of Internal Medicine
Archives of Neurology
Arthritis and Rheumatism
Australian and New Zealand Journal of Medicine
Behavior Research and Therapy
Brain
Brain Topography
Brain and Cognition
British Journal of Radiology
British Journal of Surgery
British Medical Journal
Canadian Journal of Neurological Sciences
Canadian Journal of Psychiatry
Cancer
Cancer Research
Circulation
Clinical Genetics
Clinical Orthopaedics and Related Research
Cortex
Critical Care Medicine
Developmental Medicine and Child Neurology
European Journal of Cancer
European Journal of Vascular Surgery
European Neurology
Headache
Italian Journal of Neurological Sciences
Journal of Acquired Immune Deficiency Syndromes
Journal of Bone and Joint Surgery (American Volume)
Journal of Cardiovascular Surgery
Journal of Clinical Epidemiology
Journal of Clinical Investigation
Journal of Clinical and Experimental Neuropsychology
Journal of Computer Assisted Tomography
Journal of Neurology
Journal of Neurology, Neurosurgery and Psychiatry
Journal of Neuropsychiatry and Clinical Neurosciences
Journal of Neurosurgery
Journal of Pediatric Orthopedics

Journal of Pediatric Surgery
Journal of Reproductive Medicine
Journal of Vascular Surgery
Journal of Western Pacific Orthopaedic Association
Journal of the American College of Cardiology
Journal of the American Medical Association
Journal of the American Podiatric Medical Association
Journal of the National Center Institute
Journal of the Neurological Sciences
Lancet
Mayo Clinic Proceedings
Medical Journal of Australia
Muscle and Nerve
Nature
Neuro-Chirurgie
Neurology
Neuropathology and Applied Neurobiology
Neuropediatrics
Neuropsychiatry, Neuropsychology and Behavioral Neurology
Neuropsychologia
Neuroradiology
Neurosurgery
New England Journal of Medicine
Obstetrics and Gynecology
Pain
Pediatrics
Psychological Medicine
Quarterly Journal of Medicine
Radiology
Schweizerische Medizinische Wochenschrift
Science
Seminars in Thrombosis and Hemostasis
Spine
Stroke
Surgical Neurology

STANDARD ABBREVIATIONS

The following terms are abbreviated in this edition: acquired immunodeficiency syndrome (AIDS), central nervous system (CNS), cerebrospinal fluid (CSF), computed tomography (CT), electrocardiography (ECG), electroencephalogram (EEG), human immunodeficiency virus (HIV), and magnetic resonance (MR) imaging (MRI).

Publisher's Preface

As Publishers, we feel challenged to seek ways of presenting complex information in a clear and readable manner. To this end, the 1993 YEAR BOOK OF NEUROLOGY AND NEUROSURGERY now provides structured abstracts in which the various components of a study can easily be identified through headings. These headings are not the same in all abstracts, but rather are those that most accurately designate the content of each particular journal article. We are confident that our readers will find the information contained in our abstracts to be more accessible than ever before. We welcome your comments.

NEUROLOGY

Walter G. Bradley, D.M., F.R.C.P.

Introduction

In the 91 years since the publication of the first YEAR BOOK containing neurologic literature, there have been 20 editors, including such illustrious names as Roland McKay, Percival Bailey, Russell DeJong, and Robert Currier. Now, after 10 years of editing the Neurology section of the YEAR BOOK OF NEUROLOGY AND NEUROSURGERY, Robert Currier is stepping down, and it is time to wish him much happiness in his very active retirement and to mention some of his many contributions. In reviewing Bob Currier's editorial introductions to the YEAR BOOK OF NEUROLOGY AND NEUROSURGERY again, I am struck by his common sense, his folksy style, his deep interest in the history and personalities of neurology, and his recurring concern for the question of whether we are producing enough or too many neurologists in the United States.

Neurology Training Programs in the United States

My own views on the question of the supply of neurologists in the United States are colored by my experience. I trained in Britain, where there are about 120 neurologists for some 60 million people, or one neurologist for every 500,000 of the population. Hence, in Britain, neurologists select their patients most carefully and tend to be referred only the difficult and esoteric diagnostic and management problems. British neurologists work at a much more rapid pace than do those in the United States. In Britain, in a half day I would see up to 15 new patients and 25 follow-up patients, visit the patients in a 16-bed neurologic rehabilitation unit, and do neurologic consultations in a 200-bed general hospital. This pace of work provided an enormous breadth of experience in neurologic disease. However, it also imposed its own limits. As one of my British neurologic colleagues once said, "I could not possibly look after patients with strokes! I haven't enough beds or time!"

Neurology as practiced in the United States is very different from that in Britain. First, I must reveal my prejudice that it is appropriate that *all* neurologic disease should be managed by neurologists. Second, it is a joy to spend 1 hour with a new patient, obtaining the nuances of the history, getting to know the detailed background of the patient, and explaining the important features of the diagnosis and management to the patient and family. The acceptance of these principles explains why we have almost 8,000 practicing neurologists in the United States for nearly 260 million people, approximately 1 neurologist per 32,500 of the population.

However, there still remains the lingering question whether we are training too many neurologists. After two "Manpower Retreats" arranged by the Association of University Professors of Neurology and deliberations by several committees of the American Academy of Neurology, there is still no clear answer. The predictions of Matthew Menkin that the continuing graduation of 300 or so neurologists each year will greatly increase the total number of practicing neurologists is likely to be correct. Nevertheless, Mark Dyken and many others emphasize that there continue to be many areas of the country crying out for neurologists. The excess concentration of all medical specialists on the east and west coasts and around the Great Lakes counterbalances these other areas of need.

Neurologists have increasingly taken over the care of all neurologic disease from internists, which helps to explain the increased number of neurologists in the United States. Unfortunately, this has been accompanied by a gradual decrease in the internal medicine community in terms of competency in neurology and comfort with neurologic problems. This is partly a result of the decreased amount of neurologic training received by internal medicine residents.

In my judgment, of greater concern than the number of neurologists is the question of the quality of graduates from neurologic residency programs in the United States. The majority of such graduates spend only three years in training. For someone trained in Britain, where it takes 10–15 years after medical school graduation to achieve Consultant (Attending) Neurologist status, it is astounding that a neurologist can be fully trained in only three years. Learning continues from birth to the grave, but there is clearly a good deal to be learned after the end of the three-year residency!

A crucial and unanswered question concerns the standard of today's neurology graduates compared with those of 10 or 20 years ago. The number of neurology residency positions in the United States has steadily increased, more in relation to work load than to educational requirements. The competition for neurology residency positions has steadily decreased, and there are now fewer applicants than there are positions available. Although some of the brightest minds still go into neurology, I ascribe to the widely held belief that the average standard of the graduating neurology resident is progressively worsening. The neurologic profession in the United States needs to police itself in the same way that the neurosurgeons did many years ago. We need to improve the quality and competitiveness of neurology training by rigorously applying criteria of excellence both to the incoming resident candidate and to the training program.

Crisis in Health Care Funding

The problem of the supply of neurologists may seem relatively minor when we consider the problems of the United States health care system as a whole. Nearly 90% of the population of the United States is dissatisfied with the system and believes that it needs to be changed. No one can be happy with a system that fails to provide adequate care to 40 million individuals, that can potentially bankrupt another 40 million if they have a major illness, and that can destroy the life savings of almost everyone needing long-term institutional care. This United States health care system, which used to be the envy of the world, now costs more than 12% of the gross national product. The rate of increase of health care costs is more than twice that for all other commodities.

We have now reached a situation in which neither the government nor commercial insurers can afford the full cost of health care. Hence, they are putting more of the expenses onto the individuals and the employers, while decreasing the extent of reimbursement to health care providers. Employers and industry are being destroyed by the increasing health insurance premiums for their workers. For many firms, these premiums now gobble up between one third and one half of their profit margin. In turn, employers are trying to pass on some of the health insurance premiums to their workers. This is occurring at a time when both employers and workers are suffering increasingly from the economic recession. Bankruptcies, closures of businesses, unemployment, and industrial strife are the consequences. Large employers in the health care arena, such as hospitals and medical schools, are having to react to the same escalating health insurance premiums for their employees, which leads both to employee stress and to a vicious cycle of increased health care fees.

What is the cause of these spiraling health care costs in the United States? The finger can be pointed at many causes. The cost of administration and regulatory controls may be as high as 30% compared with Canada, where it is less than 5%. This regulatory superstructure was introduced by the United States government to reduce health care expenditures. It has probably been counterproductive with regard to total costs, and it certainly has impaired the quality of service and life for patients and health care providers alike. On the one hand, high technology advances have considerably improved the quality of life and diagnostic capabilities for patients, but the costs of technology have added greatly to the inflation of health care costs. The tort system, with resultant defensive medicine and high malpractice premiums, also increases health care costs, perhaps by 10% to 20% according to some estimates.

Entrepreneurship remains the backbone of the United States and the capitalist system. It has been responsible for most of the technological and therapeutic advances that distinguish medical treatment today from that of 30 years ago. However, entrepreneurship in the delivery of medical diagnosis and care may be responsible for a significant part of the increase in the number of health care services provided and, hence, in health care costs, although there is little reliable information on this point. It is widely believed that doctors with financial involvement in diagnostic facilities to which they refer usually request several more diagnostic procedures than do those doctors with no such financial involvement.

Perhaps of even greater significance to the health care budget is the high level of expectation of patients and physicians in the United States. This is particularly striking to anyone like me who has practiced outside of the United States. In the United States, the physician and the patient share in the belief that *every attempt* must be made to preserve life, whatever the costs and consequences. Marketplace economics clearly do not apply to the health care industry. If it is *your health,* you are prepared to spend any amount to regain it! If a doctor says that twice as many tests or a new expensive test is going to help, the patient is generally not sufficiently sophisticated to raise the questions of cost-effectiveness or to consider the national need for cost containment. To physicians coming from outside the United States, at times this looks like gross profligacy.

How can we get the spiraling costs of health care under control? How can this be achieved in a way acceptable to the American public, patients, and doctors, and how can it be achieved through the American political process at a time of severe budgetary constraints? It seems clear that health care reform will be an important issue in the next year or two in the United States. However, I have difficulty in believing that the outcome will be a clear and universally acceptable plan to correct all of the ills of our current health care system. The political process desperately needs input from those of us who see the problems and needs. Neurologists, by virtue of their role in some of the most life-threatening (and life-terminating) diseases have a potentially unique insight. The collective voice of neurologists could help direct the health care revolution that is coming.

Many are calling for the adoption of universal health insurance, rather like that in Canada. Although this would be an answer to the problem of those who are currently uninsured and also might answer questions about the cost of administration, it would do little to control costs. Canada is currently suffering a rate of inflation of health care costs similar to that of the United States, and the Canadian provinces are attempting to introduce a variety of controls to limit the provision of services and the number of physicians in the system. Socialized medicine with salaried physicians and universal health coverage might seem to be the ideal, but this removes the entrepreneurial drive to improve technology, quality of care, and treatment. Moreover, in a socialized system, the government regulation of total expenditure on health care is politically driven rather than responsive to the needs of patient care. This leads to impossible swings of funding for health care at the patient level.

What is needed is a totally new way of looking at the provision of medical care, its regulation, and its financing. We need a strong, well-funded primary care (family doctor) service throughout the country. We need a new system of budgeting that will make the public and physicians equally responsible for prioritization and choice in the use of the much restricted dollars that will be available for health care. We should regionalize this decisional process to make it responsive to local needs. We must develop an educational process for the public and health care professions that will make our expectations rational and our decisions cost-effective.

Neuroscience Advances in the Third Year of the Decade of the Brain

Congress declared the 1990s as the Decade of the Brain. In doing so, it responded to the clear belief of the leaders of the neurologic community that this decade will see an explosion of knowledge in the basic neurosciences and in our understanding and ability to treat neurologic disease. This explosion of information will result from new techniques of molecular neurobiology, especially those based on genes, namely the discipline of molecular genetics. Unfortunately, the congressional declaration has not resulted in significant new monies being directed to neuroscience research. Rather, there has simply been a shifting around of existing money. The competition for research dollars becomes ever stiffer, with increasing time and effort wasted on writing unsuccessful grant proposals. If we wish to see this changed, we shall have to accept cutbacks in other programs or new taxes. An improvement in the economy might help put more dollars into neuroscience research, reverse this trend, and rekindle the fire that is beginning to sputter in the neurosciences.

Nevertheless, the expansion of our current understanding of the workings of the nervous system seems to be exponential. Advances in neurobiology have steadily accumulated during the past decade, and a recent rapid growth has come from the new field of molecular genetics. The selections for this YEAR BOOK OF NEUROLOGY AND NEUROSURGERY include a number of such papers, and I have also introduced a new section of invited reviews to broaden the presentations for the reader. Three excellent reviews are provided by Dr. Franz Hefti and his colleagues on neurotrophic factors, by Dr. Phillip Chance on recent advances in molecular genetics in the field of nuclear DNA, and by Dr. Donald Johns on diseases associated with abnormalities of mitochondrial DNA.

The Neurologic Literature in Review

The basis of the YEAR BOOK OF NEUROLOGY AND NEUROSURGERY is the review of some of the most important papers published in the world's literature over the previous year. The selection of these papers and the editorial comments that provide a brief analysis of each paper require an expertise beyond that of one person. For this reason, I have invited 12 Associate Editors to assist me in the selection and review of the papers: Dr. Joseph Berger for the neurologic complications of general medical diseases, including AIDS; Dr. John Blass for neurorehabilitation; Dr. Robert Davidoff for headaches and pain; Dr. Gerald Fenichel for pediatric neurology; Dr. Albert Galaburda for behavioral neurology; Dr. Myron Ginsberg for cerebral vascular disease; Dr. Jerome Posner for neuro-oncology; Dr. Robert Quencer for neuroimaging; Dr. Eugene Ramsay for epilepsy and central electrophysiology; Dr. Peter Spencer for neurotoxicology; Dr. Subramaniam Sriram for neuroimmunology and multiple sclerosis; and Dr. William Weiner for movement disorders. The quality of the material in the 1993 YEAR BOOK OF NEUROLOGY AND NEUROSURGERY is in large part a result of their selfless efforts.

Walter G. Bradley, D.M., F.R.C.P.

The Role of Molecular Genetics in Clinical Neurology: Recent Advances

PHILLIP F. CHANCE, M.D.*

Assistant Professor of Pediatrics, Division of Medical Genetics and the MDA Muscle Clinic, University of Utah Medical Center, Salt Lake City, Utah

Taken individually, most neurogenetic disorders are rare; however, collectively they constitute an important and frequently encountered group of diseases in both pediatric and adult neurology. Approximately one third of known human disease phenotypes involve the nervous system, as is revealed by scanning the approximately 3,000 disorders listed in Dr. Victor A. McKusick's *Mendelian Inheritance in Man*. Additionally, there is strong evidence that the majority of the human genome may encode proteins and polypeptides required for normal development and maintenance of function of the nervous system. Studies of rodent-brain messenger RNA populations have determined that approximately two thirds of the RNAs are neuron-specific. In theory, then, by analogy to rodent studies, mutations affecting any two-thirds of an estimated 50,000–100,000 human genes could produce clinical neurogenetic conditions.

Given the sheer number of neurogenetic disorders and their frequent occurrence, it is not surprising that, among medical disciplines, neurology has benefited heavily by the introduction of molecular genetic methodology. Still, the biochemical abnormalities at the protein level remain unknown in the majority of genetic neurologic disorders. Rational therapy for most neurogenetic conditions will await the elucidation of a protein abnormality and the successful reintroduction of a normally functioning protein into the patient.

During the past decade, the application of molecular biologic techniques, including genetic mapping of diseases to specific chromosomes and positional gene cloning, has brought about a genesis in neurology. Through positional cloning, also known as "reverse genetics," it is possible to localize the position of a genetic disorder by linkage analysis or, in some instances, cytogenetic studies to a particular chromosomal region and then search that region for candidate genes relating to the condition of interest. After successful gene isolation, the DNA and amino acid sequences can be determined in the normal and abnormal genes. Using a computer database, the sequence information can be compared to that of known proteins, providing clues as to the nature of function of the normal and mutant proteins. This approach sharply contrasts that of time-honored methods in which the mutant protein first must be identified, its amino acid sequence determined, and then the DNA sequence isolated. The power of positional cloning lies in the ability to identify and characterize abnormal proteins in disorders with unknown biochemical defects. Triumphs of positional cloning strategies in neurologic diseases include Duchenne and Becker muscular dystrophies, neurofibromatosis I, and, more recently, myotonic dystrophy.

* Dr. Chance receives support from the Muscular Dystrophy Association, the March of Dimes (Basil O'Connor Starter Scholar Research Award, 5-667) and the NINDS (Clinical Investigator Development Award, NSO1341).

Historically, without knowledge of specific protein or molecular genetic abnormalities, most studies of clinical neurogenetic disorders remained descriptive and focused on the clinical sorting-out, known as nosology. The clinical nosology continues, but with the much greater precision now afforded by the tools of molecular biology. Are there other immediate benefits to clinical neurology that result from the application of molecular methods to neurogenetic problems? There are numerous benefits, including methods for improved accuracy of diagnosis and greater certainty of genetic counseling given to patients and their families. The loci of virtually all the major neurogenetic disorders have now been assigned to a specific chromosome, and for a few diseases the mutant gene has been isolated. Therefore, something can be offered to almost any patient with a neurogenetic illness, whether it be an examination of their DNA with a specific gene probe to confirm a suspected diagnosis, or the application of probes to other family members to determine their disease status. General reviews outlining recombinant DNA strategies in neurologic disorders may be found elsewhere (1, 2).

During the past year, 2 new and exciting molecular mechanisms causing neurologic disorders have been described. These mechanisms include the inheritance of unstable trinucleotide repeat regions in myotonic dystrophy and fragile X syndrome and the autosomal trisomy resulting from chromosomal duplication in Charcot-Marie-Tooth disease (hereditary motor and sensory neuropathy). In the next sections these recent advances will be discussed, with an emphasis on their usefulness in clinical neurology.

Myotonic Dystrophy

Myotonic dystrophy is an autosomal dominant disorder causing progressive muscular weakness, myotonia, cataracts, and other systemic manifestations. The clinical spectrum is amazingly wide and ranges from asymptomatic gene carriers to a severe neonatal presentation with respiratory distress and mental retardation. Approximately 1 in 8,000 people worldwide has this condition, which has been mapped to chromosome 19q13.3 in many linkage studies with DNA probes. Probes mapping to the proximal long arm of chromosome 19 have been used extensively in clinical settings for both prenatal and presymptomatic diagnosis.

More recently, the myotonic dystrophy gene was isolated, and the mutation-causing myotonic dystrophy was found to result from a series of trinucleotide (CTG) repeats located in the 3' untranslated region of the gene (3). Whereas normal persons have an average of 5 copies of this trinucleotide repeat, persons with myotonic dystrophy have been found to have at least 52 copies, and some patients with myotonic dystrophy have more than 1,000 copies. A higher number of copies is associated with a more severe phenotype and, conversely, a lower number of repeat copies is associated with a milder clinical presentation. The region of repeats demonstrates meiotic instability and can increase as a result of crossing over. This feature of the repeat can explain a worsening of presentation (genetic anticipation) sometimes observed in family members showing an earlier and more severe presentation as the myotonic dystrophy gene is passed down through the family. The myotonic dystrophy gene (designated myotonin-protein kinase) has similarities with a cyclic adenosine monophosphatase-dependent protein kinase and is encoded by a 3,186 base-pair complementary DNA. Although patients with severe congenital myotonic dystrophy have a high number of repeats, it remains unclear whether other molecular mechanisms are involved in the determination of which offspring of an affected mother will have the severe neonatal presentation. More work is needed to clarify how the CTG repeat affects expression of the myotonic dystrophy gene, but it is thought to perturb regulatory elements located in the 3' region.

A number of clinical applications of these recent breakthroughs in myotonic dystrophy can be envisaged. Gene identification will now remove diagnostic uncertainty, permit the direct examination of patients at risk, and possibly eliminate the need for extensive electromyography and slit-lamp screening to detect mildly affected cases. When evaluating persons at risk for having myotonic dystrophy in the future, diagnostic testing may include a determination of the number of CTG repeats in the myotonic dystrophy gene. The number of repeats found will predict the affected status and is likely to give prognostic information with regard to anticipated severity of illness. In addition to postnatal applications, similar uses of myotonic dystrophy probes can be applied to prenatal diagnosis. Eventually, it may be practical to predict whether an affected fetus will present with severe congenital myotonic dystrophy.

Fragile X Syndrome

Fragile X syndrome is recognized to be the most common form of inherited mental retardation, affecting approximately 1 in 1,000 males and 1 in 2,000 females. The disorder is associated with a constriction or fragile site at the tip of the long arm of the X chromosome (Xq27.3). The phenotype in males may include severe mental retardation, macro-orchidism and facial dysmorphia. Carrier females may have normal intelligence or mild mental retardation. Patients with fragile X syndrome are frequently encountered by pediatric neurologists, and this disorder ranks highly in the differential diagnosis of developmental delay and mental retardation of unknown cause. The physical signs of the fragile X syndrome may not be present in childhood, making early diagnosis difficult. A high degree of suspicion will lead the clinician to obtain a special chromosome analysis with cells cultured in folate-deficient media necessary to reveal the presence of the fragile X. Unfortunately, fragile X expression in cultured cells is not complete, and cytogenetic methods for detecting the fragile X identify only approximately 80% of affected males with this condition. Identifying at-risk carrier females may also be very difficult by cytogenetic methods.

Recently the fragile X gene (FMR-1) was cloned and found to contain an unstable region of trinucleotide repeats (CGG), similar to that previously discussed in myotonic dystrophy (4). As in myotonic dystrophy, expansion of this CGG trinucleotide within the FMR-1 gene increases the size of certain restriction fragments detected with FMR-1 probes and correlates with expression of the fragile X syndrome. For example, after digestion of leukocyte DNA with the restriction enzyme EcoRI and blotting and hybridization with probe StB12.3, a fragment of 5.2 kb (kb: 1,000 base pairs) is seen in normal persons. On the other hand, in males with the fragile X syndrome, fragments ranging from 5.7 to 8 kb or more are obtained, indicating an increase of .5 to > 3 kb resulting from an increase in the size of the trinucleotide repeat. Interestingly, some individuals display a small increase of 100–500 base-pairs, suggesting an intermediate, or premutation, state. Again, as in myotonic dystrophy, expansion of the trinucleotide repeat present in a premutational carrier may expand and give rise to an individual with the full-blown syndrome. However, this meiotic expansion occurs only in the offspring of carrier females, because the exchange between two X chromosomes is required.

For clinical diagnostic purposes, the detection of the CGG repeat offers far greater simplicity and sensitivity compared with cytogenetic methods for detecting the fragile X. The test using DNA probes to detect the expanded trinucleotide can be obtained on cultured amniotic cells, permitting more reliable prenatal diagnosis. Indeed, the test for trinucleotide expansion in the FMR-1 gene is likely to become a very widespread screening test for males and females with unexplained developmental delay and mental retardation.

Charcot-Marie-Tooth Neuropathy

Charcot-Marie-Tooth neuropathy (CMT), or hereditary motor and sensory neuropathy, is the most common inherited disorder of the peripheral nervous system and, with an estimated 125,000 patients with CMT in the United States alone, is possibly the most frequently occurring neurogenetic disease. Based on electrophysiologic evaluation, CMT is subdivided into demyelinating (CMT1) and axonal (CMT2) types. Generally, the two types cannot be distinguished by clinical examination alone. Type 1 has proven genetic heterogeneity and has forms that map to chromosome 1 (CMT1B), chromosome 17 (CMT1A), an unknown autosome (CMT1C) and the X chromosome (5). It has been estimated that 70% to 80% of all CMT1 patients have CMT1A, which has recently been found to be associated with a large DNA duplication on chromosome 17p, band 11.2, spanning approximately 1–2 million DNA base-pairs (6, 7). This observation suggests that a "CMT1A gene" has been interrupted at a chromosomal breakpoint or, even more likely, that the CMT1A phenotype is the result of a trisomic overexpression of one or more genes contained within the duplicated region. Interestingly, rare patients with trisomy 17p have been found to have a demyelinating neuropathy consistent with CMT1A (8). The trembler mouse (*Tr*) has a hypomyelinating neuropathy and, because of phenotypic similarities, is thought to be a mouse mutant that is homologous to CMT1. The *Tr* locus maps to mouse chromosome 11, which has conserved evolutionary homology to human chromosome 17p in the region of the CMT1A locus. Recently, the *Tr* locus was found to be a point mutation in a growth arrest-specific gene (gas3) (9). The gas3 gene is a strong candidate for being the CMT1A locus as it is now known to map in humans to chromosome 17 in the region of the 17p11.2 duplication associated with CMT1A.

Patients frequently wish to know if they have inherited CMT1 before the onset of clinical symptoms. By nerve conduction testing the CMT1A gene is penetrant by age 5 years. The 17p11.2 duplication provides an additional powerful tool for diagnosis and counseling in families with CMT1A. The duplication is easily detected by analysis of leukocyte DNA samples from patients with CMT1A and can serve as a marker for this disorder both presymptomatically and prenatally. If an estimated 70% to 80% of all CMT1 patients have CMT1A, then the duplication can serve as a diagnostic reagent in the majority of cases. Some consideration might be given to obtaining the 17p11.2 duplication study in any patient presenting with a phenotype suggesting CMT1, especially in sporadic cases.

Through the application of X-linked DNA probes and linkage studies, it has been confirmed that, in many families, CMT segregates as an X-linked disorder (CMTX); CMTX should be suspected in pedigrees where there is no male-to-male transmission, where males are more severly affected than females, and where all female offspring of affected males are affected. Both CMT1 and, CMT2 forms have been observed, and linkage to the region of Xq13-21 has been reported, suggesting that there are two different X-linked loci or different mutations at the same locus. It is important to recognize that CMTX, as genetic counseling for families, is different from that given for autosomal forms of CMT1 or CMT2. A search for the 17p11.2 duplication in suspected X-linked kindreds may be helpful. If found, the possibility of CMTX is eliminated.

References

1. Payne CS, Roses AD: The molecular genetic revolution: Its impact on clinical neurology. *Arch Neurol* 45:1366, 1988.
2. Wexler NS, Rose EA, Housman DE: Molecular approaches to hereditary diseases of the nervous system: Huntington's disease as a paradigm. *Ann Rev Neurosci* 14:503, 1991.
3. Mahadevan M, Tsilifidis C, Sabourin L, et al: Myotonic dystrophy mutation: An unstable CTG repeat in the 3″ untranslated region of the gene. *Science* 255:1253, 1992.
4. Rousseau MD, Heitz D, Biancalana V, et al: Direct diagnosis by DNA analysis of the fragile X syndrome of mental retardation. *N Engl J Med* 325:1673, 1991.
5. Vance JM: Hereditary motor and sensory neuropathy. *J Med Genet* 28:1, 1991.
6. Lupski JR, Montes de Oca-Luna R, Slaugenhaupt S, et al: DNA duplication associated with Charcot-Marine-Tooth disease type IA. *Cell* 66:219, 1991.
7. Raeymaekers P, Timmerman V, Nelis E, et al: Duplication in chromosome

17p11.2 in Charcot-Marie-Tooth neuropathy type 1A (CMT1A). *Neuromusc Disorders* 1:93, 1991.

8. Chance PF, Bird TD, Matsunami N, et al: Trisomy 17p is associated with Charcot-Marie-Tooth Neuropathy 1A. *Neurology* 42:1427, 1992.

9. Suter U, Welcher AA, Ozcelik T, et al: Trembler mouse carries a point mutation in a myelin gene. *Nature* 356:241, 1992.

Molecular Genetics of Mitochondrial Encephalomyopathies

DONALD R. JOHNS, M.D.

Assistant Professor of Neurology, Johns Hopkins University School of Medicine, Baltimore, Maryland

The mitochondrial encephalomyopathies are a diverse group of disorders that have in common functional, structural, or genetic abnormalities of mitochondria (1). There has been tremendous progress in determining the molecular basis of these diseases in the past four years. The purpose of this review is to update the molecular genetic advances in the mitochondrial encephalomyopathies and to illustrate the impact these advances have had on these diseases for the neurologist.

Each of the mitochondrial diseases is a relatively rare entity, but the availability of specific molecular genetic assays for many of these diseases has revealed that they are present at a higher incidence than was previously suspected on clinical grounds alone. Moreover, they represent some of the first molecularly proven examples of many cardinal neurologic diseases (Table 1): myopathy [chronic progressive external ophthalmoplegia (CPEO)], stroke [mitochondrial encephalomyopathy, lactic acidosis, and stroke-like episodes (MELAS)], seizures [myoclonic epilepsy and ragged red fibers (MERRF)], and optic neuropathy [(Leber's hereditary optic neuropathy (LHON)]. Thus, information gleaned from the detailed study of the pathophysiological basis of these diseases may further our understanding of much more prevalent diseases such as stroke and epilepsy.

TABLE 1.—Common Neurologic Manifestations of
Mitochondrial Encephalomyopaties

1. Myopathy with prominent fatiguability

2. Sensorineural deafness

3. Atypical pigmentary retinopathy

4. Cerebellar ataxia

5. Seizures

6. Vascular headache

7. Dementia

8. Myoclonus

(Courtesy of Dr. Johns.)

TABLE 2.—Laboratory Abnormalities in Mitochondrial Encephalomyopathies

1. Myopathic potentials on electromyography

2. "Ragged red fibers" in skeletal muscle biopsy

3. Sensorineural hearing loss on audiogram

4. Cardiac conduction defects

5. Elevated serum and CSF lactate concentration

6. Oxidative phosphorylation defects on biochemical studies

7. Molecular genetic demonstration of mtDNA mutation

(Courtesy of Dr. Johns.)

Mitochondria function to produce sufficient adenosine triphosphate (ATP) to fuel the myriad energy-requiring cellular processes. Mitochondria contain their own DNA, mitochondrial DNA (mtDNA); therefore, mitochondrial energy production can be deranged genetically by mutations in the nuclear DNA or mtDNA genes that are involved in oxidative phosphorylation. Mitochondrial DNA has a number of properties that make it a unique genetic element, including its exclusively maternal inheritance. The human mitochondrial diseases have been associated with a variety of pathogenetic mutations involving mtDNA-encoded genes.

Deletions of mtDNA, as opposed to point mutations, are not transmitted from one generation to the next. For this reason, diseases that are caused by mtDNA deletions (CPEO) are usually sporadic, whereas diseases that result from point mutations of mtDNA (MELAS, MERRF, and LHON) may demonstrate a maternal pattern of inheritance. Not all persons who harbor a pathogenetic mtDNA point mutation will express the disease. Therefore, these mitochondrial diseases often will appear to occur sporadically, despite the existence of the mutation in previous generations. The mitochondrial diseases exhibit variable penetrance and expressivity, as well as marked intrafamilial and interfamilial variation.

Initiation of a diagnostic work-up in patients with suspected mitochondrial disease depends on recognition of the phenotypic manifestations of the disease and referral for appropriate specialized testing (Table 2). The simplest tests for mitochondrial dysfunction are serum or cerebrospinal fluid lactate concentrations that often are increased in patients with mitochondrial disease. Unfortunately, this increased concentration is rather insensitive and may only be present intermittently. Skeletal muscle, a relatively accessible tissue, is clinically involved in many of these disorders and is the focus of most diagnostic procedures. Electromyography can document the presence of a myopathy, even in the absence of clinically overt symptoms. In vivo phosphorus MR spectroscopy of resting muscle is a powerful tool that may detect associated metabolic abnormalities, but it is not 100% specific and is not yet widely available.

Skeletal muscle biopsy, with appropriate histochemical stains, has remained the gold standard in the diagnosis of most mitochondrial diseases. Light microscopy may reveal "ragged red fibers" on Gomori trichrome stain or focal cytochrome oxidase negative fibers. Ultrastructural analysis may reveal more direct evidence of abnormal, proliferating mitochondria. Skeletal muscle is suitable for biochemical analysis by enzymatic, spectrophotometric, or oxygen electrode polarographic techniques that are available at a number of specialized centers. Most importantly, skeletal muscle biopsy provides appropriate material for the molecular genetic assays that have revolutionized the diagnostic work-up of these diseases.

We will review the basic clinical features of each of the major mitochondrial encephalomyopathies, with an emphasis on the molecular genetic testing now available for each of them and on how the study of molecularly defined groups of patients has influenced our clinical conceptualization of these diseases.

Chronic Progressive External Ophthalmoplegia (CPEO)

One of the cardinal manifestations of human mtDNA disorders is CPEO, which manifests as a slowly progressive disorder of skeletal eye muscle that is typically symmetric and unaccompanied by diplopia. The initial manifestation of this disorder is usually ptosis, but the ophthalmoparesis is progressive and eventually results in total ophthalmoplegia. Chronic progressive external ophthalmoplegia may occur in isolation or may be accompanied by a number of other ophthalmologic, neurologic, and systemic features: "ophthalmoplegia plus." One subset of the "ophthalmoplegia plus" disorders is the Kearns-Sayre syndrome, a disorder characterized by ophthalmoplegia with onset before 20 years of age and pigmentary retinopathy plus at least one of the following: cardiac conduction defects, elevated CSF protein concentration (> 100 mg/dL), or cerebellar ataxia. Many of the neurologic signs in CPEO, other than ophthalmoplegia and ptosis, also are seen in other mtDNA diseases (Table 1).

Molecular genetic analysis of mtDNA from skeletal muscle will demonstrate large deletions in most patients with CPEO. The frequency of demonstrable mtDNA deletions depends on the presence of other features: 50% of patients with isolated CPEO harbor a deletion, whereas 80% of patients with CPEO and pigmentary retinopathy and 90% of patients with the Kearns-Sayre syndrome have deletions. At least some of the deletion-negative patients have pathogenetic mtDNA point mutations in transfer RNAs (tRNAs), including the same tRNA-leucine (UUR) mutation seen in the majority of patients with MELAS syndrome. These deletions, which were the first proven examples of mtDNA abnormalities causing human disease, can be detected by Southern blot analysis or by widely interspaced primer polymerase chain reaction. The deletions vary markedly in size and location, but 25% to 40% occur in the exact same location at a "hot spot" for mtDNA deletion formation.

There is a poor correlation between size, location, and proportion of deleted mtDNA with the phenotypic expression or associated biochemical abnormalities (2).

Mitochondrial Encephalomyopathy, Lactic Acidosis, and Stroke-Like Episodes (MELAS) Syndrome

The MELAS syndrome is another mitochondrial disease that brings patients to neurologic attention. The stroke-like episodes tend to occur in the setting of prolonged focal seizures or prolonged vascular headache. Episodic nausea and vomiting are noted intercurrently and are particularly severe at the time of the stroke-like events. The strokes do not follow vascular territories, but they have a definite posterior preponderance so that many patients develop cortical visual field defects. The strokes appear to be caused by an overwhelming defect in substrate utilization rather than the usual defect in substrate availability operative in occlusive vascular disease. The neurologic deficits may be reversible despite demonstrable signal abnormalities on MRI studies.

The availability of molecular genetic testing has broadened the clinical parameters of MELAS syndrome. The age of onset ranges from infancy to 45 years. Developmental delay and short stature may be noted in the early onset cases, whereas dementia may predominate in older patients. Seizures are virtually always present, and vascular headache occurs commonly. A host of other neurologic accompaniments common to many mitochondrial diseases also are seen (Table 1), and these may precede the development of stroke-like episodes.

Computed tomography may demonstrate basal ganglia calcification or evidence of tissue loss. Magnetic resonance imaging may reveal the signal abnormalities of new and old "infarcts" with a posterior predominance. Although less widely available, phosphorus MR spectroscopy may demonstrate abnormalities in high-energy phosphate metabolism.

The MELAS syndrome has been linked to 2 point mutations in the tRNA-Leucine (UUR) mtDNA gene (3). The mutation at position 3,243 accounts for 80% to 90% of patients with the MELAS phenotype, and it can be detected by molecular genetic analysis of polymerase chain reaction-amplified mtDNA that has been digested with the restriction enzyme Apa I. The mutation originally was described based on analysis of DNA extracted from muscle, but DNA derived from tissues such as blood and urine also contains a detectable proportion of the mutation.

Recognition of the MELAS syndrome in a young stroke patient may dramatically alter the extent and nature of the diagnostic work-up and management. Because many of the stroke-like episodes occur in the setting of prolonged seizures, we recommend aggressive treatment of the seizure disorder with vigilant attention to anticonvulsant levels. Genetic counseling must be individualized in each family and can be supplemented with molecular genetic testing of noninvasive tissues from maternal relatives. The majority of cases are sporadic, but mild oligosymptomatic manifestations may be seen in maternal relatives. One important goal of genetic counseling is to assure an affected male proband that he will not pass the disorder to his offspring because of the strict maternal transmission of mtDNA. His maternal relatives are at risk for the disorder, and the females also may act as carriers.

Myoclonic Epilepsy and Ragged Red Fibers (MERRF)

The third major mitochondrial encephalomyopathy to have its molecular basis identified in recent years is MERRF. The dominant clinical symptoms are progressive myoclonus epilepsy and ataxia. A peculiar form of respiratory insufficiency is seen in the most severe cases. Some of the associated neurologic manifestations of mitochondrial encephalomyopathies (Table 1) are also seen. Phosphorus MR spectroscopy has demonstrated abnormalities in skeletal muscle but not in brain tissue of these patients. The majority of patients with MERRF have a point mutation in the tRNA-lysine gene at position 8,344 that can be detected by molecular genetic methods in skeletal muscle and blood (4).

Leber's Hereditary Optic Neuropathy (LHON)

The first human disease shown to be caused by a heritable defect in mtDNA is LHON. Three primary pathogenetic mtDNA mutations and several secondary mtDNA mutations have been associated with LHON. The core clinical phenotype is that of a painless optic neuropathy occurring in an otherwise healthy young person (5, 6). Loss of central vision may occur rapidly or may progress slowly for several months. Visual symptoms often affect only 1 eye initially, but they virtually always involve both eyes within 1 year. Most patients become symptomatic in the third or fourth decade of life, with a mean age at onset of 23 years (range, 6–70 years). Men are affected much more frequently than women (male:female ratio, 2–3:1). As most patients with molecularly proven LHON have no documented family history of visual loss, one should not be dissuaded from the diagnosis of LHON in the absence of a suggestive family history.

The visual loss is severe, with a nadir of visual acuity ranging from 20/200 to hand motions, and it is accompanied by central or cecocentral scotomas. The funduscopic findings at the onset of visual loss are variable and may be entirely normal. Optic atrophy eventually supervenes in the chronic phase. Significant recovery of visual acuity is noted in some patients and is more commonly associated with certain LHON genotypes. Other neurologic accompaniments are infrequent and include peripheral neuropathy and demyelinating disease.

The major diagnostic errors made in patients who are eventually proven molecularly to have LHON include atypical optic neuritis and "toxic nutritional amblyopia." Therefore, LHON should be considered in any patient with an atypical optic neuritis (painless, bilateral, no recovery) or a presumed toxic or nutritional optic neuropathy. The most important dictum for the work-up of suspected LHON is to have a high index of suspicion and to order appropriate molecular genetic testing.

The availability of reliable molecular genetic testing has revolutionized the diagnosis of LHON. Three primary pathogenetic mtDNA mutations have been described to date in LHON, and each can be detected readily with molecular genetic techniques. The first mutation at nucleotide position 11,778 ("11,778 mutation") in the ND-4 gene accounts for 55% of cases and can be detected with 100% sensitivity and specificity by molecular genetic analysis of polymerase chain reaction-amplified mtDNA that is extracted from a routine blood sample. Although rare exceptions have been noted, the 11,778 mutation is a very poor prognostic sign for significant recovery of visual acuity.

The second pathogenetic mtDNA mutation occurs at nucleotide 3,460 in the ND-1 gene and accounts for 8% of cases of LHON. The clinical phenotype associated with this mutation differs in 3 major respects when compared with the phenotype of patients with the 11,778 mutation (6). Patients with the 3,460 mutation have a much better prognosis for visual recovery (21% vs. 4% of eyes), are more likely to have a positive family history of visual loss compatible with LHON (86% vs. 43%), and have a high incidence of tobacco and alcohol abuse. Indeed, tobacco–alcohol amblyopia was the major source of diagnostic confusion in these patients. The use of tobacco and alcohol are the only known potentially modifiable risk factors for visual loss in this disease, although other environmental factors may also play a role.

A third pathogenetic mtDNA mutation has been identified at nucleotide 15,257 in the cytochrome b gene; it accounts for 8% of LHON cases. Patients with this mutation appear to have a better prognosis for visual recovery than patients with the more common 11,778 mutation, and they have a higher incidence of neurologic accompaniments, particularly spinal cord and peripheral nerve involvement.

Molecular genetic testing for each of the 3 primary mtDNA mutations is 100% specific, but it currently is only approximately 70% sensitive. This testing has proven useful in a number of different settings, including confirmation of the diagnosis in probable cases and establishment of the diagnosis in atypical or obscure cases. In addition to expediting the diagnostic work-up of LHON, molecular genetic testing has implications for family counseling, risk factor intervention, prognosis for visual recovery, and therapy.

Co-existent systemic abnormalities that are occasionally associated with LHON, such as cardiac conduction defects, migraine, and peripheral neuropathy, should be recognized and treated appropriately. Referral for genetic counseling and low vision assessment also are important in management of LHON patients.

Novel Mitochondrial Disease Phenotypes

The 4 disorders discussed above were thought to have a mitochondrial origin for many years because of inheritance patterns and morphological and biochemical characteristics. Recent advances in molecular genetics established their precise origin. More recently, a number of novel mitochondrial disease phenotypes have been identified on the basis of mtDNA defects. These include a family from England with a syndrome of peripheral neuropathy, ataxia, retinitis pigmentosa, seizures, developmental delay, and dementia as a result of an mtDNA mutation at nucleotide 8,993 in the adenosine triphosphatase 6 gene. This mutation is readily detected in polymerase chain reaction-amplified mtDNA from blood or muscle by the creation of an AvaI restriction site. We have identified a family with a syndrome of subacute optic neuropathy and myelopathy that harbored mtDNA mutations in the cytochrome oxidase II gene and in the tRNA-aspartate gene. An Italian family with maternally inherited myopathy and cardiomyopathy has been shown to harbor an mtDNA mutation at position 3,260 in the tRNA-leucine (UUR) gene.

Summary

Molecular genetic analysis of mtDNA in human disease has had a rapid and profound impact on a number of different diseases that are of primary interest to the neurologist. These molecular genetic advances have been translated rapidly from the laboratory bench to the bedside of the patient with neurologic disease. Although the diseases covered in this review were discussed as separate entities, many of the patients have clinical and laboratory features that overlap (Tables 1 and 2). The neurologist is in a pivotal position to recognize these patients and guide their diagnosis and management. Many patients with mitochondrial diseases will present with partial or novel phenotypes and will require a high index of suspicion from an astute clinician. We anticipate that molecular genetic advances in the near future will allow us to definitively diagnose more of these challenging patients and will eventually guide their effective treatment.

References

1. Kosmorsky G, Johns DR; Neuro-ophthalmological manifestations of mitochondrial DNA disorders. *Neurol Clin* 9:147, 1991.
2. Holt IJ, Harding AE, Cooper JM, et al; Mitochondrial myopathies: Clinical and biochemical features of 30 patients with major deletions of muscle mitochondrial DNA. *Ann Neurol* 26:699, 1989.
3. Goto Y-I, Nonaka I, Horai S: A mutation in the tRNS Leu (UUR) gene associated with the MELAS subgroup of mitochondrial encephalomyopathies. *Nature* 348:651, 1990.
4. Shoffner JM, Mott MT, Lazza AMS, et al: Myoclonic epilepsy and ragged red fibers (MERRF) is associated with a mitochondrial DNA tRNA Lys mutation. *Cell* 61:931, 1990.
5. Newman NJ, Lott MT, Wallace DC: The clinical characteristics of pedigrees of Leber's hereditary optic neuropathy with the 11778 mutation. *Am J Ophthalmol* 111:750, 1991.
6. Johns DR, Smith KH, Miller NR: Leber's hereditary optic neuropathy: Clinical manifestations of the 3460 mutation. *Arch Ophthalmol* (in press).

Neurotrophic Factors: Prospects for Future Use in the Treatment of Neurodegenerative Diseases

DALIA M. ARAUJO, PH.D., PAUL A. LAPCHAK, PH.D., AND FRANZ HEFTI, PH.D.
Department of Gerontology, University of Southern California, Ethel Percy Andrus Gerontology Center, Los Angeles, California

Currently, the list of substances that are being considered for the treatment of several neurodegenerative diseases includes such diverse molecules as growth factors (GFs) and anti-inflammatory agents (1-4). Clearly, however, much of the attention has focused on the potential of GFs to be used in the treatment of neurodegenerative diseases such as Alzheimer's and Parkinson's diseases (table). This emphasis has stemmed in part from experimental results showing that not only may GFs stimulate the synthesis of proteins necessary for cell survival and function, but they also may decrease vulnerability of neurons to the degenerative processes of a particular disease. Furthermore, it appears that many of these molecules may have the additional advantage of augmenting the capability of specific neurons to compensate for the degeneration of other neurons (2-5).

The Neurotrophins as Therapy for Neurodegenerative Diseases

The neurotrophin family of GFs consists of several homologous proteins that have conserved structural identities, including nerve GF (NGF), brain-derived neurotrophic factor (BDNF), neurotrophin-3 (NT-3), neurotrophin-4 (NT-4), and neurotrophin-5 (NT-5). Of these, only

Growth Factors and Their Potential Clinical Applicabilities	
GF	Therapeutic Potential
NGF	Alzheimer's disease
BDNF	Parkinson's disease
NT-3	Trauma-induced nerve damage
	Diabetes or chemotherapy-induced neuropathy
	Alzheimer's disease
CNTF	ALS
	Diabetes or chemotherapy-induced neuropathy
bFGF	Wound healing and repair
	Stroke
	Parkinson's disease

(Courtesy of Drs. Araujo, Lapchak, and Hefti.)

NGF, BDNF, and NT-3 protein, and messenger RNA (mRNA) have thus far been identified in the mammalian brain (5). In vitro studies have demonstrated that these 3 neurotrophins can augment the activity of the acetylcholine (ACh)-synthesizing enzyme choline acetyltransferase (ChAT) of septal neurons, although BDNF and NT-3 were shown to be significantly less potent than NGF. Moreover, a wealth of in vivo studies attest to the significance of NGF as a neurotrophic factor for basal forebrain cholinergic neurons. Thus, NGF enhances a variety of cholinergic parameters such as septal ChAT mRNA, as well as ChAT activity, ACh synthesis, and, in the hippocampus of rats with fimbria-fornix lesions, the major source of septal cholinergic input to the hippocampus. In addition, NGF recently has been shown to prevent lesion-induced cholinergic deficits in the primate brain as well.

Although extensive literature exists on the subject, it is not entirely clear whether levels of NGF and NGF mRNA are altered in Alzheimer's disease. Some evidence suggests that levels of NGF and its mRNA remain constant in Alzheimer tissue, despite extensive degeneration of the cholinergic neurons of the basal forebrain. However, whether this results from a compensatory response by surviving cells to increase their levels of expression has not been demonstrated conclusively. Nevertheless, it is clear that expression of the receptors for NGF, trk A (high-affinity NGF site), and p75NGFR (low-affinity NGF site), which is specific to cholinergic neurons of the basal forebrain (5, 6), is not changed in Alzheimer's tissue. Therefore, it seems reasonable to infer that, in Alzheimer's patients, the surviving cholinergic neurons of the basal forebrain may be responsive to NGF. Because the degeneration of these neurons in Alzheimer's disease has been implicated as the main cause of the progressive memory impairment, it is not surprising that NGF, with its selective and pronounced trophic action on these neurons, has been proposed as a leading candidate in the treatment of Alzheimer's disease (2).

A limited clinical trial of the effectiveness of NGF in the treatment of Alzheimer's disease is currently in progress. Reports from a single patient indicate that there was some improvement in selected memory tests, as well as in cerebral blood flow in a patient receiving NGF infusions for 3 months (7). In addition, combined NGF therapy with adrenal medullary autografts appears to result in a mild improvement of symptoms associated with Parkinson's disease.

Unlike NGF, which specifically affects cholinergic neurons of the basal forebrain in the CNS, BDNF appears to be less selective. In addition to its effect on cholinergic cells of the basal forebrain (see below), BDNF also had been shown to promote the survival and differentiation of dopaminergic mesencephalic neurons and to protect these neurons from the neurotoxic actions of MPP+ (4, 5, 8). Moreover, BDNF enhances [^{3}H]dopamine and [^{3}H]γ-aminobutyric acid uptake into mesencephalic and cerebellar Purkinje neuronal cultures, respectively. Because degeneration of the dopaminergic neurons of the substantia nigra accounts for many of the symptoms of Parkinson's disease, these in vitro findings seemed to imply that BDNF might be beneficial in the treatment of this disease. However, thus far, in vivo studies have not corroborated this; no obvious protective effects of BDNF were observed on dopaminergic neurons of the ventral mesencephalon after transection of the axons emanating from the medial forebrain bundle.

Administration of BDNF to rats with fimbria-fornix transections has been shown to increase the number of ChAT-positive cell bodies at the level of the septum, suggesting that some protection of lesion-induced degeneration is afforded by the GF (8). However, even with much higher concentrations, this effect of BDNF was modest in comparison to NGF. Moreover, this attenuation of septal ChAT levels does not appear to translate into a functional recovery of cholinergic function, because hippocampal cholinergic parameters (ChAT activity, high affinity choline uptake, ACh synthesis and release) were not noticeably altered by infusions of BDNF (6).

Neurotrophic effects of NT-3 in vivo have not yet been reported. In cultures of basal forebrain neurons, NT-3 increased ChAT activity, but this effect was modest in comparison to that of either NGF or BDNF. However, because NT-3 mRNA is heterogeneously distributed in the brain, it is possible that the neurotrophin affects other neuronal subpopulations more potently. Moreover, the neurotrophic properties of NT-3 are contingent on the presence of receptors that may be selective for NT-3 (trkC) on specific neurons.

Other Neurotrophic Factors

The fibroblast growth factors (FGFs) belong to a family of growth factors that includes several oncogene products (1, 9). Of these, the most commonly studied are the structurally related acidic and basic FGFs, both of which are known to function as neurotrophic factors. The more potent of the two factors, basic FGF, has been shown to protect cholinergic cell bodies in adult rats from degenerative changes induced by fimbrial transections. However, basic FGF was less potent in this effect than NGF. In addition, intracerebral administration of basic FGF to adult mice treated with MPTP, the metabolic precursor of MPP+, promoted the recovery of dopaminergic parameters. Other effects of acidic FGF and basic FGF include survival enhancement of a large variety of cultured neuronal populations, as well as angiogenic and mitogenic effects. Thus, the broad spectrum of actions of the FGFs in the CNS may preclude them from consideration as realistic candidates for the treatment of Alzheimer's and Parkinson's diseases. Nevertheless, because of its involvement in wound healing and repair, basic FGF appears to be an attractive option for the treatment of stroke and trauma-induced damage.

Other factors are known to promote the differentiation of mesencephalic dopaminergic neurons in vitro. Of these, insulin and the insulin-like GFs (IGF-I and IGF-II), transforming GF-α and epidermal GF have been tested extensively (1, 4, 10). However, it is not clear whether the tropic effects of these GFs that are evident in vitro are also manifested in vivo.

Ciliary neurotrophic factor (CNTF) has been demonstrated to have only moderate effectiveness in the prevention of degenerative changes induced by fimbrial transections. Thus, CNTF preserves p75NGFR but not ChAT, immunoreactivity (4). The most potent effect of CNTF appears to be on motor neurons; with relatively low concentrations, the factor rescues motor neurons from naturally occurring cell death during development of the chick embryo and prevents degeneration of motor neurons in axotomized rats. This finding has aroused considerable interest in its potential use for the treatment of disease-related degenerative changes of motor neurons, such as that which occurs in amyotrophic lateral sclerosis. Ciliary neurotrophic factor is also being considered as a logical therapeutic agent for the treatment of many polyneuropathies that are the consequence of chronic anti-cancer drugs. At present, there has been some preliminary confirmation of the effectiveness of CNTF in these clinical settings.

Caveats

When considering any agent for clinical use, several criteria must be met. One of the most important points to consider is the potential side effects of the compounds in question. Furthermore, a suitable route of administration and dosage regimen must be achieved. With GFs, other details that require attention include determining whether interactions with other GFs may potentiate the response or, conversely, whether they may result in undesirable side effects. At present, our understanding of these complex interactions is limited.

Because NGF is the most efficacious factor in protecting cholinergic neurons of the basal forebrain, it is currently the preferred factor for the treatment of Alzheimer's disease. However, whereas the cholinergic deficit in Alzheimer's disease has received considerable attention, only a few studies have dealt with the other populations of affected neurons. Therefore, it seems likely that combined therapy of NGF and other factors that protect various populations of vulnerable neurons may be necessary to obtain behaviorally significant effects in Alzheimer's disease. Nevertheless, several lines of evidence indicate that, with chronic administration of NGF, as with other GFs, detrimental effects may ensue. For example, hypophagia and changes in local cerebral blood flow in rats receiving NGF infusions have been reported (2–4, 6). Aberrant cholinergic sprouting and increased sympathetic innervation also may occur. In addition, NGF has been shown to increase levels of amyloid precursor protein mRNA in cultured cells and neonatal rodents. Thus, although initial studies with long-term intraventricular administration of NGF to rats have not revealed any obvious neurodegenerative changes in rats, it is evident that caution must be exercised when considering NGF therapy.

Of substantial significance when considering GF therapy is that protein GFs do not readily cross the blood–brain barrier. This predicament has necessitated some innovative pharmacological strategies. Of these, the most feasible consist of delivering GFs into the cerebral ventricles through pumps or intracerebral implants. Perhaps more unconventional is the possibility that GFs could be produced intracerebrally by implanted natural or genetically engineered cells.

Future Prospects

Because the use of GFs in a clinical setting may be hampered by various obstacles (see above), intensive investigation of a new wave of non-GF molecules that may function like their GF counterparts is now in progress. Rather than administering entire GF molecules, it may be possible to use active fragments or other non-GF molecules mimicking the active sites of neurotrophic factors. However, while fragments of some GFs apparently retain biologic activity, this approach has not been successful for NGF or the other neurotrophins to date. Alternatively, the development of new compounds that can influence neurotrophic actions, either by modulating release of neurotrophins or by modifying their interactions with specific receptors, may be a feasible approach in the treatment of certain neurodegenerative diseases.

References

1. Araujo DM, Chabot J-G, Quirion R: Potential neurotrophic factors in the mammalian central nervous system: Functional significance in the developing and aging brain. *Int Rev Neurobiol* 32:141, 1990.
2. Hefti F, Schneider L: Trophic factors and invasive procedures, in Thal LJ, Moos WH, Gamzu ER (eds): *Cognitive Disorders: Pathophysiology and Treatment.* New York, Dekker, 1992, pp 329–353.
3. Hefti F, Lapchak PA, Knusel B, et al: Correlation of molecular, cellular and behavioral effects of nerve growth factor administration to rats with partial lesions of the septo-hippocampal cholinergic pathway. *J Cogn Neurosci* 1992, (in press).
4. Hefti F, Lapchak PA, Denton TL: Growth factors and neurotrophic factors in neurodegenerative diseases, in *Alzheimer's Disease: New Treatment Strategies.* Khachaturian ZS, Blass JP (eds): New York, Dekker, 1992, pp 87–101.
5. Lapchal PA, Araujo DM, Hefti F: Neurotrophins in the central nervous system. *Rev Neurosci* 3(1):1, 1992.
6. Lapchak PA: Therapeutic potential for nerve growth factor in Alzheimer's disease: Insights from pharmacological studies using lesioned central cholinergic neurons. *Rev Neurosci* 3(2): 1, 1992.
7. Olson L, Blacklund EO, Ebendahl T, et al: Intraputaminal infusion of nerve growth factor to support adrenal medullary autografts in Parkinson's disease: One-year follow-up of first clinical trial. *Arch Neurol* 48:373, 1991.
8. Knusel B, Beck KD, Winslow JW, et al: Brain-derived neurotrophic factor administration protects basal forebrain cholinergic but not nigral dopaminergic neurons from degenerative changes after axotomy in the adult rat brain. *J Neurosci* 1992 (in press).
9. Walicke PA: Novel neurotrophic factors, receptors, and oncogenes. *Annu Rev Neurosci* 12:103, 1989.
10. Sara VR, Carlsson-Skwirut C: The role of insulin-like growth factors in the regulation of brain development. *Prog Brain Res* 73:87, 1988.

1 Cerebrovascular Disease

The Decline of Mortality Due to Stroke: A Competitive and Deterministic Perspective
Riggs JE (West Virginia Univ)
Neurology 41:1335–1338, 1991   1–1

Background.—Death caused by stroke has been decreasing since the early part of the twentieth century, especially since the early 1970s. This decrease often is credited to the management of risk factors, especially hypertension, but there is some question as to whether risk factors alone account for the magnitude of the most recent decline.

Deterministic Mortality Dynamics.—Age-specific general mortality rates have deterministic dynamics; thus, the mortality rate from 1 disease may affect the mortality rate from another disease. According to longitudinal Gompertzian analysis of human mortality, the age-specific mortality for men at age 87.4 years has remained constant in this century, whereas the mortality rate at birth has decreased considerably in this century. Age-specific mortality distributions for a variety of conditions, such as ischemic heart disease, Parkinson's disease, and lung cancer, conform to deterministic dynamics.

Decline of Stroke.—Quantitative comparison of the relative risk of mortality from all causes demonstrates the competitive basis for the decline in stroke mortality. This analysis shows that stroke has become a less competitive cause of mortality in 1985 than it was in 1965 for most ages. This has lowered stroke mortality and resulted in deterministic compensatory increase in other causes of death. Improved survival also decreases overall mortality from some disorders and increases overall mortality from others.

Conclusions.—The decline in stroke mortality is best viewed from a deterministic and competitive perspective. The competitive nature of mortality must be understood to appreciate the dangers of making conclusions based on mortality data of a single disease. This idea also explains the increasing mortality associated with cancer and degenerative disease.

▶ Stroke mortality in the United States declined by 7% per year between 1973 and 1981. The refreshing (but initially perhaps foreboding) insight of

27

this article, using a model of competitive and deterministic mortality dynamics, is that a major responsible factor for this decline is that stroke has come to compete less well (whereas cancer and degenerative diseases, correspondingly, are becoming increasingly competitive) as a cause of mortality. This paper thus encourages our awareness of how disease *compete* for mortality. Alas, we must all die of something!—M.D. Ginsberg, M.D.

Benefit of a Stroke Unit: A Randomized Controlled Trial

Indredavik B, Bakke F, Solberg R, Rokseth R, Haaheim LL, Holme I (Univ Hosp of Trondheim, Norway; Ullevaal Hosp, Oslo)
Stroke 22:1026–1031, 1991   1–2

Background.—No effective treatment has been found to limit the neuronal damage associated with stroke, and investigations of the value stroke rehabilitation have been inconclusive. Intensive care for stroke patients has not limited morbidity or mortality, although some trials reported a benefit to team care and early rehabilitation. This randomized trial evaluates the clinical outcome of a maximum of 6 weeks' treatment in a stroke unit compared with treatment in general medical wards.

Methods.—A group of 110 acute stroke patients were allocated to treatment in a stroke unit and a second group of 110 received treatment in general medical wards. Treatment differed between the 2 groups only in the first 6 weeks. Characteristics of sex, age, marital status, medical history, and functional impairment on admission were similar in the 2 groups. Outcome at 6 and 52 weeks after the stroke was measured by the proportion of patients at home, the proportion of patients in an institution, patient mortality, and the functional state of the patient.

Results.—After 6 weeks, there was a significant difference in all reported outcomes; after 1 year, all the differences except mortality were still significant. The combination of acute medical treatment and early systematic rehabilitation in a stroke unit increased the proportion of patients able to live at home, improved functional outcome, reduced the need for institutional care, and reduced early mortality.

Conclusions.—Care for patients with acute stroke in a stroke unit improved clinical outcome compared with treatment in general medical wards. The acute care in a stroke unit significantly improved all patient outcomes. Mortality also was improved in the stroke unit group, but the difference was not significant. The reduced need for institutional care in patients treated in a stroke unit is an economic benefit.

▶ The important findings of this well-conducted study should be taken to heart by clinicians involved in acute stroke care. The marked increase (63% vs. 45%) in patients able to live at home when assessed even 1 year after early treatment in a dedicated stroke unit is very impressive. However, this study does not analyze which components of acute care are specifically responsible for this improved outcome. The early avoidance of glucose infusion, the nonmanipulation of increased blood pressure in the acute phase, the early anticoagulation of patients with embolic infarction or progressive ischemic deficits, or the prompt institution of a systematic program of functional recovery are all possible candidates in this regard. It would be of great importance to subject this issue to critical analysis in a future study, so as to be able to optimize those components of acute care delivery specifically responsible for enhanced functional outcome.—M.D. Ginsberg, M.D.

Lacunar Infarcts: Pathogenesis and Validity of the Clinical Syndromes
Boiten J, Lodder J (Univ Hosp Maastricht, The Netherlands)
Stroke 22:1374–1378, 1991   1–3

Background.—There is still some question as to the clinical value of the lacunar hypothesis, which suggests that symptomatic lacunar infarcts cause specific lacunar syndromes and usually result from a distinct vasculopathy of the small perforating arteries. An investigation was conducted to establish the validity of the lacunar syndrome in diagnosing lacunar infarction, to compare the frequency of potential cardiac vs. carotid embolic sources, and to assess the frequency of vascular risk factors in patients with lacunar vs. cortical infarct.

Patients.—The patients were drawn from a prospective registry of 252 patients with a first brain infarct of greater than 24 hours' duration during a 2-year period. Of this group, 103 were classified as having a lacunar infarct, and 144 were classified as having a cortical infarct. Routine investigations included standard blood and urine tests, ECG, chest radiography, noninvasive carotid studies, and CT, usually within 2 weeks of admission.

Findings.—The lacunar syndromes had a sensitivity of 95% and a specificity of 93% in diagnosing lacunar infarction. The positive predictive value of lacunar syndromes in diagnosing lacunar infarction was 90%, and the negative predictive value was 97%. The 2 groups had no differences in risk factors. Patients with lacunar infarction had a significantly lower frequency of a cardiac source of embolism (odds ratio, .32). They also had a lower frequency of significant carotid stenosis (odds ratio, .35).

Conclusions.—Lacunar syndrome is a very good clinical test for the diagnosis of lacunar infarction. This type of infarction is likely to result not from cardiac and carotid embolism but rather from small vessel disease. Otherwise, patients with cortical vs. lacunar infarction have the same risk factors for ischemic stroke.

▶ In this important study, cardiac sources of embolism were about three times less common in lacunar infarction than in cortical infarction; non-rheumatic atrial fibrillation was, correspondingly, three times higher in the cortical infarct group. Ipsilateral internal carotid artery stenosis of 50% or greater was also about three times more frequent in the cortical infarct cases. These data make it rather improbable that lacunar infarcts are caused by cerebral emboli.—M.D. Ginsberg, M.D.

Headache in Transient or Permanent Cerebral Ischemia

Koudstaal PJ, van Gijn J, Kappelle LJ, for the Dutch TIA Study Group (Univ Hosp Rotterdam; Univ Hosp Utrecht; Univ Hosp Amsterdam; Univ Hosp Maastricht; De Wever Hosp Heerlen, The Netherlands; et al)
Stroke 22:754–759, 1991   1–4

Background.—Headache is a common feature in acute cerebrovascular disease. Patients with acute cerebral ischemia of variable duration were examined to determine the relationship among the occurrence and nature of headache and the presence of vascular risk factors, the probable site of neurologic symptom origin, the time course of the attack, and CT findings.

Methods.—All 3,126 patients included in this multicenter treatment trial had acute cerebral or retinal ischemia. A checklist was used to record symptoms.

Results.—Headache occurred in 18% of the patients. It was mostly continuous in all types of attacks. Of the patients with monocular visual symptoms, 16% had headache. Headache occurrence was unrelated to mode of onset, mode of disappearance, and duration of attack. Patients reporting headache more often had heart disease. Headache was less common among patients with small deep infarcts, who were more often hypertensive. It was also less frequent in patients with infarcts in the anterior circulation. Headache was more frequent in those with cortical infarcts and with infarcts in the posterior circulation. Patients with a relevant small deep infarct on CT and accompanying headache relatively often had symptoms compatible with cortical ischemia.

Conclusion.—Headache is frequent in patients with acute cerebral and retinal ischemia. The occurrence of headache appears to be partly related to the underlying cause of the ischemic lesion.

▶ Headaches are among the primary symptoms of a number of cerebrovascular afflictions. The authors are to be congratulated for precisely defining many of the factors that predispose to headache in patients with cerebrovascular disease. This paper is a major prospective contribution, but the characteristics of the headaches were not sufficiently specified. It would have been valuable to determine the localizing and lateralizing value of the headache and its attributes, such as associated symptoms and sensitivity to movement. Such information is necessary to distinguish the transient and permanent vascular events that accompany some migraine headaches from cerebrovascular occlusive disease.—R.A. Davidoff, M.D.

Early Spontaneous Hematoma in Cerebral Infarct: Is Primary Cerebral Hemorrhage Overdiagnosed?
Bogousslavsky J, Regli F, Uské A, Maeder P (Centre Hospitalier Universitaire Vaudois, Switzerland)
Neurology 41:837–840, 1991   1–5

Introduction.—The diagnosis of intrainfarct hematoma usually is based on the compatibility of the first CT scan with ischemic infarction and on the presence of a hematoma in the presumed site of infarction on a second CT scan, typically after anticoagulant treatment is initiated. However, when hemorrhagic transformation occurs within the first hours of stroke, CT scans may already show hemorrhage and may wrongfully suggest primary cerebral hemorrhage (PCH). This is especially true in patients with known hypertension who are not undergoing anticoagulant treatment.

Patients.—Data on 15 patients in whom intrainfarct hematoma developed less than 1 day after stroke onset in the absence of antithrombic therapy were reviewed. There was no bleeding seen on CT scans within 6 hours of stroke onset in any patient, but basal ganglionic or lobar hemorrhage appeared less than 18 hours later without visible underlying infarct. None of the patients had antithrombotic treatment or a coagulation disorder; 8 had hypertension.

Results.—In 10 patients, the second CT scan was prompted by rapid worsening. A second CT was performed in the remaining 5 patients because the first scan was not available. Previous transient ischemic attacks, silent infarcts on CT scan, and a potential cardiac source of embolism were more frequent in patients with early spontaneous intrainfarct hematoma than in a comparison group of 200 patients with PCH admitted at the same time. There were distal occlusions in 4 of 5 patients undergoing intracranial studies in the first 2 days. Most patients probably had embolism with extensive early bleeding in the ischemic region.

Conclusion.—These findings suggest that early spontaneous intrainfarct hematoma may be underdiagnosed, whereas PCH is overdiagnosed. The possibility of early spontaneous intrainfarct hematoma must be considered in patients with the clinical radiologic diagnosis of PCH before further studies are performed.

▶ This thought-provoking study raises the old question of the separation of ischemic stroke from primary intracerebral hemorrhage. The authors suggest that a secondary intrainfarct hematoma develops in embolic infarcts more commonly than is recognized, and that many such cases are misinterpreted as primary intracerebral hemorrhage. An alternative explanation, that stroke symptoms arise with very small primary intracerebral hemorrhage that later extends, might be considered. Resolving this question is of importance for thrombolytic studies for the future.—W.G. Bradley, M.D., F.R.C.P.

Antibodies to Cardiolipin in Stroke: Association With Mortality and Functional Recovery in Patients Without Systemic Lupus Erythematosus
Chakravarty KK, Byron MA, Webley M, Durkin CJ, Al-Hillawi AH, Bodley R, Wozniak J (Stoke Mandeville Hosp, Aylesbury, England)
Q J Med 79:397–405, 1991   1–6

Background.—A syndrome of thrombosis, cerebral disease, thrombocytopenia, and recurrent fetal loss has been associated with increased serum levels of antibodies to negatively charged phospholipids such as cardiolipin. Anticardiolipin antibody is associated most obviously with

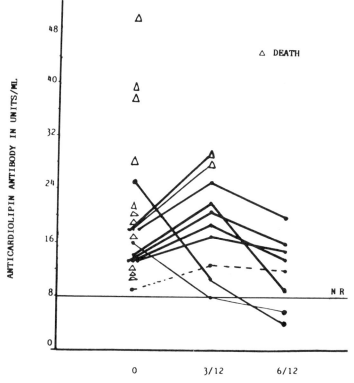

Fig 1–1.—Natural history of anticardiolipin antibody levels in 21 patients with stroke. The *dashed line* indicates a patient who had intracerebral hemorrhage. NR refers to normal range. (Courtesy of Chakravarty KK, Byron MA, Webley M, et al: *Q J Med* 79:397–405, 1991.)

thrombosis in patients with systemic lupus erythematosus or related conditions.

Methods.—The prevalence of anticardiolipin antibody was determined in 100 consecutive patients aged 60–94 years who were admitted with a first acute stroke. None had evidence of connective tissue disease, malignancy, active or recent infection, or recent myocardial infarction. A control group of 100 healthy elderly persons was used.

Findings.—Twenty-one stroke patients and no controls had a serum anticardiolipin antibody titer 5 SD above the laboratory control mean. Mortality within 3 months was 62% in patients with increased antibody and 21.5% in those without antibody elevation. Six of the 8 stroke survivors with persistent antibody elevation had significant disability, compared with 11 of 62 patients who lacked persistently increased anticardiolipin antibody. Antibody titers tended to decline after 3 months in surviving patients (Fig 1–1).

Conclusions.—It appears that anticardiolipin antibody in increased titer is an independent prognostic marker in patients with acute stroke. It remains unclear whether the antibody causes the clinical features or is an epiphenomenon.

▶ Anticardiolipin antibodies have been reported in association with stroke in patients with systemic lupus erythematosus and in young individuals without other risk factors. This study suggests that these antibodies are significantly associated with stroke in about 20% of older patients with stroke. Moreover, high antibody titers correlated both with mortality and with residual disability. It still remains to be determined whether these associations are secondary and whether the antibodies cause the stroke.—W.G. Bradley, D.M., F.R.C.P.

Acute Cerebrovascular Episodes in Systemic Lupus Erythematosus
Eustace S, Hutchinson M, Bresnihan B (St Vincent's Hosp, Dublin)
Q J Med 81:739–750, 1991   1–7

Background.—Acute cerebrovascular disorders occur rarely in patients with systemic lupus erythematosus (SLE). The neurologic, clinical, and laboratory features, as well as the clinical course and outcome, were recorded for an unselected cohort of patients with SLE who later contracted a major acute cerebrovascular disorder.

Patients.—During a 10-year period, 12 women with SLE or lupus-like syndromes had acute cerebrovascular episodes. The mean patient age was 43 years; the mean duration of SLE was 9.3 years (range, 1 month to 22 years).

Clinical Aspects and Outcome.—All patients had clinical and laboratory evidence of active systemic disease, despite therapy with corticosteroids and azathioprine. Only 3 patients had previous neuropsychiatric disorders. Acute cerebrovascular episode was the initial neurologic manifestation in 9 patients. Cerebral infarction was confirmed by CT in 8 patients. Transient retinal ischemia occurred in 2 patients with associated transient spinal cord ischemia in 1 patient. The remaining 2 patients had acute cerebral hemorrhage. Six patients had clinical and serologic features of antiphospholipid antibodies, and all 6 had cerebrovascular occlusion. Five patients died of stroke, 2 other patients died within 1 year, and 3 of the 5 survivors had major residual neurological deficits.

Conclusions.—Acute infarction is the most frequently observed acute cerebrovascular episode in SLE. The occurrence of these episodes invariably represents an exacerbation of incompletely controlled systemic disease. It appears that, in some patients, cerebrovascular occlusion is associated with the presence of antiphospholipid antibodies. Outcome after cerebrovascular episodes in SLE is poor.

▶ This clinical report of 12 patients, although of restricted scope, reinforces the view that focal cerebral ischemic infarction is a predominant neurologic complication in patients with SLE, and that antiphospholipid antibody-related features are commonly observed.—M.D. Ginsberg, M.D.

Neurological Disease Associated With Anticardiolipin Antibodies in Patients Without Systemic Lupus Erythematosus: Clinical and Immunological Features

Chancellor AM, Cull RE, Kilpatrick DC, Warlow CP (Western Gen Hosp; Blood Transfusion Service, Edinburgh)
J Neurol 238:401–407, 1991   1–8

Background.—Anticardiolipin antibodies are 1 of a group of antiphospholipid antibodies that includes the lupus anticoagulant. Anticardiolipin antibodies and lupus anticoagulant may appear in the same individuals, and anticardiolipin antibodies may occur in association with systemic lupus erythematosus. The spectrum of disease associated with abnormal anticardiolipin antibody levels in 39 patients was examined.

Methods.—Testing for anticardiolipin antibodies was offered as part of an immunology profile on standard laboratory request forms; thus, the included patients were preselected by their physicians. The 39 patients with abnormal anticardiolipin antibody activity were identified from 748 consecutive patients tested. The hospital records of these 39 patients were examined.

Findings.—Systemic lupus erythematosus was diagnosed definitively in 12 patients. Of the rest, 13 had non-neurologic associations with anticardiolipin antibodies. Seven of them had a history of deep venous thrombosis, pulmonary embolism, a poor obstetric history, or some combination of these. Two had lupus-like disease, and 2 others had infections. The remaining 14 (12 women and 2 men; mean age, 44 years) had neurologic disease. Six of them had no evidence of lupus anticoagulant. Neurologic disease—cerebrovascular disease, migraine, or epilepsy—was the presenting or only complication in all patients but 1. Four patients had peripheral venous thrombosis, and 3 had peripheral arterial thrombosis. Another 3 had livedo reticularis, and the mother of 1 patient had 6 spontaneous abortions before delivering a term infant while taking corticosteroids for an allergic condition. Severity of disease and anticardiolipin antibody level were not clearly related.

Conclusions.—A primary antiphospholipid syndrome may exist, seen mainly with stroke and migraine; however, in some cases it is seen with features of a hypercoagulable state. Serious complications could be prevented by early recognition and treatment of anticardiolipin antibody-associated stroke. Randomized, multicenter trials are needed to find sufficient numbers of patients with anticardiolipin antibodies as their primary immunologic abnormality.

▶ This retrospective review of neurologic abnormalities associated with anticardiolipin antibodies reinforces the need for prospectively designed, randomized, multicenter studies of therapy to prevent the multisystem thrombotic complications associated with this immunologic abnormality.—M.D. Ginsberg, M.D.

Antiphospholipid Antibodies in Cerebral Ischemia

Montalbän J, Codina A, Ordi J, Vilardell M, Khamashta MA, Hughes GRV (Hosp Gen "Vall d'Hebron," Barcelona, Spain; St Thomas' Hosp, London)
Stroke 22:750–753, 1991   1–9

Background.—A grave and prominent feature associated wiith antiphospholipid antibodies is cerebral ischemia. This association is well-documented in patients with autoimmune disorders. However, there are few investigations of this association in a general population with thrombotic stroke. The importance of antiphospholipid antibodies in the cause of stroke was determined.

Methods.—Plasma was collected from 146 consecutive patients (mean age, 51.4 years) during a 2-year period. Different antiphospholipid antibodies were assessed in these patients with cerebral ischemia. Vascular risk factors were compared with clinical and laboratory findings.

Results.—Ten patients (6.8%) were positive for at least 1 antiphospholipid antibody. One of these patients had systemic lupus erythematosus; 1 had rheumatoid arthritis; and 8 had primary antiphospholipid syndrome. These patients were mostly men and were not necessarily young. Half of them did not have any other vascular risk factors. No significant clinical or paraclinical differences could be found between these patients and patients without antiphospholipid antibodies. These 10 patients had good outcomes. Platelet antiaggregating drugs were beneficial in preventing further cerebrovascular ischemic events.

Conclusions.—A considerable proportion of patients with cerebral ischemia have antiphospholipid antibodies. Most of these patients fulfill criteria for the diagnosis of primary antiphospholipid syndrome. Measuring the antiphospholipid antibody concentration may be useful in patients with cerebral ischemia, because the prognosis may be good for patients with these antibodies.

▶ This report confirms the not inconsequential presence of antiphospholipid antibodies in 10 of 146 consecutive patients (6.8%), aged 27–59 years, presenting with cerebral ischemia, the great majority of whom had no immunologic disorder. However, three patients had previous stroke, pulmonary embolism, or myocardial infarction. A series of concurrently studied healthy blood donors was negative for these antibodies. Future studies of the proper treatment and the prognostic implications of this serologic abnormality are needed.—M.D. Ginsberg, M.D.

Inherited Protein C Deficiency and Nonhemorrhagic Arterial Stroke in Young Adults

Camerlingo M, Finazzi G, Casto L, Laffranchi C, Barbui T, Mamoli A (Ospedali Riuniti, Bergamo, Italy)
Neurology 41:1371–1373, 1991   1–10

Background.—It is widely accepted that protein C deficiency can lead to venous thrombosis. However, few reports on the relationship between protein C and arterial thrombosis exist. Three young adults with nonhemorrhagic arterial stroke and protein C deficiency were encountered.

Patients.—Of 1,333 patients with acute cerebrovascular disease hospitalized at 1 center between 1985 and 1990, 50 were younger than 45 years. Those patients were extensively evaluated. Three met the criteria for the diagnosis of inherited protein C deficiency.

Findings.—Results of all other coagulation tests in the 3 patients were normal. Assessment of the patients' families revealed other persons with protein C deficiency. All relatives with the same coagulation abnormality were asymptomatic. In the 3 patients, CT showed hypodense areas consistent with the clinical picture. Angiography showed occlusion of some intracranial arterial vessels. One patient had a transient ischemic attack and a peripheral venous thrombosis before the stroke. The other 2 were completely asymptomatic before the actual cerebrovascular event.

Conclusion.—In a consecutive series of 50 young patients with nonhemorrhagic arterial stroke, 3 had inherited protein C deficiency. Protein C should be assessed in all young adults suffering ischemic stroke, especially when major risk factors are excluded.

▶ Protein C is a vitamin K-dependent glycoprotein with anticoagulant (by virtue of activating factors V and VII), as well as profibrinolytic properties. This report offers further evidence of an association of inherited protein C deficiency and ischemic stroke in young adults. However, even in this age group it is uncommon—6% in this series. In future reports, it would be reassuring to know the incidence of the disorder in age-matched controls.—M.D. Ginsberg, M.D.

Symptomatic and Asymptomatic High-Grade Carotid Stenoses in Doppler Color-Flow Imaging

Steinke W, Hennerici M, Rautenberg W, Johr JP (Columbia Presbyterian Med Center, New York; Univ of Heidelberg, Mannheim, Germany)
Neurology 42:131–138, 1992   1–11

Background.—Many reports have examined the pathogenesis of cerebral ischemia from carotid atherosclerosis. However, the significance of distinct morphologic features, such as plaque composition, degree of luminal narrowing, and plaque surface configuaration, is still debated. Doppler color-flow imaging (DCFI) was used to assess morphologic features of plaque and blood flow patterns in symptomatic and asymptomatic patients with high-grade carotid stenoses, in an attempt to identify the echomorphologic and hemodynamic features distinguishing the 2 groups.

Methods.—Sixty-three patients with 31 symptomatic and 44 asymptomatic carotid stenoses were examined. Conventional Doppler duplex examinations had demonstrated a hemodynamic obstruction in all cases.

Findings.—Plaque surface morphologic analysis revealed more ulcerated plaques in the symptomatic than in the asymptomatic stenoses (43% vs. 23%). The frequency of homogeneous and heterogeneous plaques did not differ, but calcific lesions were more frequent in asymptomatic cases. Echolucent plaques, probably indicating mural thrombi, were more frequent in symptomatic cases. Color-coded hemodynamic patterns, such as jet flow, post-stenotic turbulence, or reversed flow, did not differ. When DCFI findings were compared with those of 30 angiograms, plaque surface analysis agreed in only 70%. In 85%, DCFI measurements of area reduction in cross-sections correlated with angiography. Doppler color-flow imaging tended to underestimate the degree of stenosis from diameter reduction in longitudinal cuts.

Conclusions.—Improved plaque analysis by DCFI in a study of high-grade carotid stenosis showed that ulcerations and echolucent plaques occurred more often in symptomatic stenoses, whereas smooth and calcific plaques occurred more often in asymptomatic stenoses. Thus, morphologic changes in plaque may be relevant in the pathogenesis of cerebrovascular events. However, treatment of patients with hemodynamically relevant stenoses should be based on the patient's clinical presentation.

▶ These interesting findings obtained by (DCFI) would be strengthened by correlation with pathologic material. The 30% incidence of discordant results obtained on comparing DCFI to conventional angiography would suggest that, although DCFI is an intriguing research tool, there is need for caution in drawing definitive diagnostic conclusions from it.—M.D. Ginsberg, M.D.

Vascular Risks of Asymptomatic Carotid Stenosis
Norris JW, Zhu CZ, Bornstein NM, Chambers BR (Univ of Toronto; Repatriation Gen Hosp, Melbourne, Australia)
Stroke 22:1485–1490, 1991   1–12

Background.—Recent evidence suggests that the asymptomatic neck bruit is a risk factor for later stroke, myocardial infarction, and death. The risk of stroke is, however, low.

Methods.—A group of 696 patients with an initial diagnosis of asymptomatic carotid stenosis underwent follow-up for a mean period of 41 months. The mean age was 64 years. Patients were evaluated clinically and by carotid Doppler ultrasound examinations.

Findings.—Seventy-five patients had transient ischemic attacks, and 29 had a stroke. A total of 132 patients had ischemic cardiac events during follow-up. Five patients died of stroke, and 59 died of cardiac causes. The annual rate of stroke was 1.3% in patients with 75% or less carotid stenosis and 3.3% in those with more marked stenosis (table). Patients with severe stenosis had an annual rate of cardiac events of 8.3% and an annual mortality of 6.5%.

Conclusions.—Even moderate carotid stenosis increases the combined risk of cardiac ischemia and vascular death to almost 10%. The risk of

Annual Percentage Rate of Vascular Events Over a Period of Follow-Up			
Degree of stenosis	TIA	Stroke	Cardiac	Vascular death
<50% (mild)	1.0	1.3	2.7	1.8
50–75% (moderate)	3.0	1.3	6.6	3.3
>75% (severe)	7.2	3.3	8.3	6.5

Abbreviation: TIA, transient ischemic attack.
(Courtesy of Norris JW, Zhu CZ, Bornstein NM, et al: *Stroke* 22:1485–1490, 1991.)

stroke is increased in the presence of more than 75% stenosis, even in the absence of symptoms.

▶ The important messages of this paper are, first, the confirmation that higher grades of asymptomatic carotid stenosis are a marker for both increased stroke risk, heightened risk of cardiac events, and greater mortality. Not surprisingly, patients in the severely stenotic group were also older, more commonly hypertensive, and more often afflicted with symptomatic peripheral vascular disease than were those with lower grades of stenosis. Second, that the annual risk of ipsilateral stroke was only 2.5%, even in the most highly stenotic group, would tend to make it, perhaps, improbable that carotid surgery would be beneficial. This latter issue must, of course, be settled by controlled trials.—M.D. Ginsberg, M.D.

The Prevalence of Ulcerated Plaques in the Aortic Arch in Patients With Stroke

Amarenco P, Duyckaerts C, Tzourio C, Hénin D, Bousser M-G, Hauw J-J (Hôpital de la Salpêtrière; Hôpital Saint-Antoine, Paris; Institut Natl de la Santé et de la Recherche Médicale, Villejuif, France)
N Engl J Med 326:221–225, 1992   1–13

Background.—In many cases of cerebral infarction, the cause is undetermined. Ulcerated plaques protruding into the lumen of the aortic arch can cause strokes, but this is considered a rare event. The frequency of ulcerated plaques in the aortic arch and the role of these plaques in the formation of cerebral emboli were investigated.

Methods.—Autopsy records on 500 consecutive patients with neurologic disease from a Paris hospital were reviewed. Of the 500, 239 patients had cerebrovascular disease (ischemic stroke or hemorrhagic stroke), and the remaining 261 patients had neither cerebrovascular disease nor history or pathologic evidence of stroke.

Findings.—Ulcerated plaques were found in the aortic arch of 26% of patients with cerebrovascular disease, significantly more than the 5% found in patients with other neurologic diseases. Strong correlations were found between the presence of ulcerated plaques in the aortic arch and increasing age and heart weight. After controlling for these confounding factors, the prevalence of ulcerated plaques in patients with cerebrovascular disease was 16.5%, significantly more than the 5.1% prevalence in patients without cerebrovascular disease. No definite cause was found in 28 of 183 patients with cerebral infarcts. Of these 28 patients, 61% had ulcerated plaques in the aortic arch, significantly more than the 22% of the 155 patients in whom a cause of cerbral infarction could be identified. The difference between these groups remained significant after adjustment for age, sex, and heart weight. The presence or degree of extracranial internal carotid artery stenosis was not related to the prevalence of ulcerated plaques in the aotic arch.

Conclusions.—Ulcerated plaques in the aortic arch are common. They occur more frequently in patients with cerebrovascular disease, especially in those with cerebral infarctions of unknown cause. Ulcerated plaques of the aortic arch might serve as a source of cerebral emboli, thereby accounting for some cases of cerebral infarction with unknown cause.

▶ The conclusion of this retrospective, nonblinded, autopsy databank-based study is a cautious one: namely, that ulcerated plaques in the aortic arch may "play a part" in causing cerebral infarction. The odds ratio of 5.7 (after adjustment for covariates) convincingly distinguishes the prevelance of this finding in patients with no known cause of cerebral infarction (58%) vs. that in those with known causes (20%). Tantalizingly, all ulcerations lay "around the origin of the cerebral arteries." One would like to know the comparative details of the clinical stroke pictures of these 2 groups. As ulcerated plaques would seem to pose a risk primarily of cerebral embolism, the similar prevelance of aortic arch plaques in patients with cerebral infarcts of "no identifiable cause" and patients with brain hemorrhage supports the notion that, in those patients, this finding may represent only an incidental stigma of atherosclerosis.—M.D. Ginsberg, M.D.

Neurovascular Complications of Cocaine Abuse

Peterson PL, Roszler M, Jacobs I, Wilner HI (Wayne State Univ School of Medicine and Detroit Receiving Hosp)
J Neuropsychiatry Clin Neurosci 3:143–149, 1991   1–14

Background.—An estimated 5 million Americans abused cocaine regularly in 1985; in 1986, 15% of the population reportedly had used it at least once. Neurovascular complications were examined prospectively in a large group of patients from a single institution.

Patients.—More than 30,000 admissions to Detroit Receiving Hospital, an inner-city emergency trauma center, were reviewed. Thirty-three patients with cocaine-related neurologic episodes were identified. They were aged 45 years or younger and were admitted with an acute neurologic deficit that lasted at least 24 hours and appeared to be caused by vascular pathology. Those using cocaine intravenously at the time of the event were excluded. The 33 patients, with 35 acute neurovascular events related to cocaine abuse, represented 3% of all cocaine-related admissions during the same time period.

Findings.—Thirteen of the 33 patients admitted to intravenous drug abuse, but 10 of them reported no longer using intravenous drugs; all had changed to crack cocaine. A majority of patients were hypertensive when admitted, but only 1 required treatment. Eighteen patients had ischemic infarcts, and 15 had hemorrhagic neurovascular events. One patient had a recurrent infarct and died. Five patients with hemorrhage died in hospital, and 1 died after a recurrent event.

Conclusions.—A great majority of these neurovascular events were related to the abuse of crack cocaine. Young persons with such events should be asked about the use of cocaine and should have urine screening for cocaine metabolites. Those having a hemorrhagic event related to cocaine abuse should have angiography.

▶ Cocaine abuse, unfortunately, is relatively widespread in the United States at present. The association of neurologic complications with vasculitis in intravenous cocaine abusers is well known. This study demonstrates that abusers of crack cocaine also have a significant risk of both cerebral infarction and cerebral hemorrhage.—W.G. Bradley, D.M., F.R.C.P.

Prognostic Value of the Dense Middle Cerebral Artery Sign in Patients With Acute Ischemic Stroke

Ricci S, Caputo N, Aisa G, Celani MG, Chiurulla C, Mercuri M, Guercini G, Scaroni R, Senin U, Signorini E (Università di Perugia, Perugia, Italy)
Ital J Neurol Sci 12:45–47, 1991   1–15

Background.—It has been suggested that the appearance of a dense middle cerebral artery sign (DMCAS) on an unenhanced CT scan taken 24 hours or less after the onset of ischemic stroke is a poor prognostic sign. A large series of patients was examined to confirm this association.

Methods.—Participants were drawn from the Italian Acute Stroke Study—Hemodilution. Ninety consecutive patients who had experienced their first stroke within 12 hours were included. Patients with hemorrhagic stroke were not included. All patients had a CT scan within 48 hours, most within 12 hours. At 3 weeks, all surviving patients were ranked for residual disability on a modified Rankin scale.

Results.—Fourteen patients (15.6%) had the DMCAS. Outcome was good in 29% of these patients compared with 63% of those without the sign. The odds ratio of a poor outcome in patients with the DMCAS was 4.3. Twenty-nine percent of sign-positive patients died within 3 weeks, compared with 11% of sign-negative patients, although the difference was not significant.

Conclusions.—The DMCAS appears to be a useful prognostic variable in the acute phase of an ischemic stroke. These results should be verified by data from stroke registries.

▶ Previous studies have confirmed angiographically that acute arterial thromboembolism may be detected as a high-density appearance on noncontrast CT scans. This retrospective study suggests that the sign connotes a poor outcome. These preliminary results arouse our interest but require further substantiation.—M.D. Ginsberg, M.D.

Hyperdense Middle Cerebral Artery CT Sign: Comparison With Angiography in the Acute Phase of Ischemic Supratentorial Infarction

Bastianello S, Pierallini A, Colonnese C, Brughitta G, Angeloni U, Antonelli M, Fantozzi LM, Fieschi C, Bozzao L (Univ of Rome "La Sapienza")
Neuroradiology 33:207–211, 1991   1–16

Background.—The early CT finding of a hyperdense portion of the middle cerebral artery in patients with supratentorial stroke often indicates embolic occlusion. An investigation was conducted. A study was done to verify the incidence and reliability of the hyperdense middle cerebral artery sign (HMCAS) and its possible correlation with early CT findings and the extent of late brain damage.

Methods.—Thirty-six patients with symptoms of stroke in the middle cerebral artery territory underwent CT and angiography within 4-6 hours of presentation. Follow-up CT scans were done 1 week and 3 months after the ischemic event.

Results.—Half of the patients had the HMCAS. In these patients, the sign always correlated positively with the finidng of occlusion on angiography. These patients also had a high incidence of early CT hypodensity (88%). The HMCAS appeared to be a negative prognostic sign for the development of extensive brain damage.

Conclusions.—The HMCAS on early CT indicates an arterial occlusion and possibly, its angiographic location as well. It may be important in predicting the severity of ischemia. However, the absence of this sign should not be interpreted as indicating the absence of middle cerebral artery occlusion. The HMCAS is closely related to early CT hypodensity; both are early indicators of brain injury.

▶ This report offers further evidence that an HMCA observed by CT scan in the first few hours after onset of symptoms denotes arterial occlusion. This occlusion was, in fact, documented in *all* patients studied angiographically within six hours in this series. As the authors hasten to add, however, the converse is not true: some cases of HMCA stem or trunk occlusion that are angiographically verified may nonetheless lack this CT sign. Nonetheless, the presence of the sign appears to be reliable and may, in the future be used as part of a therapeutic decision-making process.—M.D. Ginsberg, M.D.

Enhanced Detection of Intracardiac Sources of Cerebral Emboli by Transesophageal Echocardiography

Lee RJ, Bartzokis T, Yeoh T-K, Grogin HR, Choi D, Schnittger I (Stanford Univ)
Stroke 22:734–739, 1991   1–17

Introduction.—Intracardiac pathology can promote cerebral embolic ischemia and infarction; as many as one fourth of all cerebral ischemic events have been ascribed to a cardiac origin. Predisposing factors in-

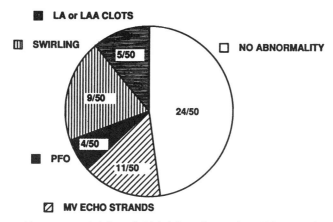

Fig 1–2.—*Abbreviations:* LA, left atrial; *LAA*, left atrial appendage; *PFO*, patent foramen ovale; MV, mitral valve. Distribution of potential intracardiac sources of emboli. Three patients had more than 1 abnormality. (Courtesy of Lee RJ, Bartzokis T, Yeoh T-K, et al: *Stroke* 22:734–739, 1991.)

clude left atrial enlargement, interatrial shunting, atrial fibrillation, valve disease, and abnormal ventricular wall motion. A trial was conducted comparing the sensitivity of transesophageal echocardiography with transthoracic echocardiography in detection of intracardiac sources of embolism.

Methods.—Transesophageal echocardiography was performed in 50 consecutive hospitalized patients with a recent stroke or transient ischemic attack of embolic origin. The patients were experiencing an abrupt onset of focal deficit in the anterior or middle cerebral territory and had no evidence of a mass or bleeding on cranial CT examination. Transthoracic echocardiography also was carried out within a week of the onset of symptoms.

Findings.—Twenty-one patients had cerebral infarction, and 29 had transient ischemic attacks. Transthoracic studies showed mild mitral valve changes without a definable mass in 23 patients. Twenty-six patients had at least 1 intracardiac abnormality on transesophageal echocardiography (Fig 1–2). Eleven patients with no other potential embolic source had very mobile filamentous strands on the mitral valve, which may represent a fissured surface or fibrosis.

Conclusions.—Transesophageal echocardiography is significantly more sensitive than the transthoracic study for detecting possible intracardiac sources of cerebral embolism. The 2 methods are viewed as complementary.

▶ The frequency of cardiac causes of ischemic neurologic deficits remains controversial. Transesophageal echocardiography is a more sensitive mechanism for detecting cardiac abnormalities than is the classic transthoracic study. More than half of the patients in this study had a cardiac abnormality, and a frequent new finding was filamentous strands on the mitral valve. Unfortunately, this study cannot tell whether such abnormalities are the cause of the stroke. A controlled study is needed.—W.G. Bradley, D.M., F.R.C.P.

Detection of Paradoxical Cerebral Echo Contrast Embolization by Transcranial Doppler Ultrasound

Teague SM, Sharma MK (Univ of Oklahoma, Oklahoma City)
Stroke 22:740–745, 1991   1–18

Background.—In embolic stroke, the detection of patent foramen ovale by contrast echocardiography implies paradoxical embolization. However, some 2-dimensional echocardiographic studies are not of diagnostic quality, and there is still no direct evidence for paradoxical cerebral embolization. Transcranial Doppler ultrasound and contrast echocardiography were compared as to sensitivity and concordance in the detection of right-to-left vascular shunting.

Methods.—Forty-six consecutive patients (average age, 41 years) who had been referred for contrast echocardiography for evaluation of interatrial shunting, were examined. Exclusion of atrial defect was the indication in 48%, fixed neurologic deficit in 26%, and transient neurologic deficit in 26%. Transcranial Doppler ultrasound and contrast echocardiography were performed simultaneously, with video displays of both signals continuously displayed (Fig 1–3). Resting studies were done in all patients, and 39 patients were tested during the Valsalva strain. Echocar-

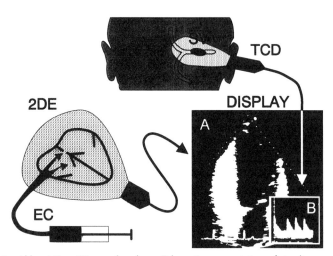

Fig 1–3.—*Abbreviation: SV,* sample volume. Schematic representation of simultaneous 2-dimensional echocardiographic (2DE) and transcranial Doppler (TCD) studies of cardinal cardiac chambers and middle cerebral artery during peripheral venous injection of echo contrast (EC). The 2 video images (A and B) are superimposed and displayed on a common screen. (Courtesy of Teague SM, Sharma MK: *Stroke* 22:740-745, 1991.)

diography was considered positive if contrast microcavitations were seen in the left atrium or ventricle, with appearance of microbubbles in the cerebral circulation indicated by a chirp in the acoustic signal and a corresponding video spike from the middle cerebral artery.

Results.—Interatrial shunting was detected by echocardiography in 26% of patients at rest and 15% during Valsalva strain. On Doppler study, venous-injected contrast was seen in the middle cerebral artery in 41% of both groups. All patients who had echocardiographic evidence of interatrial shunting had a positive Doppler examination. Concordances were 82% for resting studies and 75% for Valsalva studies. When findings were discordant, there was almost always Doppler evidence of paradoxical embolization but indeterminate echocardiographic findings.

Conclusions.—In patients suspected of having paradoxical embolization, transcranial Doppler can sensitively detect interatrial shunting, anatomic substrates, and target organ involvement. Transesophageal study may be reserved for patients with uninterpretable Doppler or echocardiographic studies. Cardiac catheterization appears for less sensitive to patent foramen ovale than these 2 ultrasonic studies.

▶ The frequency with which paradoxical emboli cause neurologic ischemic deficits is uncertain. This study of a selected group of patients found evidence of paradoxical embolization in as many as 41% of cases studied by bubble contrast echocardiography. The transcranial Doppler was significantly better than the echocardiogram in detecting paradoxical embolization. It appears likely that contrast transcranial Doppler studies will come to play a large role in the investigation of patients with possible paradoxical embolism.—W.G. Bradley, D.M., F.R.C.P.

Stroke Prevention in Atrial Fibrillation Study: Final Results
Stroke Prevention in Atrial Fibrillation Investigators
Circulation 84:527–539, 1991   1–19

Background.—The Stroke Prevention in Atrial Fibrillation Study was begun in 1985 to determine the efficacy and safety of warfarin and aspirin compared with placebo in preventing ischemic stroke and systemic embolism. Late in 1989, the placebo arm was terminated, as the superiority of both warfarin and aspirin was established. The preliminary results of this trial were reported previously. The final results in the entire population are described.

Methods.—This multicenter, randomized trial compared administration of 325 mg/day of aspirin or warfarin with administration of placebo in 1,330 inpatients and outpatients with constant or intermittent atrial fibrillation. Mean follow-up was 1.3 years.

Results.—The rate of primary events in patients receiving placebo was 6.3% per year, which was reduced by 42% in those receiving aspirin. In the subgroup of patients eligible for warfarin, most of whom were younger than 76 years, warfarin that was dose-adjusted to prolong prothrombin time to between 1.3-fold and 1.8-fold that in controls decreased the risk of primary events by 67%. Warfarin reduced primary events or death by 58%, and aspirin reduced them by 32%. Patients receiving warfarin, aspirin, or placebo had a risk of significant bleeding of 1.5%, 1.4%, and 1.6% per year, respectively.

Conclusions.—Both aspirin and warfarin effectively reduce ischemic stroke and systemic embolism in patients with atrial fibrillation. Because patients who are eligible to receive warfarin comprise a subset of aspirin-elibible patients, the magnitude of event reduction by warfarin and aspirin cannot be compared. Warfarin-eligible patients had too few events to evaluate directly the relative benefit of aspirin compared with warfarin. Patients with nonrheumatic atrial fibrillation who can take either warfarin or aspirin safely should receive prophylactic antithrombotic treatment to decrease their risk of stroke.

▶ This landmark study has shown that both low-intensity warfarin and aspirin markedly diminish the rates of ischemic stroke and systemic embolism in patients with nonvalvular atrial fibrillation, and that they do so with relative freedom from side effects. The present paper incorporates 86 additional patients randomized after publication of the preliminary results of this highly important study in 1990 (1). Thus, this study establishes firm indications for therapy, which now should be transferred to the realm of routine clinical practice. The relative merits of warfarin and aspirin will be addressed in the ongoing second phase of this study, SPAF II.—M.D. Ginsberg, M.D.

Reference

1. Stroke Prevention in Atrial Fibrillation Investigators: N *Engl J Med* 322:863, 1990.

The Risk of Cerebral Infarction in Nonvalvular Atrial Fibrillation: Effects of Age, Hypertension and Antihypertensive Treatment

Tohgi H, Tajima T, Konno T, Towada S, Kamata A, Yamazaki M (Iwate Med Univ; Iwate Health Service Assoc, Japan)
Eur Neurol 31:126–130, 1991   1–20

Background.—The prevalence of atrial fibrillation without valvular disease is 2% to 5% in persons older than 60 years. About 15% of those having ischemic strokes are patients with nonvalvular atrial fibrillation (NVAF). Stroke risk in patients with NVAF was compared with that of the general population.

Methods.—The development of stroke in a population undergoing annual mass examination beginning in 1974 was analyzed. The relationship of stroke risk to age and sex, the duration of atrial fibrillation, the effects of hypertension and its treatment, and high- or low-risk subgroups among patients with NVAF were documented. A total of 600 patients with NVAF were included.

Results.—Persons aged 41–50 years had the greatest age-matched relative risk of stroke (12.6). The risk decreased with age. It was 8.2 for persons aged, 51–60 years, 3.6 for persons aged 61–70 years, and 2.6 for those aged 71–80 years. These decreases were a result of the increase in stroke incidence with age in the general population. There was no particularly vulnerable period for stroke until the fifteenth year after NVAF diagnosis. Stroke incidence was higher in persons with hypertension than in normotensive persons. The incidence was comparable in treated and untreated patients with hypertension.

Conclusions.—These findings confirm that there is an increased risk of stroke associated with NVAF in patients aged 41–80 years. This is true for both sexes, except for men aged 71–80 years.

▶ Atrial fibrillation of rheumatic origin is well established as a major cause of cerebral embolism and stroke. This study demonstrates a similar risk for NVAF. The relative risk appears to decrease with age, although this is an artifact of the increasing frequency of stroke in the elderly population. These patients also frequently have hypertension, and a study of anticoagulants in the prevention of stroke in NVAF is awaited with interest.—W.G. Bradley, D.M., F.R.C.P.

The United Kingdom Transient Ischaemic Attack (UK-TIA) Aspirin Trial: Final Results

UK-TIA Study Group (Western Gen Hosp, Edinburgh)
J Neurol Neurosurg Psychiatry 54:1044–1054, 1991   1–21

Background.—Taken together, previous trials have shown that no antiplatelet drug or combination of drugs is definitely more effective in reducing the risk of serious vascular events than aspirin, 300 mg, given daily. A direct, randomized comparison of dosage of aspirin of 300 mg daily vs. a dosage of 1,200 mg daily was conducted.

Methods.—A total of 2,435 patients at 33 centers in the United Kingdom and Ireland who had transient ischemic attacks or minor ischemic strokes were randomized into 3 treatment groups, receiving either 600 mg aspirin twice daily, 300 mg aspirin once a day, or placebo. During a mean follow-up of about 4 years, the occurence of serious vascular events, deaths, and adverse effects were noted.

Results.—At entry, the 3 groups were well matched for all the known and important prognostic variables for stroke and myocardial infarction. The mean patient age was about 60 years; 73% were male. A significant increase in upper gastrointestinal symptoms was seen in the high-dose group compared with the low-dose and placebo groups. Both aspirin groups together had less dizziness and tinnitus and more complaints of bruising than the placebo group. There was a clear dose–response effect of gastrointestinal hemorrhages resulting from aspirin, but these hemorrhages often did not require hospitalization and rarely led to death. Most gastrointestinal symptoms induced by aspirin were mild and reversible. The efficacy was the same with high-dose and low-dose aspirin. The benefit of aspirin on reducing the incidence of major stroke, myocardial infarction, or vascular death was clearer and more significant in men than in women, but the difference between the sexes was not definite. The largest benefit from aspirin was a reduction in the odds of nonvascular death, mainly cancer deaths. The survival benefit of aspirin was first seen after 3 months and increased for the next few months, after which time the aspirin survival curve and placebo survival curve remained fairly parallel.

Conclusions.—These findings indicate that dosages of 300 mg/day of aspirin are as effective as dosages of 1,200 mg/day in reducing the risk of major stroke, myocardial infarction, or vascular death. The larger dose of aspirin was more gastrotoxic.

▶ In this rather large study in which no patients were lost to follow-up (but in which roughly one quarter of patients had discontinued their trial medication by 4–5 years), no statistically significant differences in effectiveness could be ascertained between the 300 mg per day and 1,200 mg per day aspirin dosages (although the numbers were insufficient to exclude a type II error). Perhaps surprisingly, when the 2 dose-groups were combined and compared with placebo, only the lumped outcome measure of major stroke, myocardial infarction or vascular death achieved statistical significance. As noted, the statistically best substantiated finding was the apparent reduction of nonvascular death (largely from cancer) in aspirin-treated patients! Taken in isolation, this trial is not conclusive; however, its major trends are consonant with the findings of other studies indicating that aspirin is partially preventative of stroke and is chiefly so in males.—M.D. Ginsberg, M.D.

Swedish Aspirin Low-Dose Trial (SALT) of 75 mg Aspirin as Secondary Prophylaxis After Cerebrovascular Ischaemic Events
The SALT Collaborative Group (Danderyd Hosp, Sweden)
Lancet 338:1345–1349, 1991   1–22

Background.—Many studies have confirmed the benefit of administering 300 mg or more of aspirin a day as prophylactic treatment for cerebrovascular disorders. The Swedish Aspirin Low-dose Trial (SALT) was conducted to determine whether 75 mg of aspirin a day could prevent stroke, death after a minor stroke, or a transient ischemic attack.

Methods.—Included in the trial were patients from 16 centers across Sweden seen from 1984 to 1989. Patients received 75 mg of aspirin or placebo as film-coated tablets according to a randomization schedule.

Clincial assessments were made at the initial visit and every 4 months thereafter for an average of 32 months.

Results.—Of the 1,363 patients selected, 3 with tumors were excluded. Of the remainder, 684 received placebo and 676 received aspirin. About two thirds of the patients had a minor stroke. Follow-up for those taking aspirin averaged 30.6 months; for those taking placebo it averaged 27.5 months. Ten percent of the patients missed more than 10% of the doses. Aspirin use was significantly related to an 18% decrease in the risk of primary events (stroke or death). Aspirin use also reduced the relative risks of stroke (fatal and nonfatal) and myocardial infarction (fatal and nonfatal), but not significantly. Side effects from the treatment occurred in 147 patients taking aspirin and in 123 taking placebo. Bleeding episodes happened significantly more often in aspirin patients. The 5 fatal hemorrhagic strokes that occurred during the treatment phase were in the group receiving aspirin.

Conclusions.—Although the low dose of 75 mg of aspirin a day decreased the risk of stroke or death in cerebrovascular ischemic patients, the significant number of bleeding episodes in the group receiving aspirin offers a warning against the automatic prescription of aspirin to these patients.

▶ This is the first placebo-controlled trial of secondary stroke prevention to show a benefit from an aspirin dose of less than 300 mg/day. This study was well designed. Its results, considered in the context of previous controlled trials, support the view that the degrees of risk reduction provided by various aspirin doses do not differ greatly from one another, but that gastrointestinal side effects are diminished at lower doses. Interestingly, all fatal hemorrhagic strokes in this series occurred in the aspirin group. However, as the authors note, aggregate data from secondary prevention trials show that this increase in hemorrhagic stroke (about .5 per 1,000 patients per year) is very small compared with the risk reduction in ischemic strokes associated with antiplatelet therapy (about 15 per 1,000 patients per year).—M.D. Ginsberg, M.D.

The European Stroke Prevention Study (ESPS): Results by Arterial Distribution

Sivenius J, Riekkinen PJ, Smets P, Laakso M, Lowenthal A (Univ of Kuopio, Finland; Universite Libre de Bruxelles, Brussels; Algemeen Ziekenhuis Middelheim, Antwerp, Belgium)
Ann Neurol 29:596–600, 1991   1–23

Background.—Antiplatelet treatment is a widely accepted prophylaxis against thromboembolic cerebrovascular diseases. The significance of the arterial distribution of cerebrovascular disease for the success of treatment has never been assessed in patients with ischemic atherothrombotic cerebrovascular accidents using acetylsalicylic acid (ASA) or

ASA and dipyridamole combined. A secondary subgroup of the European Stroke Prevention Study was analyzed to determine the effect of dipyridamole–ASA on the secondary prevention of stroke or death in patients with recent ischemic cerebral attack in the carotid or vertebrobasilar territory.

Methods.—The effect of dipyridamole, 75 mg, and ASA, 330 mg, 3 times a day was compared with that of placebo in 2,500 patients in a multicenter trial. Outcomes considered were stroke or death after 1 or more transient ischemic attacks, reversible ischemic neurologic deficits, or strokes of atherothrombotic origin. One third of the patient population had vertebrobasilar events at entry.

Results.—During the 2-year follow-up, the overall total incidence of stroke or death in the group receiving placebo was lower in the patients with vertebrobasilar events than in those with carotid events (14% and 24%, respectively). The dipyridamole–ASA combination markedly reduced the incidence of stroke or death in patients with vertebrobasilar and carotid events. When only stroke was used as an end point, the dipyridamole-ASA combination appeared to be more effective in decreasing the risk for both vertebrobasilar and carotid patients who were entered into the trial because of transient ischemic attacks than in those with stroke as the cause of entry. The trends for men were significant; those for women were similar but did not reach statistical significance.

Conclusion.—Combined dipyridamole-ASA is effective in preventing cerebrovascular events secondarily regardless of the anatomical location of the events.

▶ This important extension paper from the European Stroke Prevention Study reports significant benefit for patients with previous ischemic episodes in either the vertebrobasilar or the internal carotid territory. The dose of aspirin and dipyridamole was higher than is used in most studies. Although the number of women included was similar to that of men, the level of benefit for women was slightly lower and did not reach statistical significance.—W.G. Bradley, D.M., F.R.C.P.

Prevention of Stroke With Ticlopidine: Who Benefits Most?
Grotta JC, Norris JW, Kamm B, TASS Baseline and Angiographic Data Subgroup (Univ of Texas, Houston; Univ of Toronto; Syntex Research, Palo Alto, Calif)
Neurology 42:111–115, 1992   1–24

Background.—Medical treatment can reduce the frequency of subsequent stroke in patients with transient ischemic attacks. A recent multicenter, randomized trial compared ticlopidine, a new platelet antiaggregant drug that inhibits the adenosine diphosphate pathway of platelet aggregation, with aspirin. Baseline and carotid lesion characteristics of patients in this earlier trial were examined to determine which factors might differentiate response to ticlopidine vs. aspirin.

Methods and Findings.—Patients received ticlopidine, 250 mg twice daily, or aspirin, 650 mg twice daily. Patients doing less well on aspirin had elevated creatinine, hypertension, or diabetes requiring treatment, or they had treatment with anticoagulant or antiplatelet drugs before their transient ischemic attacks or stroke. Women and patients with vertebrobasilar symptoms responded especially well to ticlopidine. Arteriography was done on 1,188 of the 3,034 participants. The frequency of stroke in patients with abnormalities on arteriograms ipsilateral to their symptoms was slighter greater than in patients with normal carotid arteries. Ticlopidine was more effective in those without carotid stenosis.

Conclusions.—In patients with warning transient ischemic attacks, ticlopidine is more effective than aspirin in preventing subsequent stroke. Patients benefitting most from ticlopidine appear to be women, patients with vertebrobasilar symptoms, patients with cerebral ischemic symptoms while taking aspirin or anticoagulant treatment, and patients with diffuse atherosclerotic disease as opposed to high-grade carotid stenosis.

▶ The large Ticlopidine Aspirin Stroke Study convincingly demonstrated that ticlopidine reduces the risk of stroke or death by 12% and the risk of fatal or nonfatal stroke by 21% compared with aspirin in high-risk patients (1). This article, which is essentially a subgroup meta-analysis of that study, is admittedly not definitive, but it offers suggestions as to particular subgroups that might possibly benefit from ticlopidine over aspirin. Clinicians will have to struggle with these choices on a case-by-case basis, taking into account not only the increased efficacy of ticlopidine, but also its substantially greater cost and its slight propensity to induce reversible neutropenia.—M.D. Ginsberg, M.D.

Reference

1. Hass WK, Easton JD, Adams HP, et al: N *Engl J Med* 321:501, 1988.

Early Computed Tomographic Findings for Thrombolytic Therapy in Patients With Acute Brain Embolism
Okada Y, Sadoshima S, Nakane H, Utsunomiya H, Fujishima M (St Mary's Hosp, Kurume, Japan; Kyushu Univ, Fukuoka, Japan)
Stroke 23:20–23, 1992   1–25

Background.—Some clinical trials of thrombolytic treatment for acute brain infarction have resulted in unfavorable outcomes. In such cases, conversion to hemorrhagic infarction or frank hemorrhage caused clinical worsening or death. Recombinant tissue plasminogen activator (rt-PA) has been shown to be effective in patients with acute myocardial infarction; it was administered to patients with acute brain embolism to assess the clinical indications for this therapy.

Methods.—Ten patients received rt-PA, 20–30 MU for 1 hour, intravenously. Neurologic outcomes and findings on CT and angiography were assessed.

Results.—In 4 patients, symptoms ameliorated within 24 hours after onset. In 2 patients, occluded arteries reopened just after rt-PA infusion. Initial CT scans in 4 patients showed early indications of brain ischemia—an obscure margin of the lentiform nuclei, reduced tissue attenuation, or effacement of cortical sulci. In three of those 4 patients, occluded arteries did not reopen; 1 had a massive brain hemorrhage with clinical deterioration. Of the remaining 6 patients, 2 improved clinically with recanalization soon after treatment, suffering slight hemorrhagic complications. One-month outcomes were favorable in 5 patients and poor in 3. Two patients died.

Conclusions.—These findings suggest that thrombolytic treatment with rt-PA may be safe and effective in patients with no early CT findings within 3 hours of embolic stroke onset. However, the number of patients in this series was too small to draw definitive conclusions. Further hemodynamic and follow-up studies are needed.

▶ This small pilot study raises 2 interesting issues: the first concerns the possible value of early ischemic changes (or their absence) on CT scan in predicting the degree of responsiveness to acute thrombolytic therapy. The second issue relates to the suggestion offered by this study that the susceptibility of an occlusive thrombus to thrombolysis may relate in part to its location. In this study, occlusions at the top of the internal carotid artery failed to reopen. Definitive information on these points will come from large randomized trials.—M.D. Ginsberg, M.D.

Intracranial Hemorrhage in Association With Thrombolytic Therapy: Incidence and Clinical Predictive Factors
De Jaegere PP, Arnold AA, Balk AH, Simoons ML (Univ Hosp, Rotterdam-Dijkzigt, The Netherlands)
J Am Coll Cardiol 19:289–294, 1992   1–26

Background.—Thrombolytic therapy for patients with evolving myocardial infarction increases both survival and the risk of bleeding complications such as intracranial hemorrhage. The incidence of intracranial hemorrhage has varied from 0% to 1.4% in reported medium and large trials. It would be desirable to be able to identify patients at increased risk for bleeding. An investigation was conducted to determine the incidence of intracranial hemorrhage associated with thrombolytic therapy and to identify clinical predictive factors.

*Methods.—*A total of 2,469 patients with acute myocardial infarction treated with a thrombolytic agent were prospectively registered in 61 hospitals during an 18-month period beginning in 1988. Patients sustaining intracranial hemorrhage within 48 hours after the start of thrombolytic therapy were identified. To define clinical predictive risk factors, a case-control investigation was conducted in which 2 control patients who received thrombolytic therapy at the same hospital at the same period (but without the development of intracranial hemorrhage) were selected. These control patients were compared with patients who sustained intracranial hemorrhage.

*Results.—*Twenty-four of 2,469 patients sustained intracranial hemorrhage, for an incidence rate of 1%. The median time to first clinical manifestation of acute hemorrhage was 16 hours after thrombolytic treatment. Sixteen (66%) of these patients died (median time, 7.5 hours after diagnosis). A comparison of patients who sustained intracranial hemorrhage with control patients revealed that the former were significantly older, with a significantly greater likelihood of having a body weight of < 70 kg and a significantly greater dose index for patients treated with streptokinase. Patients who sustained intracranial hemorrhage also were more likely to have hypertension at admission, to have diabetes, and to be using oral anticoagulant drugs before admission. Multivariate analysis showed that the independent clinical predictors for intracranial hemorrhage were use of anticoagulant drugs before admission, body weight of < 70 kg, and age greater than 65 years.

*Conclusion.—*If a limited benefit of thrombolysis is expected in a patient with a low body weight, whose age is greater than 65 years, or who is using oral anticoagulants before admission; thrombolytic therapy should not be administered.

▶ The findings of this case-control study tend to confirm one's intuition; namely, that hypertension on admission, use of anticoagulants before admission, and diabetes and lower body weight are among the important independent predictive risk factors of intracranial hemorrhage in conjunction with thrombolysis. (The last factor may have led to relative overdosing.) This study, in which all patients with acute myocardial infarction received a thrombolytic agent, of course provides no data as to the expected incidence of intracranial hemorrhage in similar patients *not* so treated. Although this study does not establish *concurrent* anticoagulant therapy as an important risk factor for intracranial hemorrhage in patients receiving thrombolytic agents, this issue deserves further scrutiny.—M.D. Ginsberg, M.D.

Clinical Trial of Nimodipine in Acute Ischemic Stroke

The American Nimodipine Study Group (New York Neurological Inst)
Stroke 23:3–8, 1992   1–27

Background.—Calcium antagonists are promising for reducing the severity of acute ischemic stroke. Previously published trials of the use of nimodipine in acute ischemic stroke have yielded inconclusive or contradictory results. A randomized, double-blind, multicenter clinical trial was conducted to assess the safety and efficacy of nimodipine in patients who had sustained an acute ischemic stroke.

Methods.—A total of 1,064 patients were randomized to receive either placebo or 60 mg, 120 mg, or 240 mg of nimodipine daily for 21 days. Treatment began within 48 hours of stroke. Survival after 21 days of treatment, at 3 months posttreatment, and at 6 months posttreatment was assessed. Clinical deficit severity was assessed using the Toronto Scale and the motor strength scale from the Stroke Data Bank of the National Institute of Neurological Disorders and Stroke on days 4, 10, and 21 of treatment.

Results.—Overall, no significant effects of nimodipine on mortality, worsening, or clinical outcome measures were seen. Nimodipine was well tolerated. Among the subgroup receiving 120 mg of nimodipine daily who were treated within 18 hours of stroke onset, a small but significantly decreased frequency of worsening on day 4 was seen compared to patients receiving placebo. Among this same subgroup, those who had an initially negative CT scan had significantly better results than those who were were initially CT-positive.

Conclusions.—This trial did not demonstrate any overall benefit from nimodipine therapy begun within 48 hours of acute ischemic stroke. Further trials of its effect at a dosage of 120 mg per day on patients treated within 18 hours of stroke and having negative CT scans might clarify the meaning of the improved outcome for this subgroup.

▶ One notes with disappointment that the average time to start-of-treatment after stroke onset in this study was 28 ± 13 hours (mean ± SD), and that only 2.4% of patients were treated within 6 hours. Only 15.3% were treated within 12 hours. It is mystifying to this reviewer why costly and laborious clinical stroke trials continue to be designed in which times-to-treatment of 18, 24 or even 48 hours are permitted. A vast literature on the pathophysiology of cerebral ischemia has demonstrated rather convincingly that degradative changes in ischemically threatened neural tissue become irreversible by 4–6 hours. Thus, any therapy hoping to achieve metabolic salvage should be instituted within a time-window of 3–4 hours at the very latest.—M.D. Ginsberg, M.D.

Neurological Deterioration Under Isovolemic Hemodilution With Hydroxyethyl Starch in Acute Cerebral Ischemia
Mast H, Marx P (Freie Universität Berlin)
Stroke 22:680–683, 1991   1–28

Background.—Because hemodilution therapy for acute ischemic stroke remains controversial, a prospective, randomized trial was designed to assess isovolemic hemodilution with 10% hydroxyethyl starch in patients with acute ischemic stroke. This material appears preferable to dextran for hemorrheologic reasons.

Methods.—Seventy patients who had acute neurologic symptoms less than 48 hours before admission and who had a neurologic deficit were entered into the trial after a CT study confirmed ischemia. A group of 33 patients were randomized to undergo bloodletting and infusion of hydroxyethyl starch to produce a hematocrit of 35%. A second group of 37 patients did not undergo hemodilution. Cardiovascular risk factors were comparable in the 2 groups.

Results.—The mean hematocrit fell from 44.4% to 37.7% in the hemodilution group. Neurologic scores improved nearly twice as much in control as in those having hemodilution. No benefit from hemodilution was evident in patients seen within 12 hours or those with a marked reduction in hematocrit. Eight of the patients in the hemodilution group deteriorated clinically; many of them had a greater than 15% fall in hematocrit.

Conclusion.—Hemodilution below a hematocrit of about 45% is a potentially dangerous measure in patients with acute ischemic stroke and confers no clear clinical benefit.

▶ This study lends further weight to the view that hemodilution should be abandoned as a potential therapy for acute stroke. The improved cerebral blood flow is offset by the diminished oxygen-carrying capacity of the blood. Both isovolemic and hypervolemic forms of hemodilution have now been shown to lack clinical benefit, and each has been associated with a worsening of clinical outcome. Efforts to enhance cerebral perfusion after stroke must now take another form. One awaits the results of thrombolysis in acute stroke with anticipation and interest.—M.D. Ginsberg, M.D.

Cerebrovascular Instability in a Subset of Patients With Stroke and Transient Ischemic Attack

Friberg L, Olsen TS (Bispebjerg Hosp, Copenhagen)
Arch Neurol 48:1026–1031, 1991   1–29

Background.—Because they rarely are seen on cerebral angiograms, vasospasms have been rejected as a possible mechanism of focal cerebral ischemia in patients with transient ischemic attacks and stroke.

Methods.—The regional cerebral blood flow (rCBF) findings in 6 patients, suggesting that vasospasm may cause focal cerebral ischemia in some patients, were reviewed. The patients, 4 women and 2 men (aged 61–73 years) were taking part in a prospective consecutive investigation of 53 patients with stroke and transient ischemic attacks. All patients underwent cerebral angiography and repeated rCBF measurement no later than 48 hours after the onset of symptoms.

Findings.—Stable rCBF values, flow patterns, and clinical condition were noted in 47 patients. However, the remaining 6 patients had pronounced regional hypoperfusion and hyperperfusion during the examination, with variable rCBF values and extension of the abnormally perfused regions. Hypoperfusion was associated with transiently reduced flow consistent with ischemia; 4 patients had accompanying transient neurologic deficits. No large arterial spasms or thromboembolisms could be seen on arteriography or isotope angiography. The examination probably induced cerebrovascular instability on the arteriolar level. The patients, whether habitually or because of previous ischemic events, appeared to be hypersensitive to the provoking stimuli.

Conclusions.—The primary cause of some cases of focal cerebral ischemia could be spasm of the smallest resistance vessels rather than thromboembolism. The severity and duration of symptoms may be proportional to the number and duration of periods in which ischemic flow values occur. This type of hypersensitivity probably is much more frequent in patients with previous transient ischemic attacks and stroke than in the general population, particularly in those with classic and hemiplegic migraine.

▶ The authors of this study confront the classic dilemma that it is impossible to observe a phenomenon without also influencing it. In these patients studied within 48 hours of onset of their cerebral ischemic symptoms, a subgroup of 11% evolved patterns of regional cerebral hypoperfusion and hyperperfusion during carotid cannulation, contrast angiography, and repeated intracarotid ^{133}Xe-saline injections—procedures that may have affected platelets, vascular endothelium, or the neuromuscular elements of the vessel wall. Whether this cerebrovascular instability would have occurred in this (overly susceptible) subgroup of patients in the absence of these procedures cannot be answered, of course. These studies underscore the need for caution when applying invasive intracarotid procedures in patients with acute cerebral ischemia.—M.D. Ginsberg, M.D.

The Clinical Course of Perimesencephalic Nonaneurysmal Subarachnoid Hemorrhage
Rinkel GJE, Wijdicks EFM, Vermeulen M, Hasan D, Brouwers PJAM, van Gijn J (Univ Hosps, Utrecht and Rotterdam, The Netherlands)
Ann Neurol 29:463–468, 1991   1–30

Background.—Patients with perimesencephalic subarachnoid hemorrhage can be distinguished radiologically from other patients with subarachnoid hemorrhage by extravasation of small amounts of blood, primarily in the midbrain cisterns (Fig 1–4), and a normal angiogram. In a previous report, 13 patients with perimesencephalic hemorrhage with no

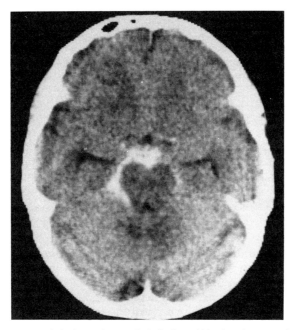

Fig 1–4.—Perimesencephalic hemorrhage with thick clots of blood in the interpeduncular and left ambient cistern, without extension to the frontal interhemispheric or sylvian fissures. (Courtesy of Rinkel GJE, Wijdicks EFM, Vermeulen M, et al: *Ann Neurol* 29:463–468, 1991.)

rebleeding or delayed cerebra ischemia (DCI) were described. These findings were tested in a much larger series.

Patients and Outcomes.—The early clinical course of 65 patients with perimesencephalic subarachnoid hemorrhage was documented. None had rebleeding and none had DCI. Only 3 patients (5%) had clinical signs of acute hydrocephalus; 2 of these patients needed ventricular shunting. These patients had hyponatremia and (ECG) changes in the same proportions as patients with aneurysmal rupture. All outcomes were good after 3 months. A control group of 49 patients with aneurysmal subarachnoid hemorrhage was examined; 4 of these patients developed DCI.

Conclusions.—The relatively small amount of blood does not account for the absence of DCI in perimesencephalic hemorrhage. Patients with a perimesencephalic pattern of bleeding and a normal angiogram should be viewed as having a distinct subset of subarachnoid hemorrhage and should be excluded from future treatment trials of patients with subarachnoid hemorrhage.

▶ All large series of patients with subarachnoid hemorrhage contain a small proportion with no demonstrated aneurysm or arteriovenous malformation. This paper recognizes the subgroup of these idiopathic cases with CT findings of small amounts of blood particularly concentrated around the midbrain. These patients clearly have a better prognosis than aneurysmal subarachnoid hemorrhage. The origin of the bleeding is still a puzzle.—W.G. Bradley, D.M., F.R.C.P.

Outcome in Patients With Subarachnoid Haemorrhage and Negative Angiography According to Pattern of Haemorrhage on Computed Tomography
Rinkel GJE, Wijdicks EFM, Hasan D, Kienstra GEM, Franke CL, Hageman LM, Vermeulen M, van Gijn J (Univ of Utrecht; Univ of Rotterdam; Univ of Amsterdam; St Elisabeth Hosp, Tilburg; De Wever Hosp, Heerlen, The Netherlands)
Lancet 338:964–968, 1991   1–31

Background.—Cerebral angiography is normal in 15% of patients with spontaneous subarachnoid hemorrhage. Although these patients do better than those with positive angiograms, patients with negative angiograms still can have rebleeding and cerebral ischemia. Patients with the perimesencephalic nonaneurysmal hemorrhage variant, who have a normal angiogram and accumulation of blood in the cisterns around the midbrain, have an excellent outcome.

Methods.—Outcome in 113 patients with and without the perimesencephalic pattern on CT were compared. The patients were treated for angiogram-negative subarachnoid hemorrhage during a 7½ year period. All patients were evaluated by CT using a third-generation scanner within 72 hours of the event. Follow-up was conducted for a minimum of 6 months (mean, 45 months). The perimesencephalic pattern was demonstrated by CT in 77 patients, and a pattern indistinguishable from that of proven aneurysmal bleeding was shown in 36 patients.

Results.—There were no deaths or disabilities resulting from hemorrhage in the patients with the perimesencephalic pattern. Of patients with the aneurysmal pattern, 4 had rebleeding, and 9 died or were disabled as a result of the hemorrhage. Overall, 97% of the perimesencephalic group had a good outcome (the other 2 patients died of carcinoma) compared with 75% of the aneurysmal group.

Conclusions.—The 2 distinct subgroups of patients wtih angiogram-negative subarachnoid hemorrhage that can be identified are those with a perimesencephalic pattern on CT, in whom the prognosis is excellent, and those with an aneurysmal pattern, who are prone to rebleeding, cerebral ischemia, and residual disability. Only patients with the latter pattern should have repeated angiographic studies in search of an occult aneurysm.

▶ Although the majority of patients with subarachnoid hemorrhage and negative angiography will prove to have an aneurysm on repeat angiography, in a proportion of patients this is not the case. Some of these have the perime-sencephalic distribution of blood that has been reported in this and several other recent papers. This paper indicates a significantly better prognosis for patients with this distribution of blood on the CT scan compared with the more typical aneurysmal type of blood distribution. Repeat angiography does not appear to be indicated. An unresolved question is the source of the perimesencephalic hemorrage.—W.G. Bradley, D.M., F.R.C.P.

2 Behavioral Neurology and Alzheimer's Disease

The Influence of Stimulus Properties on Visual Neglect
Tegnér R, Levander M (Karolinska Hosp, Stockholm)
J Neurol Neurosurg Psychiatry 54:882–887, 1991   2–1

Background.—Line bisection often is used to test unilateral neglect, but little is known about stimulus properties. A trial was conducted to determine how patients with unilateral neglect bisect objects other than lines, and to determine whether the performance of a particular task by an individual patient is related to a single neglect factor.

Methods.—Twenty-five right-handed patients with unilateral neglect after right cerebral hemisphere damage were included. Their performance on various bisection tasks was compared with that of control groups of 13 patients with right brain damage, 14 patients with left brain damage without neglect, and 10 persons without neurologic disease.

Results.—Whereas patients with right brain damage and neglect usually bisected lines of 100 and 200 mm to the right of the objective midpoint, 24 of 25 patients bisected 25 mm lines to the left of midpoint (Fig 2–1). Bisection of black filled rectangles and white lines on black paper was generally the same as with ordinary lines. When patients bisected white paper strips, rightward errors were usually less than with ordinary lines, and in 6 patients they even became leftward errors. Two patients bisected large circles accurately, although they made large rightward er-

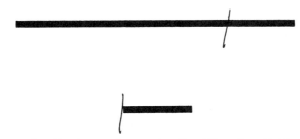

Fig 2–1.—Examples of line bisection from a patient. *Top*, 100-mm line with rightward error. *Bottom*, 25-mm line with subjective midpoint outside the presented line. (Courtesy of Tegnér R, Levander M: *J Neurol Neurosurg Psychiatry* 54:882–887, 1991.)

rors with long lines with lengths equal to the diameters of the circles. These patients made similar leftward errors with 25-mm lines and circles. When patients with neglect were asked to draw a line perpendicular to and the same length as a stimulus line 200 mm long, they drew erroneously short lines, as did the controls. With 25-mm lines, however, neglect patients drew erroneously long lines, whereas controls still drew erroneously short lines. The bisection of 25-mm lines by the only 2 patients with neglect who could perform the task at all varied with the apparent distance of the lines from the patient.

Conclusion.—Stimulus properties affect bisection performance by patients with visual neglect. In these patients, neglect may be the outcome of 2 independent mechanisms, 1 pushing to the left and 1 pushing to the right.

▶ This is an interesting study because it illustrates that many of our ideas about lateralization (and localization, for that matter) come from results of testing done with arbitrary stimuli used when syndromes were first being described. If the nature of the stimulus changes the type of deficit one observes, then this should be of importance not only to theoretical cognitive neuroscientists but also to workers in the field of rehabilitation.—A.M. Galaburda, M.D.

Left-Handedness, Homosexuality, HIV Infection and AIDS

Marchant-Haycox SE, McManus IC, Wilson GD (Univ College; St Mary's Hosp Med School; Inst of Psychiatry, London)
Cortex 27:49–56, 1991   2–2

Background.—In 1982, Geschwind and Behan proposed that high fetal testosterone levels may slow development of the left hemisphere, allowing the right hemisphere and, thus, the left hand to become dominant. It has also been suggested that homosexuality, left-handedness, and AIDS might be related through the same mechanism. Previous studies of lateralization in homosexual men have yielded conflicting results. This association was examined in a large group of male homosexuals and male and female heterosexuals.

Methods.—Included were 774 persons, 665 men and 109 women (mean age, 33.7 years). Of the men, 396 (51.2%) were heterosexual, 346 (44.7%) were homosexual, and 32 (4.1%) were bisexual. All responded to a questionnaire that asked whether they had ever been tested for HIV or had AIDS, whether they had a variety of conditions of relevance to the Geschwind hypothesis, and whether they were left or right handed.

Findings.—Of 1,204 questionnaires distributed, 791 (65.6%) were returned. In response to the question about HIV, 365 persons (47.2%) reported they had never been tested, 112 (14.5%) tested negative, 103 (13.3%) tested positive, and 194 (25.1%) had AIDS. There was a trend toward and an association between handedness and homosexuality, but it was nonsignificant after HIV and AIDS status was taken into account. A significant association was noted between left-handedness and having been tested for HIV infection, regardless of whether the test was positive or negative. There was no association between left-handedness and any of the conditions of relevance to the Geschwind hypothesis, including migraine, dyslexia, and stuttering.

Conclusions.—Left-handedness does not appear to be associated with homosexuality, but it is associated with having been tested for HIV infection. This may result from response bias by left-handers who are aware of the Geschwind hypothesis; an association between AIDS and left-handedness, and an excess mortality in left-handed patients with AIDS; or an increased likelihood of left-handers to acquire HIV infection but a reduced likelihood of AIDS developing. This investigation is incapable of distinguishing among these explanations.

▶ This is not the first study to report conflicting data on the association between immune characteristics, left-handedness, homosexuality, and HIV disease, and it is not the last. Since its publication, another paper did show a relationship between left-handedness and homosexuality, but no relationship between the latter and immune disorders. Both studies suffer from the pitfalls of ascertainment bias, and this alone may explain the conflicting results. Until a community-based epidemiologic study is carried out, with appropriate measures of handedness and reliable markers for the various immune disorders in question, no new light will be shed on this aspect of the Geschwind hypothesis.—A.M. Galaburda, M.D.

Reduced Natural Killer Cell Activity in Patients With Dementia of the Alzheimer Type
Araga S, Kagimoto H, Funamoto K, Takahashi K (Tottori Univ, Yonago, Japan)
Acta Neurol Scand 84:259–263, 1991   2–3

Background.—A previous trial reported abnormal natural killer (NK) cell activity in patients with Down's syndrome. Some characteristics of Down's syndrome are similar to those seen in Alzheimer's disease; however, NK cell activity in dementia of the Alzheimer type (DAT) has not been investigated.

Methods.—Heparinized peripheral blood samples were collected from 50 patients with DAT and 37 age-matched normal controls. Three patients with DAT had a clinical diagnosis of Alzheimer's disease. All assays for NK cell activity were performed in triplicate.

Results.—The NK cell activity in DAT was significantly less than that in controls. The NK cell activity induced by either interferon-α (IFN-α) or interleukin-2 (IL-2) was also significantly less than that in controls. Thus, NK cell activity and augmented NK cell activity in DAT were both less than in controls. Serum IL-2 and IFN-α levels in patients with DAT and controls were not significantly different.

Conclusions.—A conclusive diagnosis of DAT can only be made by examination of autopsied brain tissue. Increasing attention is therefore being focused on abnormalities of non-neuronal tissue, including circulation cells and fibroblasts. The molecular basis of reduced NK cell activity in DAT is still unknown, but the NK cells may have functional abnormalities that could provide valuable clues to fundamental cellular and molecular aberrations.

▶ Neuroimmunomodulation is the term given to the interaction between nervous and immune structures. There is growing interest in the relationship between immune disorders and neurologic disorders. Of special relevance to this article is the finding that, in rodents, NK cell activity is differentially affected by left hemisphere and right hemisphere lesions. Left hemisphere lesions depress this activity, whereas those on the right do not change it. There may be sex differences, too. In Alzheimer's disease, the question is: Do the brain lesions affect immunity, or do changes in immunity affect the brain lesions? Given the rodent model, I would suggest that the former is likely to be playing the main role in the changes in NK cell activity.—A.M. Galaburda, M.D.

The Medial Temporal Lobe Memory System
Squire LR, Zola-Morgan S (VA Med Ctr, San Diego; Univ of California, San Diego)
Science 253:1380–1386, 1991   2–4

Background.—Anatomical components of human memory are located in the medial temporal lobe, which is comprised of the hippocampus, amygdala, and adjacent anatomically related cortical regions, including the entorhinal, perirhinal, and papahippocampal cortices. Because the medial temporal lobe is a large region, it has been difficult to pinpoint which structures and connections within it make up the medial temporal lobe memory system that processes declarative memory. The development of a model of human amnesia in the monkey has made it possible to systematically investigate which anatomical structures are important for memory.

Methods.—A large bilateral lesion of the medial temporal lobe approximating the damage sustained by amnesic patients was produced surgically in the hippocampus, amygdala, and surrounding cortical cortices of monkeys. This lesion reproduced many important features of the memory impairment seen in amnesic patients.

Findings.—The monkeys were severely impaired on a number of memory tasks, but they were entirely normal in terms of acquiring and retaining new skills, confirming that the ability to acquire new memories

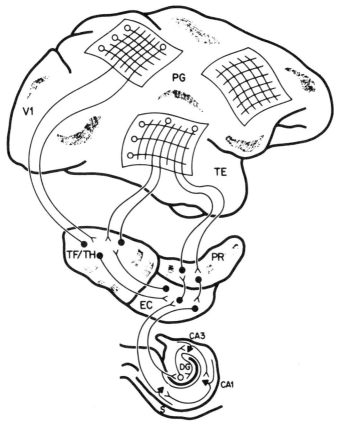

Fig 2–2.—Schematic drawing of primate neocortex plus the components of the medial temporal lobe memory system believed to be important in the transition from perception to memory. Networks in cortex show representations of visual object quality (in area *TE*) and object location (in area *PG*). If this distributed activity is to develop into a stable long-term memory, neutral activity must occur at the time of learning along projections from these regions to the medial temporal lobe, first to the parahippocampal gyrus (*TF/TH*), perirhinal cortex (*PR*), and entorhinal cortex (*EC*), and then in the several stages of the hippocampus (the dentate gyrus [*DG*] and the CA3 and CA1 regions). Fully processed input eventually exits this circuit by way of the subiculum (*S*) and EC, where widespread efferent projections return to neocortex. The hippocampus and adjacent structures bind together or otherwise support the development of representations in the neocortex, so that subsequently memory for a whole event (for example, represented in *TE* and *PG*) can be reactivated (even from a partial cue). (Courtesy of Squire LR, Zola-Morgan S: *Science* 253:1380–1386, 1991.)

is a distinct cerebral function separable from other perceptual and cognitive abilities. The studies also showed that the amygdaloid complex is not a component of the medial temporal lobe memory system and does not contribute to declarative memory. Thus, the medial temporal lobe memory system comprises the hippocampus and the adjacent anatomically related cortex, but not the amygdala. These structures, presumably by virtue of their widespread and reciprocal connections with neocortex, are crucial to the rapid acquisition of new information about fact and events. Although the medial temporal lobe memory system is fast, it has only limited capacity and its role in the establishment of long-term memory at the time of learning is only temporary. Its role in establishing long-term memory after learning continues during a long period of reorganization and consolidation during which memories stored in neocortex eventually become independent of the medial temporal lobe memory system. As time passes, the burden of long-term memory storage is gradually taken over by neocortex to ensure that the medial temporal lobe system is always available for the acquisition of new information (Fig 2–2). This explains why very remote memory is unaffected by damage restricted to the medial temporal lobe.

Conclusion.—As time passes after learning, permanent memory in the neocortex becomes independent of the medial temporal lobe, and remembering eventually becomes possible without the participation of the medial temporal lobe memory system.

▶ Clinicians will recall their patients wtih Korsakoff's syndrome and the discrepancy between severe involvement of recent memories but sparing of remote memories. However, emphasis is placed on the fact that 1 form of memory (declarative), but not the other (procedural), is affected by the medial temporal lesions. This work also may help resolve the age-old question about whether injury to the amygdala is necessary before the memory syndrome emerges. The authors strongly believe that it is not.—A.M. Galaburda, M.D.

Memory Loss Due to Transient Hypoperfusion in the Medial Temporal Lobes Including Hippocampus

Tanabe H, Hashikawa K, Nakagawa Y, Ikeda M, Yamamoto H, Harada K, Tsumoto T, Nishimura T, Shiraishi J, Kimura K (Osaka Univ, Japan)
Acta Neurol Scand 84:22–27, 1991   2–5

Objective.—A patient with typical transient global amnesia (TGA) who was examined with single-photon emission CT (SPECT) during and after an amnesic episode was described.

Case Report.—Woman, 63 years, was seen with a severe but transient inability to form new memories without other higher cortical dysfunctions. Retrograde memory loss also was evident, but remote past and immediate memory were preserved. During the amnesic episode, SPECT showed a marked decreased of cerebral blood flow in the areas confined to the territory of the bilateral posterior cerebral arteries including the hippocampus. With resolution of the amnesia, the hypoperfusion disappeared and cerebral blood flow returned to normal. One month after the TGA attack, MRI showed a focal lesion in the middle portion of the CA 1 field of the left hippocampus that could not be detected by CT scan.

Conclusion.—A transient reduction of cerebral blood flow in both medial temporal lobes, including the hippocampal formation, was demonstrated during an episode of TGA, which disappeared on resolution of the amnesia. These findings provide direct evidence that the medial temporal structures ae involved in the establishment of new memories as well as in the process of recalling recently acquired memories but not in retrieval of memories acquired long ago. The finding on MRI indicates the necessity of performing high-resolution MRI on the hippocampus of patients with TGA.

▶ The first point that must be stressed is that TGA is not global, but instead preserves remote memories, much like the Korsakoff syndrome. Amnesia for all memories is seen only in advanced neurologic disorders (in which severe elementary neurologic findings are evident) and in psychiatric disorders such as fugue states. The second point is that bilateral perfusion deficits may not be needed for the amnesic disorder to occur. Left-sided infarcts can produce transient memory disorders, but the latter usually last weeks.—A.M. Galaburda, M.D.

A Dyscalculic Patient With Selectively Impaired Processing of the Numbers 7, 9, and 0

Weddell RA (Morriston Hosp, Swansea, England)
Brain Cogn 17:240–271, 1991   2–6

Background.—Brain damage can selectively disrupt the component subprocesses involved in calculation. The study of patients with brain damage may help in identifying number processes that do not involve comprehension. A patient was encountered who had impaired arithmetic fact retrieval for the numbers 7, 9, and 0 only.

Case Report.—Man, 45, had a mild head injury followed 2 years later by a stroke, which left him with mild work-finding problems and paragrammatism for several months. Initially, he was incapable of doing simple number tasks. Neurologic testing showed only brisk reflexes in the left arm and leg, and CT showed mild dilation of the left lateral ventricle and possible hyperdensity in the right parietal region. Scores on the Wechsler Intelligence Scale, revised subtests involving numbers were selectively impaired, and he could not write the number 1–10, stopping after 6 because he did not know what came next. Further psychometric testing revealed special difficulties with the numbers 7, 9, and 0 in calculations presented both aurally and visually. The patient underwent a series of investigations of his abilities to perform addition, subtraction, multiplication, and division; acoustic analysis, including auditory input and phonologic output lexicons; and visual analysis, including orthographic input and output lexicons. The patient's difficulties were explained by a modification of the McCloskey, Caramazza, and Basili model of calculation processes. The patient had degraded sematic representations of the numbers 7 and 9, and he had lost knowledge of the rules pertaining to calculations involving the number 0. The problem was not found at the level of acoustic analysis, auditory input lexicon, phonologic output lexicon, visual analysis, or orthographic output lexicon.

Conclusion.—This patient reported use of visual imagery during single digit addition, but there is considerable interindividual variation in use of imagery.

▶ This paper is selected to demonstrate the power of modern cognitive science approaches for comprehension of the organization of the human mind. Cognitive science approaches, with their processing boxes and connections, are visually reminiscent of anatomical schemes with brain areas and axonal connections, although the similarity ends there. The justification for the boxes in the former is still, to a large extent, strengthened by the discovery of individual patients who lose one function while leaving another, seemingly proximate function, intact. The modularity of organization, that is, the evidence for remarkably independent processes, is often striking, as in the case in this patient, who has an inability to understand operations relating to the number 0 and the meaning of the numbers 7 and 9 only.—A.M. Galaburda, M.D.

Distribution of Cortical Neural Networks Involved in Word Comprehension and Word Retrieval
Wise R, Chollet F, Hadar U, Friston K, Hoffner E, Frackowiak R (Hammersmith Hosp, London; Charing Cross Hosp, Lond; Tel Aviv Univ, Israel)
Brain 114:1803–1817, 1991   2–7

Background.—Increasingly complex models of language processing have been proposed based on the assumption that the performance of an aphasic patient reflects the whole sequence of normal language processing minus the damaged components. If there is neurologic specificity in these models, then each step in a model based on symptom dissociation in patients with focal lesions must have a specific anatomical representation in the brain. The distribution of cortical neural networks involved in word comprehension and work retrieval was examined using positron emission tomography (PET) to measure activity-related changes in regional cerebral blood flow (rCBF).

Methods.—Six healthy men aged 29–48 years volunteered for the investigation. Activity-related changes in rCBF were measured in each man on 6 occasions—2 while the participant was at rest and 4 while single word language tasks were being performed. Data from each volunteer were standardized for brain shape and size, reconstructed parallel to the intercommissural line, and normalized for global flow differences. They were then averaged for each activation condition across the volunteers. Significant areas of rCBF change between task and rest conditions were referenced to the coordinates of a standard neuroanatomical atlas.

Results.—Categorical judgments on heard pairs of real words activate neural networks along both superior temporal gyri, but with an anatomical distribution comparable to that observed when the volunteers listened to nonwords. These tasks, which appear to be very different in cognitive demands, are apparently not different in the distribution of activation. During a verb generation task that required the volunteers to think of verbs appropriate to heard nouns presented slowly, the only temporal region activated was the left posterior superior temporal association cortex. Although activation in other superior temporal areas, both right and left, correlated with rates of work presentation during the 4 tasks, there was no such correlation in Wernicke's area. During verb generation, the left premotor and prefrontal cortex also were activated. Since the volunteers did not speak during the task, it appears that the act of retrieving words from semantic memory activates networks concerned with the production of speech sounds.

Conclusions.—Single word comprehension and retrieval activate very different distributed regions of cerebral cortex. Wernicke's area is the only area engaged by both processes. During silent word generation, networks involved in vocalization also participate.

▶ Most PET studies, including this one, are averaged over a series of subjects that have been matched for age, sex, and handedness. However, exact matching for the latter is not possible, particularly without the use of handedness questionnaires. This results in some sample heterogeneity that tends to lead to underestimation of the regions of the brain that participate in a given task. This reader believes that significant underestimation of right hemisphere participation is common is these studies and that the right hemisphere participation is common is these studies and that the relative size of areas in the left hemisphere that participate in language functions is also underestimated. This problem will be solved when technological advances permit sufficient signal detection from single cases.—A.M. Galaburda, M.D.

Positron Emission Tomographic Studies During Serial Word-Reading by Normal and Dyslexic Adults

Gross-Glenn K, Duara R, Barker WW, Loewenstein D, Chang J-Y, Yoshii F, Apicella AM, Pascal S, Boothe T, Sevush S, Jallad BJ, Novoa L, Lubs HA (Univ of Miami; Mt Sinai Med Center, Miami Beach, Fla; Toaki Univ Hosp, Kanagawa, Japan)
J Clin Exp Neuropsychol 13:531–544, 1991   2–8

Background.—The origin of the familial form of dyslexia is presumed to be neural. The first study to apply positron emission tomography (PET) to brain functioning during reading in dyslexics is reported.

Methods.—Twenty-five right-handed men were included. Eleven had a childhood history of reading and spelling problems severe enough to warrant remedial treatment, to disrupt their educational process, or

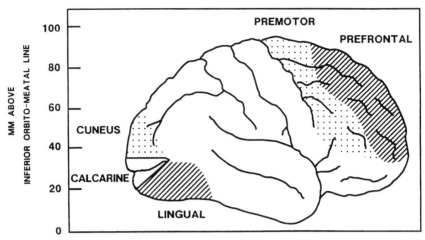

Fig 2–3.—Lateral projection of the brain, shown for anatomic localization only. Normalized rCMRglc differed between dyslexic and normal readers only in prefrontal and lingual regions (*shaded area*). *Dotted areas* indicate regions in which comparable differences between hemispheres were observed for both groups. (Courtesy of Gross-Glenn K, Duara R, Barker WW, et al: *J Clin Exper Neuropsychol* 13:531–544, 1991.)

both. In addition, these dyslexic men also had a positive family history of reading disability in at least 1 first-degree relative. The other 14 men did not have such histories and served as normal controls. Regional cerebral metabolic activity during oral reading was examined using PET.

Results.—The 2 groups differed signifiantly in normalized regional metabolic values in the prefrontal cortex and the lingual region of the occipital lobe. Dyslexic men had bilaterally greater lingual values than normal readers. Nondyslexic men had asymmetric findings in the prefrontal and lingual regions during reading, whereas the dyslexic pattern was more symmetric (Fig 2–3).

Conclusions.—These findings suggest that neural activity accompanying oral reading in dyslexics differs from that of normal persons in the lingual and prefrontal cortex regions. The location of these anomalies differs from the lesion sites previously found in persons with acquired dyslexia.

▶ Martha Denckla reported on differences in regional blood flow between dyslexics and controls and noted abnormalities in the frontal lobes, which this paper did not cite. The finding of greater symmetry in dyslexics is in accordance with anatomical and MRI studies published in recent years. Moreover, Galaburda and colleagues have reported minor cortical malformations in the dyslexic brain's cortex, many of which affect the prefrontal cortex anterior to Broca's speech area. Finally, the findings in the lingual gyrus may be related to recent data showing visual perceptive deficits in dyslexics.—A.M. Galaburda, M.D.

Transcortical Aphasia: Importance of the Nonspeech Dominant Hemisphere in Language Repetition

Berthier JL, Starkstein SE, Leiguarda R, Ruiz A, Mayberg HS, Wagner H, Price TR, Robinson RG (Inst of Neurological Research 'Dr Raul Carrea,' Buenos Aires; Johns Hopkins Univ; Univ of Maryland)
Brain 114:1409–1427, 1991   2–9

Background.—In transcortical aphasia (TA), relative preservation of repetition has traditionally been associated with functional integrity of the speech dominant (left) perisylvian (right) area. However, recent amytal data indicate that the nondominant (right) hemisphere plays a fundamental role in language repetition. The neuroradiologic correlates of repetition were examined in 21 patients with acute TA.

Methods.—The patients all had an acute focal brain lesion in the absence of previous brain injury and less than 2 months of evolution after the brain lesions. Each patient underwent language examination using the Western Aphasia Battery. Further tests of language processing also were done to more closely evaluate the mechanism subserving repetition. Neuroradiologic studies, including CT, MRI, or both were done 2–6 weeks after the stroke.

Results.—Nine patients had perisylvian lesions and 12 had lesions limited to the extraperisylvian areas; these frequencies were considered similar. The 2 groups had no significant differences in motor, sensory, or visual field deficits, or in neglect. Two of the patients in the perisylvian group had abolishment of repetition on injection of amytal in the hemisphere contralateral to the lesion. In another patient with a basal ganglia lesion, positron emission tomography showed marked hypometabolism across the entire left cortical mantle ipsilateral to the lesion. This indicated that structures in the right hemisphere were responsible for the preservation of repetition. This conclusion was confirmed in another patient with left extraperisylvian disease when a second lesion in the right hemisphere caused impairment of repetition.

Conclusions.—In some patients with TA who have lesions within or outside the speech-dominant perisylvian area, residual repetition may be subserved by the spared contralateral hemisphere. Further, more detailed studies of the brain areas associated with preserved repetition in TA are needed.

▶ The authors suggest that the right hemisphere may participate importantly in the fluent and intact repetition seen in transcortical aphasias. This would imply the radical notion that the nondominant hemisphere has the full complement of phonologic, semantic, and syntactic structures but is separated from thought, hence its inability to generate speech or comprehend language. It is also possible to think that in the event of the typical left hemisphere lesion causing TA, it is the right supplementary speech area, and not the left, that activates the standard left hemisphere speech area. I wonder what would happen if the left hemisphere got the amytal injection in the same patients? I would suggest that the ability to repeat would again stop.—A.M. Galaburda, M.D.

The Aphasic Isolate: A Clinical-CT Scan Study of a Particularly Severe Subgroup of Global Aphasics
De Renzi E, Colombo A, Scarpa M (Univ of Modena, Italy)
Brain 114:1719–1730, 1991   2–10

Objective.—Seventeen patients who appeared completely bereft of the possibility of entering into any form of communication after a stroke were examined to elucidate the clinical features of this subtype of global aphasia, its evolution, and its pathologic correlates as assessed by CT.

Patient.—The patients were completely unable to communicate with people who were addressing them 3–4 weeks after a left hemisphere stroke. Their willingness to interact with the environment differed, but they were all characterized by complete loss of speech output and inaccessibility to any kind of message, either verbal or through gestures. Twelve patients survived to the 6-month follow-up, and 11 survived to the 1-year examination. One patient was lost to follow-up before the 6-month assessment. Half of the patients reassessed were still in a state of complete communicative isolation. The rest had improved somewhat but were still globally aphasic.

Results of CT Scanning.—A CT scan basis for the aphasic picture could not be found. Only 35% of the patients had a lesional pattern consistent with the traditional view that ascribes global aphasia to the involvement of Broca's and Wernicke's areas. In the other patients, location of the lesion ranged from the anterior cortex to the posterior cortex to deep nuclei damage. None of the lesions that have been proposed to explain subcortical global aphasia were observed consistently.

Conclusions.—The reason for some patients' severe global aphasia cannot be found in a consistent anatomical pattern, at least using CT scanning. Studies with MRI, single-photon emission computed tomography, and positron emission tomography may show patterns of brain impairment specific for this picture. An alternative hypothesis is that the differences are the result of individual variability in the localization of cortical sites essential for language, as suggested by electrical stimulation mapping studies.

▶ It would not be prudent to abandon classical models of global aphasia as yet, based on the findings of the present study. All but one of the patients (patient 14) show involvement of a substantial portion of the perisylvian cortex, cortical or subcortical, or both. We also know that, even compared with MRI, CT tends to miss parenchymal involvement, and recent research with positron emission tomography has shown that areas of functional depression often are much larger than those shown to be structurally affected.—A.M. Galaburda, M.D.

Progressive Aphasia: A Case With Postmortem Correlation

Benson DF, Zaias BW (Univ of California, Los Angeles; City of Hope Natl Med Ctr, Duarte, Calif; Sheriff-Coroner, County of Orange, Santa Ana, Calif)
Neuropsychiatry Neuropsychol Behav Neurol 4:215–223, 1991   2–11

Background.—A small series of patients undergoing a slowly progressive aphasia was described in 1982. Their disease course was similar to that of the degenerative dementias, but their clinical signs and symptoms involved language almost exclusively. An additional case of progressive aphasia was described, including postmortem findings.

Case Report.—Man, 62, had a history of 4–5 years of progressively increasing difficulty finding words. He was still working as a manager of business development for an engineering firm but was having increasing difficulty explaining proposals to potential clients. He denied having problems with anything other than language. Language assessment showed a fluent, only mildly aphasic output. His word-finding problems were most notable, resulting in a hesitant, empty verbal output. Although his understanding of spoken language was excellent, his ability to repeat spoken language was limited. His ability to name on confrontation was extremely disturbed. He could accurately point to objects when named but often could not name these items. He had a significant calculation disorder; his insights were acute. Physical and neurologic examinations were not helpful in diagnosing this patient. About 1 year later, he underwent a detailed extensive research battery of neuropsychological and language tests. All defects found were directly referrable to his language disorder. An 18-fluorodeoxyglucose positron emission tomography scan showed asymmetric uptake with reduced metabolism in the left temporal-parietal region, with lesser degrees of hypometabolism in frontal and thalamic areas on the left. The progression of his language impairment was evident in the following 1½ years. His verbal output became almost unintelligible, and he could no longer read or write. The last 8 months of his life were marked by progressive physical and mental deterioration. He contracted a serious case of pneumonia and had a series of grand mal seizures. He died about 3 years after his initial neurobehavior examination. At postmortem, he was found to have bilateral and widespread distribution of plaques and tangles.

Conclusions.—This case was characterized by a slowly progressive mental disorder that appeared as an almost pure aphasia in its initial 6 years with a broader dementia developing in the end stage. These findings are best described as progressive aphasia.

▶ This case, like the previously reported cases of progressive aphasia, illustrates the difficulty with establishing clinicopathologic correlations in this disorder. My reading here is that the demonstrated neuropathologic changes would not have permitted a secure diagnosis of Alzheimer's disease, and that it is possible that the language systems of this brain were particularly vulnerable to relatively small degrees of pathology. One explanation may involve the presence of a cryptic developmental language disorder in this patient, and it may be important to characterize language development in future case studies.—A.M. Galaburda, M.D.

Apperceptive and Associative Forms of Prosopagnosia

De Renzi E, Faglioni P, Grossi D, Nichelli P (Università di Modena, Italy; Università di Napoli, Italy)
Cortex 27:213–221, 1991   2–12

Background.—Agnosia is further subclassified into an apperceptive and an associative form based on the stage at which impairment occurs. In apperceptive agnosia, impairment occurs at the stage where the physical characteristics of the stimulus are processed into a fully structured description. In associative agnosia, the stimulus is properly processed into a fully structured description, but associations that render the description meaningful cannot be recalled from semantic memory. Agnosia for faces, or prosopagnosia, is still considered a single disorder. However, subclassification into an apperceptive and an associative form would seem reasonable. A trial was conducted to determine whether prosopagnosia covers distinct forms of deficit similar to those recognized for agnosia.

Methods.—Three prosopagnosic patients each underwent 2 sets of visual tests, 1 set to evaluate object recognition and the other to assess face recognition. The set of agnosia tests included the object-naming test, picture-naming test, street completion test, and coin discrimination. The set of prosopagnosia tests included the unknown face matching and age-estimation tests to assess perception, and the familiarity check and famous face recognition tests to assess memory. The inner and outer tolerance limits of normal performance for the set of face-recognition tests were obtained from giving the tests to 100 normal volunteers, correcting the scores for age and educational level.

Results.—The first patient failed both the perceptual and the mnestic tests. In this patient, agnosia for faces was only 1 aspect of a more general disorder in processing shape information, resulting in apperceptive agnosia for every category of stimuli. The second patient also scored poorly on both perceptual and memory tests, but perception was more impaired. In contrast, the third patient had no perceptual deficit, but failed the memory tests. In this patient, the recognition impairment was restricted to faces, and recognition of objects in any other categories of stimuli was not impaired.

Conclusion.—Similarly to object agnosia, prosopagnosia also manifests different types of impairment covering distinct forms of perception and memory deficits.

► It is not surprising that deficits of face recognition could occur from the breakdown of any of the necessary psychological components necessary for this complex function. This article emphasizes the difference between the perceptual and memory deficits that contribute to face recognition difficulties. Unfortunately, we are not given enough anatomical detail to separate the size or location, or both, of the lesions in the two situations. However, it appears that some occipital dysfunction is needed for the apperceptive form. Of interest is the finding in the third patient of isolated face recognition difficulty, which brings to mind the face-sensitive cells described in the monkey.—A.M. Galaburda, M.D.

Denial of Visual Perception
Hartmann JA, Wolz WA, Roeltgen DP, Loverso FL (Univ of Missouri; Hahnemann Univ, Philadelphia; Braintree Hosp)
Brain Cogn 16:29–40, 1991   2–13

Background.—Patients with cortical blindness usually remain aware of both their deficit and their preserved visual ability, but some individuals have exhibited visual perception within a blind visual field. One patient totally denied intact visual perception in the absence of conversion disorder. He has inverse Anton's syndrome, Anton's syndrome being a condition in which patients with no visual perception deny blindness.

Case Report.—Man, 56, reported that 2 years earlier he had suddenly lost all vision and had regained no vision since. Bilateral cerebral infarction had been diagnosed. He was largely independent in living skills, taking care of his own affairs without the help of a housekeeper and walking in unfamiliar surrounds without help. He had never applied for services for the blind or attempted to obtain benefits. A stroke producing speech impairment had occurred about 15 years earlier. Examination showed a very well-oriented patient with normal pupillary responses and ocular motility. There were left-sided weakness, sensory loss, and moderate hypokinesis as well as a Babinski sign. Short term memory was slightly reduced, and a mild anomic aphasia was evident. Comprehension was mildly impaired at the level of complex syntactic commands. Responses depended heavily on the circumstances of stimulation. Occasional visual fixation was apparent, although the patient reported being unable to see. Testing for optokinetic nystagmus confirmed residual visual ability. On confrontation visual field testing, there was preserved vision in a 30-degree wedge-shaped region in the right upper quadrant. Several visual tasks were administered to confirm the presence of visual function; these tasks included confrontation naming, recognition of colors and faces, and reading single words. Separate lesions in the lower right occipital lobe, in the left parietal–occipital region, and involving the right frontal and parietal opercula were revealed on CT.

Conclusions.—This patient's denial of visual perception can be explained by a disconnection of parietal lobe attentional systems from visual perception. In prosopagnosia, visual perception is disconnected from memory systems.

▶ Clinicians are familiar with cases of denial of deficit, e.g., denial of hemiplegia and denial of blindness (Anton's syndrome). Such cases usually are seen in association with right hemisphere or bilateral lesions. The present case is particularly unusual because of denial of intact function, which in a way represents a neurologic lesion causing a conversion symptom. The authors propose an attentional disconnection to explain the phenomenon, as if the patient could only attend to the functions that are missing and not to those that are preserved.—A.M. Galaburda, M.D.

Musical Hallucinations: Report of Two Unusual Cases
Fisman M (Victoria Hosp, London, Canada)
Can J Psychiatry 36:609–611, 1991   2–14

Background.—Although rare musical hallucinations usually occur in females and are associated with age, deafness, and brain disease of the nondominant hemisphere. Data on 2 elderly patients with musical hallucinations were reviewed.

Case 1.—Woman, 65, had auditory hallucinations of sirens, ringing, hissing, and humming for 8 months. After taking lorazepam as an anxiolytic and temazepam as a hypnotic, she experienced musical hallucinations. She heard various songs in the left ear, but had no evidence of hallucinosis in any other sensory modality. She appeared alert although tense, without evidence of psychosis or personality disorder. Results of a neurologic examination including EEG were within normal limits. After discontinuation of temazepam and substitution of chloral hydrate for lorazepam, the musical hallucinations stopped, but tolerable tinnitus and hyperacusis in the left ear remained.

Case 2.—Woman, 87, had heard songs in her right ear for 3 years, which had been deaf as a result of childhood trauma. The songs were enjoyable tunes that she heard as a child. They had been more frequent in the evening for the last year. She had no hallucinations in any other modalities, no delusions, and no evidence of depression. She was alert and oriented but tended to isolate herself from the other residents of the home for the elderly in which she lived. She was diagnosed with mild organic brain syndrome and, because she functioned well, was not treated.

Conclusion.—These patients resemble those in the literature in most respects. Patient 1 is unusual in that hallucinations were associated with administration of rather than withdrawal from benzodiazepines. Benzodiazepine-precipitated musical hallucinations do not seem to have been previously reported. Patient 2 appeared to have Charles Bonnet syndrome, with musical hallucinations and auditory pathology replacing visual hallucinations and ocular pathology. Both patients had evidence of ear disease and CNS involvement. Appropriate tests should be performed so that musical hallucinations are not misdiagnosed as schizophrenia.

▶ This interesting but uncommon problem occurs in the setting of hearing loss and advanced age. It tends to affect women, but cases in men have been reported. It is important to look for a hidden depression, the treatment of which often resolves the hallucinations.—A.M. Galaburda, M.D.

Contributions of Occipital and Temporal Brain Regions to Visual and Acoustic Imagery—A SPECT Study
Goldenberg G, Podreka I, Steiner M, Franzen P, Deecke L (Neurologische Universitätsklinik, Vienna)
Neuropsychologia 29:695–702, 1991   2–15

Background.—Cognitive theories of visual imagery implicitly suggest that visual imagery is based on the activity of modality-specific visual cortex. If visual imagery is based on the activity of modality-specific visual brain areas, its cerebral correlate should be different from that of nonimaginal visual thinking and from imagery in other modalities, e.g., acoustic. Regional cerebral blood flow (rCBF) patterns elicited by imagery of the visual appearance of objects were compared with those of rCBF patterns elicited by imagery of the sounds made by those objects.

Methods.—Regional cerebral blood flow was assessed using ^{99m}Tc-hexamethyl-propylene-amine-oxime single photon emission computerized tomography. Two experimental groups were examined. In the control condition, both groups listened to abstract words. In th experimental condition, they heard 5 names of objects. One group was asked to visually imagine these objects; the other, to imagine the sounds made by these objects.

Findings.—Questionnaires completed after the experiment indicated that most of the participants in the acoustic imagery condition had visual images along with acoustic images. Both imagery conditions resulted in about equal increases of rCBF in the left inferior occipital region and the left thalamus. Participants in the acoustic condition had greater flow increases in both hippocampal regions and the right inferior and superior temporal regions than the participants in the visual imagery condition.

Conclusions.—Only the flow increases in the left inferior occipital region and the left thalamus fulfill criteria for being recognized as depending on modality-specific visual components of imagery. Flow increases in both hippocampal and the right inferior temporal region appear to depend on the total amount of information use for imagery rather than on the modality-specific visual aspect of imagery.

▶ The subtraction method illustrated by the present study is commonly used for determining minimum regions participating in a function of interest. However, from these results, I would also have concluded that the right superior temporal gyrus participates in acoustic imagery, because it is difficult to exclude the possibility that subjects undergoing visual imagery do not also image the objects, at least partly, in the acoustic modality.—A.M. Galaburda, M.D.

Brain Injury and Neurologic Sequelae: A Cohort Study of Dementia, Parkinsonism, and Amyotrophic Lateral Sclerosis
Williams DB, Annegers JF, Kokmen E, O'Brien PC, Kurland LT (Mayo Clinic, Rochester, Minn; Univ of Texas, Houston)
Neurology 41:1554–1557, 1991   2–16

Background.—Head trauma has been reported as a risk factor for Alzheimer's disease; it has also been linked to Parkinson's disease and amyotrophic lateral sclerosis (ALS).

Methods.—Data on 821 head trauma victims were reviewed to determine their incidence of dementia, parkinsonism, and ALS. The patients were treated for 859 episodes of head trauma with presumed brain injury in 1935–1974, and all were aged 40 years or older at their last medical assessment. Follow-up of more than 15,000 person-years was done until patients died, moved out of the study area, or contracted one of the target disorders.

Results.—There were no significant increases in the incidence of dementia and AD; the standard morbidity ratio (SMR) as 1.06 for dementia and 1 for Alzheimer's disease. There was no significant increase in the incidence of parkinsonism or ALS; the SMR was 1.04 for parkinsonism, .94 for Parkinson's disease, and 1.05 for ALS. Because of the number of patients involved, the power of these findings was weaker for parkinsonism and ALS.

Conclusions.—Contrary to previous reports, these findings suggest no association between head trauma and the development of Alzheimer's disease in mentally competent survivors. Nor does there appear to be any increase in risk of developing Parkinson's disease or ALS. Previous conclusions probably resulted from bias resulting from the use of surrogate respondents.

▶ Epidemiologic studies of risk factors based on retrospective patient-derived or relative-derived data often throw up many interesting and curious associations, but they often are unreliable. A person or a relative of someone with a disease searches back in his/her memory for antecedent events, whereas controls have no reason to do so. Only a population-based prospective study can resolve these problems. Kurland and his colleagues from the Mayo Clinic have done us a service by casting doubt on previous epidemiologic studies suggesting that head injuries predisposed to Alzheimer's disease, Parkinson's, and ALS.—W.G. Bradley, M.D., F.R.C.P.

Prospective Neuropathological Validation of Hachinski's Ischaemic Score in Dementias
Fischer P, Jellinger K, Gatterer G, Danielczyk W (Univ of Vienna; Lainz Geriatric Hosp, Vienna; Ludwig Boltzmann Inst for Clinical Neurobiology, Vienna)
J Neurol Neurosurg Psychiatry 54:580–583, 1991   2–17

Background.—Hachinski's Ischemic Score had been used as an empirical scale for differentiating between primary degenerative dementia (PDD) and multi-infarct dementia (MID) in many clinical investigations of dementia. However, its validity has been questioned and several modifications have been proposed. A prospective clinicopathologic investigation of 32 demented elderly patients was performed to validate the ischemic score.

Methods.—Autopsy specimens from each patient were examined. All of the patients had been chronically demented inpatients. The clinical diagnosis was established by complete medical and neuropsychiatric examination. Each patient was rated on the ischemic score at 1 month after admission and between 6 months and 4.1 years before death. Neuropathologic examination was done only in patients with clinical dementia.

Results.—At autopsy, 7 cases of primary degenerative dementia and 5 of MID were confirmed. Of 20 patients who were not classified unequivocally in life, 9 were found to have had primary degenerative dementia, 2 had MID, and 6 had mixed dementia (MIX). Sixteen patients had neuropathologic criteria for Alzheimer's disease. Mean ischemic score was 9.4 in MID, 11.3 in MIX, and 5 in primary degenerative dementia; the difference between MID–MIX and primary degenerative dementia was highly significant. The 2 items that were able to differentiate significantly were history of stroke and fluctuating course, both of which were more common in MID–MIX. The ischemic score correctly diagnosed MID–MIX in 92.3% of the patients, although there were a number of false positive diagnoses. Its sensitivity in diagnosing primary degenerative dementia ranged from 52.6% to 78.9%; it labeled 21% of patients with primary degenerative dementia as having a vascular cause.

Conclusions.—Hachinski's Ischemic Score is sensitive in diagnosing vascular dementia, but not in diagnosing primary degenerative dementia. It cannot define a group of patients wth purely vascular dementia. A patient with clinical and pathologic evidence of stroke does not necessarily have dementia resulting from cerebrovascular disease. The ischemic score could be useful in excluding patients with a vascular pathogenesis of dementia, but its use in epidemiologic studies could result in over-diagnosis of MID.

▶ This clinical/pathologic study underscores the limitations of Hachinski's Ischemic Score in differentiating vascular and degenerative dementias. For example, the ischemic score is completely unable to differentiate pure MID from cases in which vascular and degenerative elements co-exist (MIX). Of note is that, on the basis of *one* element of Hachinski's Score alone (history of stroke), one can correctly diagnose MID–MIX (84.6%) and degenerative dementia (89.5%) in about as high a percentage of cases as by the use of the entire score (92.3% and 78.9%)! As the authors suggest, the ischemic score may be useful in facilitating the exclusion of vascular cases from clinical drug trials of degenerative dementia, but it offers no advantage in differential diagnosis.—M.D. Ginsberg, M.D.

Estimated Prevalence of Dementia Among Elderly Black and White Community Residents

Heyman A, Fillenbaum G, Prosnitz B, Raiford K, Burchett B, Clark C (Duke Univ; Graduate Hosp, Philadelphia)
Arch Neurol 48:594–598, 1991   2–18

Background.—One study in an elderly biracial population suggested that blacks have a higher prevalence of dementia than whites, whereas another, smaller study suggested that the prevalence is equal in the 2 races, but that blacks have a higher prevalence of dementia caused by cerebrovascular disease. The prevalence of dementia was estimated in elderly blacks and whites in the Piedmont region of North Carolina.

Methods.—Participants were drawn from a longitudinal investigation of a stratified sample of 4,164 elderly residents. Of this group, a random sample of 164 persons, 83 blacks and 81 whites, were examined by a neurologist, who administered a semistructured interview. The diagnosis

Distribution of Subjects
With Dementia

	Black	White
Probable Alzheimer's disease	12	4
Mixed or multi-infarct dementia	5	1
Systemic cancer or brain tumor	2	1
Parkinson's disease	...	1
Total	**19**	**7**

(Courtesy of Heyman A, Fillenbaum G, Prosnitz B, et al: *Arch Neurol* 48:594–598, 1991.)

of dementia and Alzheimer's disease was made using the *Diagnostic and Statistical Manual of Mental Disorders, Third Edition* and the National Institute of Neurological Disorders and Stroke—Alzheimer's Disease and Related Disorders Association criteria.

Results.—Dementia was diagnosed in 26 persons (table), for an estimated prevalence of 16% for blacks and 3.05% for whites. Prevalence was 2.9% for white women and 3.3% for white men, whereas it was 19.9% for black women and 8.9% for black men. Only 26.9% of whites with impaired Short Portable Mental Status Questionnaire scores had dementia, compared with 44.4% of blacks. Standards for accepting dementia appeared to be no different between the races. Thirteen patients had a previous diagnosis of dementia, and 7 of the remainder had a diagnosis of Alzheimer's disease; the remaining 6 patients could not be evaluated. History of stroke, hypertension, and other chronic disorders was more common in blacks. Other than the higher rate of institutionalization of whites, none of the identified factors could explain the differing prevalence of dementia.

Conclusions.—There appears to be a significant difference in the prevalence of dementia in blacks and whites. The higher rate in blacks may result from a history of stroke and hypertension. Black and white patients with dementia show no significant differences in their ability to perform activities of daily living.

▶ The importance of this study lies in that at least 2 of the issues raised to explain the differences between the 2 groups are potentially capable of being changed. The first issue involves cerebrovascular disease, which, in the black population, is most often related to hypertension. The second is education. The reviewer believes that the speed of the clinical course of dementia is inversely proportional to the number of mental strategies for problem solving available to the patient at the onset of the disease, which in turn depends to a large extent on education. The more educated the patient, the longer it will take for the disease to eliminate all of the learned strategies, which will manifest clinically as dementia. This is another (socially) treatable condition, that may lead to more equivalent results in black and white populations.—A.M. Galaburda, M.D.

Is Age Kinder to the Initially More Able? A Study of Eminent Scientists and Academics
Christensen H, Henderson AS (Australian Natl Univ, Canberra)
Psychol Med 21:935–946, 1991   2–19

Background.—Whether those who are initially more able decline less rapidly in terms of mental ability remains unanswered. A substantial minority of reports have found more rapid rates of decline for those who are initially less able, but a few have reported the reverse.

Methods.—A cross-sectional analysis was undertaken in which elderly groups of academics and blue-collar workers were compared with PhD students and trade apprentices. Twenty-six academicians aged 70 and older were matched for age with retired blue-collar workers. The younger participants were mostly in their twenties. Mental activity was estimated using a scale developed by Schonfeld, which focuses on the part of each day occupied by active or passive pursuits. Various intellectual and memory tasks also were used.

Results.—Both elderly groups did less well than the younger participants on tests of perceptual–motor speed, visuospatial reasoning, inferential thinking, and memory. With 1 exception, the similarities subtest of the Wechsler Adult Intelligence Scale, rates of change in memory and intelligence did not differ between the high- and low-ability groups.

Conclusions.—This investigation strongly supports the view that high initial intelligence does not protect normal persons against an age-related decline in cognitive functioning. It nevertheless is true that the more able can compensate on tests of vocabulary and classification, which depend on previously stored information.

▶ This study concludes that, in normal aging, the previous level of achievement does not appear to affect the rate of deterioration. This is not surprising, because achievement relates only in part to intelligence. It also suggests that normal aging is diffuse enough that compensation by unaffected areas in individuals with more education and practice is not substantially better. However, this may not be the case in dementia, in which a more focal process may be involved and experience with multiple ways to solve problems may be useful for early compensation.—A.M. Galaburda, M.D.

Mild Cognitive Impairment in the Elderly: Predictors of Dementia
Flicker C, Ferris SH, Reisberg B (New York Univ)
Neurology 41:1006–1009, 1991   2–20

Background.—Clinical interviews with elderly individuals are commonly used to assess mild cognitive impairment. However, the information obtained in these interviews usually is not sufficient to classify a mildly impaired person as demented or nondemented. Psychometric tests that could distinguish between benign senescent forgetfulness and more significant conditions would be useful. This longitudinal trial was carried out to examine the potential usefulness of objective psychological tests for use as predictors of follow-up cognitive status.

Methods.—Thirty-two elderly persons (mean age, of 71.3 years) with clinically identified mild cognitive impairment and 32 normal elderly age- and education-matched controls (mean age, of 70.9 years) underwent a full diagnostic evaluation that included medical, neurologic, and psychiatric evaluation, CT of the head, and a comprehensive cognitive assessment evaluation. Follow-up involved assessment of primary degenerative dementia using the global deterioration scale (GDS) approximately 2 years after the initial work-up. The mean follow-up interval was 2.21 years for controls and 2.11 years for mildly impaired individuals.

Results.—Individuals with clinically identified mild cognitive impairment at baseline performed significantly more poorly than did normal elderly controls on tests of recent memory, remote memory, language function, concept formation, and visuospatial praxis. Twenty-three of the 32 mildly impaired individuals had an increase in GDS rating, whereas only 4 controls had such an increase. Of the 23 mildly impaired persons who showed decline on the GDS, 16 had a previous diagnosis of probable Alzheimer's disease; 5, vascular or mixed dementia; 1, brain granuloma; and 1, leukemia and CNS involvement.

Conclusions.—Objective psychological tests can be used to discriminate between mildly impaired elderly individuals who are likely to undergo significant cognitive deterioration during a 2-year period and those whose prognosis is relatively benign.

▶ This paper addresses a common and critical clinical question. Will this elderly patient with mild cognitive and memory difficulties develop frank dementia? The authors suggest that some psychometric tests are helpful for making an accurate prediction. In any case, however, most of these patients will progress to the diagnosis of dementia, and in the relatively short period of about 2 years.—A.M. Galaburda, M.D.

Memory and Attention in Patients With Senile Dementia of the Alzheimer Type and in Normal Elderly Subjects

Lines CR, Dawson C, Preston GC, Reich S, Foster C, Traub M (Merck Sharpe and Dohme Neuroscience Research Ctr, Harlow; St Thomas' Hosp, London; Queen Mary's Hosp, Sidcup, England)
J Clin Exp Neuropsychol 13:691–702, 1991   2–21

Background.—Previous trials demonstrated that cholinergic blockade in normal persons impairs vigilance and causes memory deficits. The extent to which these deficits mimic the symptoms of early Alzheimer's disease remains unknown. To test the validity of the pharmacologic model of dementia, patients with mild dementia were tested on measures of vigilance known to be sensitive to cholinergic blockade.

Methods.—Included were 6 women and 2 men with mild senile dementia of the Alzheimer's type of 8 normal age-matched controls; 8 patients with moderate dementia also were tested. The 3 broad categories of assessments were tests of overall intellectual function, sustained attention tests, and memory tests.

Results.—All patients with mild dementia and half of those with moderate dementia performed normally on tests of vigilance and demonstrated the expected memory deficits. The patients with mild dementia performed as well as controls on tasks of visual and auditory vigilance, but they showed considerable impairment in domains of cognition such as verbal free recall, delayed recall, and fluency.

Conclusions.—In patients with mild dementia, unlike in normal persons receiving scopolamine, the memory deficit observed does not involve failure of sustained attention. Thus, drugs that enhance vigilance may be of questionable value for these patients. This finding does not preclude such attentional deficits appearing as the disease progresses; the various aspects of attention at different stages of the disease should be examined in detail.

▶ The classic condition in which memory loss is not associated with disorders of vigilance or attention is Korsakoff's syndrome. On the other hand, it is clear that any cause of impaired vigilance will impair memory as well as other cognitive functions. The present results suggest that the patient with Alzheimer's disease is more like the patient with Korsakoff's syndrome, which is probably true, but problems with attention and vigilance often creep into the clinical picture of Alzheimer's disease.—A.M. Galaburda, M.D.

Evaluation of Cerebral Biopsies for the Diagnosis of Dementia
Hulette CM, Earl NL, Crain BJ (Duke Univ)
Arch Neurol 49:28–31, 1992   2–22

Background.—In most patients dementia can be diagnosed clinically, although histologic confirmation may be necessary. A series of cerebral biopsies were reviewed To identify patients most likely to benefit from this procedure.

Methods.—Fourteen unselected cerebral biopsies were performed during a 9-year period for the sole purpose of diagnosing dementia in adult patients. The patients were 7 men and 7 women (mean age, 51.6 years); the mean duration of symptoms was 2.3 years.

Results.—A definitive diagnosis was made in 7 patients: 3 had Cruetzfeldt-Jakob disease, and 1 each had Alzheimer's disease, diffuse Lewy body disease, adult-onset Niemann-Pick disease, and anaplastic astrocytoma. Of the nondiagnostic group, 2 were normal and 5 showed nondiagnostic abnormalities, especially gliosis (table). Most patients in the nondiagnostic group had hemiparesis, chorea, athetosis, or lower motor neuron signs, compared with none of the diagnostic group.

Conclusions.—A cerebral biopsy specimen can provide a definitive diagnosis for many patients with atypical dementia. Patients with certain signs are unlikely to benefit; consultation is needed to select the best patients and sites. As many patients undergoing biopsy have Creutzfeldt-Jakob disease, precautions are need in handling biopsy tissue.

Pathologic Findings at Biopsy

Case	Site of Biopsy	Type of Biopsy	Tissue Examined	Spongi-form Change	Neuritic Plaques per ×10 Field	Tangles	White-Matter Gliosis	Other
1	R temporal	Open	1 cm³	+	0	0	0	0
2	L temporal	Open	1 cm³	+	0	0	0	0
3	R temporal	Open	1 cm³	+	0	0	0	0
4	R frontal	Open	1 cm³	0	>100	+	+	Amyloid angiopathy
5	R temporal	Open	1 cm³	0	9	0	0	Lewy bodies
6	R temporal	Open	1 cm³	0	0	0	0	Neuronal storage
7	R temporal / L temporal	Needle / needle	1 × 0.3 × 0.3 cm / 1 × 0.3 × 0.1 cm	0/0	0/0	0/0	+/0	0/anaplastic astrocytoma
8	R frontal	Open	1 cm³	0	0	0	+	0
9	L parietal	Open	1 cm³	0	0	±	+	0
10	R temporal	Open	1 cm³	±	0	0	0	0
11	L temporal	Open	1 cm³	0	23	0	+	0
12	L temporal	Open	1 cm³	0	0	0	+	0
13	R frontal	Open	1 cm³	0	0	0	0	0
14	L temporal / L frontal	Open / open	1 cm³ / 1 cm³	0/0	0/0	0/0	0/0	0/0

Note: *Plus sign* indicates present; *zero*, absent; *plus-minus sign,* questionably present.
(Courtesy of Hulette CM, Earl ML, Crain BJ: *Arch Neurol* 49:28–31, 1992.)

▶ Two advances have diminished the need of biopsy for establishing a specific cause of a dementing illness: (1) a better understanding of the clinical profile associated with the different types of dementias (including blood tests and lumbar puncture, as in the case of paraneoplastic syndrome); and (2) improved anatomical classification based on the appearance seen on MRI scans. It is hoped that improving clinical sophistication, standard anatomical imaging, and functional studies done with activation MRI or positron emission tomography will be able to improve prebiopsy diagnostic ability further, with the goal of eliminating biopsy altogether.—A.M. Galaburda, M.D.

Physical Basis of Cognitive Alterations in Alzheimer's Disease: Synapse Loss Is the Major Correlate of Cognitive Impairment
Terry RD, Masliah E, Salmon DP, Butters N, DeTeresa R, Hill R, Hansen LA, Katzman R (Univ of California, San Diego)
Ann Neurol 30:572–580, 1991   2–23

Background.—Many neuropathologic and neurochemical alterations in association with Alzheimer's disease have been identified, but few investigations have found a correlation between any of these markers and cognitive deficiency. Recent reports have suggested that neuronal death in Alzheimer's disease is closely associated with the extensive loss of synapses in the neocortex. The correlation among a number of structural and neurochemical measurements in the neocortex of patients with Alzheimer's disease and 3 global neuropsychological tests was examined.

Patients.—Fifteen patients with confirmed Alzheimer's disease aged 59–91 years at the time of death and 9 normal controls aged 57–89 years at the time of death were examined. All autopsies were performed within 8 hours of death. Midfrontal, rostral superior temporal, and inferior parietal areas of the neocortex were analyzed for total plaques, neuritic plaques, tangles, large neurons, synapses, choline acetyltransferase (ChAT), and somatostatin. The Blessed Information–Memory–Concentration test, the Minimental State Examination, and the Dementia Rating Scale had been administered between 2 weeks and 3 years before death.

Results.—In all 15 patients with Alzheimer's disease, the concentrations of ChAT and somatostatin were below normal according to published values, but a statistical comparison with controls was not possible. Multivariate analysis revealed only weak correlations between psychometric test scores and the presence of plaques and tangles. The duration of disease did not correlate with psychological test scores. Age at death correlated slightly with all 3 tests. The loss of synaptic density in the midfrontal and inferior parietal areas of the neocortex was very powefully associated with all 3 psychological tests.

Conclusions.—The loss of synapses in the neocortex appears to be the most powerful factor leading to the dementia of Alzheimer's disease.

▶ This article is important in at least 2 respects. First, it illustrates that synaptic density correlates better with psychological profiles than do other neuropathologic findings in Alzheimer's disease. This is not surprising, because loss of inputs will change synaptic densities well before they lead, if ever, to cell death. Thus, synaptic density better assesses the extent of the anatomical substrate of the dysfunction. The best correlation with the inferior parietal cortex is also interesting, because this area is strongly interconnected with the hippocampal formation. Second, it is possible to demonstrate synaptic density with antibodies under light microscopy, thus making it possible to bypass electron microscopy and to apply this clinical predictor to routine biopsies.—A.M. Galaburda, M.D.

Alzheimer's Disease: The Proteoglycans Hypothesis
Celesia GG (Loyola Univ of Chicago, Maywood, Ill)
Semin Thromb Hemost 17:158–160, 1991   2–24

Introduction.—The cause of Alzheimer's disease (AD) remains uncertain, but its pathology is characterized by the presence of neurofibrillary tangles in neurons, neuritic (or senile) plaques in the gray matter, granulovacuolar degeneration of neurons within the pyramidal cell layer of the hippocampus, and amyloid angiopathy. Plaques are much more prevalent in Alzheimer's disease than in the normal aged brain. They consist of immunoglobulin and complement, inorganic aluminosylicate, and, at their core, amyloid. Immunocytochemical evidence suggests that neurites within plaques are degenerating neuronal processes.

Observations on Amyloid.—The amyloid protein precursor may be a heparan sulfate proteoglycan, and proteoglycans are important parts of the extracellular matrix and of cell membranes. Altered heparan sulfate proteoglycan might interfere with normal synaptic transmission. Sera from patients with Alzheimer's disease contain IgG antibodies that react with small vessels and capillaries of normal brain. Antibody to purified vascular heparan sulfate proteoglycan also has been identified in Alzheimer's disease sera.

Hypothesis.—Antivascular antibodies may be directed against vascular heparan sulfate proteoglycan to block antibody receptor sites of the blood–brain barrier. A defective barrier could allow the passage of injurious substances into the brain. Or, the antibodies could penetrate into the brain and react with neurons, impairing synaptic vesicle function. A defective blood–brain barrier also could disrupt normal clearance of amyloid protein precursor metabolites, leading to deposition of amyloid.

▶ In diseases in which attempts to find the underlying cause have been so difficult, as in Alzheimer's disease, we are always looking for new theories. Celesia suggests that an abnormal blood–brain barrier, perhaps related to proteoglycans, might underlie the disease. The importance of theories is that they can lead to new experiments and, hence, to the accumulation of new data.—W.G. Bradley, D.M., F.R.C.P

Segregation Analysis Reveals Evidence of a Major Gene for Alzheimer Disease
Farrer LA, Myers RH, Connor L, Cupples LA, Growdon JH (Boston Univ; Harvard Med School)
Am J Hum Genet 48:1026–1033, 1991   2–25

Background.—There is evidence from a wide variety of sources for a genetic component of Alzheimer's disease, but it has been difficult to sort out the relative effects of major genes, multifactorial heritability, and cohort effects.

Methods.—Complex segregation analysis was carried out on 232 nuclear families ascertained consecutively through a single proband referred for assessment of a memory disorder. In the analysis, the unified version of the mixed model of Morton and MacLean was used.

Findings.—Alzheimer's disease was present in 108 of 1,193 first-degree relatives of the 232 probands (9%). The mean age at onset in affected relatives was 75 years, 7.4 years older than the mean for probands. Susceptibility to Alzheimer's disease appeared to be determined in part by a major autosomal dominant allele with an added multifactorial component. The single-locus, polygenic, sporadic, and nontransmission models all were rejected to a statistically significant degree, as was recessive inheritance of the major effect. A marginally significant excess of transmission from the heterozygote may reflect the presence of phenocopies or, perhaps, the existence of 2 or more major loci for Alzheimer's disease. The estimated frequency of the Alzheimer's disease susceptibility allele was .04. The major locus accounted for 24% of variance in transmission.

Future Work.—The challenge for future research is the dissection of the non–major-locus component of Alzheimer's disease to distinguish individual genetic and environmental factors. Hopefully, accurate characterization of genetic and other risk factors will suggest ways of preventing the disease or will at least enhance the ability to predict individual susceptibility.

▶ Alzheimer's disease is clearly dominantly inherited in families with early onset of dementia and appears to be caused by a gene on chromosone 21 close to the amyloid precursor gene. However, in the general population, Alzheimer's disease becomes more frequent with age, being present in more than one third of patients surviving past age 85 years. In later onset cases, there is often a similarly affected family member, but this would be expected quite frequently by chance. This study suggests an underlying dominant gene even in the later onset cases, with many other factors playing a role in manifestation. The chromosome localization and nature of this gene remains to be determined.—W.G. Bradley, D.M., F.R.C.P.

Linkage Studies in Familial Alzheimer Disease: Evidence for Chromosome 19 Linkage
Pericak-Vance MA, Bebout JL, Gaskell PC Jr, Yamaoka LH, Hung W-Y, Alberts MJ, Walker AP, Bartlett RJ, Haynes CA, Welsh KA, Earl NL, Heyman A, Clark CM, Roses AD (Duke Univ)
Am J Hum Genet 48:1034–1050, 1991   2–26

Background.—Alzheimer's disease is the leading cause of dementia in elderly persons. Its cause remains uncertain, but a genetic component is supported by indirect evidence. Familial aggregation of affected persons has been explained by autosomal dominant inheritance with age-dependent penetrance. Linkage of familial Alzheimer's disease has been described in families with early-onset disease, but later reports have provided inconsistent results.

Methods.—A genomic search for an additional locus of familial Alzheimer's disease (other than chromosome 21) was undertaken in 293 members of 32 families with Alzheimer's disease; 87 members were affected. Of the 32 families, 28 had 3 or more affected persons in their pedigree. Most of those affected were first-degree relatives. The affected-pedigree-member method of linkage analysis was used as an initial screeen.

Findings.—Two regions suggesting linkage were identified: the chromosome 21 region described by Hyslop et al. and the proximal long arm of chromosome 19. Standard likelihood analysis supported the possibility of a familial gene for Alzheimer's disease on chromosome 19, especially in families with late-onset disease.

Conclusions.—There now is evidence supporting chromosome 19 linkage in families with late-onset Alzheimer's disease and chromosome 21 linkage in families with early-onset with disease. These findings confirm genetic heterogeneity in Alzheimer's disease.

▶ This study of a large number of families with Alzheimer's disease by the Duke group confirms the heterogeneity of the condition. Only about half the families had autopsy-proven Alzheimer's disease and almost all of them had late-onset disease. Evidence for a gene linkage on the proximal long arm of chromosome 19 was identified in this group of families, in addition to the chromosome 21 region linkage.—W.G. Bradley, D.M., F.R.C.P.

Widespread Serum Amyloid P Immunoreactivity in Cortical Amyloid Deposits and the Neurofibrillary Pathology of Alzheimer's Disease and Other Degenerative Disorders
Kalaria RN, Galloway PG, Perry G (Case Western Reserve Univ; Children's Hosp, Akron, Ohio)
Neuropathol Appl Neurobiol 17:189–201, 1991   2–27

Background.—Amyloid P component is a highly structured protein found in all systemic forms of amyloid disease. Amyloid P has also been demonstrated in cerebral amyloid lesions of Alzheimer's disease, Creutzfeldt-Jakob disease, and other related disorders exhibiting cerebral congophilic amyloid angiopathy. An investigation was conducted using immunocytochemical staining methods to characterize the spectrum of amyloid P immunoreactivity in the neurofibrillary pathology of Alzheimer's disease and other neurodegenerative disorders.

Methods.—Tissue samples were obtained at autopsy from different cortical areas of 40 patients. Five patients had no brain pathology at the time of death and served as controls. The others had died with Alzheimer's disease, Down's syndrome, diffuse Lewy body diseases, Parkinson's disease, Creutzfeld-Jakob disease, Pick's disease, multi-infarct dementia, or progressive supranuclear palsy.

Findings.—Amyloid P immunoreaction product was seen in all classic amyloid lesions, and neurofibrillary pathology was seen in a large sample of all cortical areas examined from patients who died with Alzheimer's disease or Down's syndrome. In sections from patients with Alzheimer's disease and Down's syndrome, the distribution and pattern of immunoreactivity were strikingly similar to the distinct staining of the amyloid lesions by thioflavin S and by an antiserum to A4/β protein. Electron microscopy confirmed that amyloid P immunoreactivity was associated with the abnormal filaments characteristic of neurofibrillary pathology and with the amyloid fibrils found in plaques and vessels showing congophilic amyloid angiopathy. Plaques of Creutzfeld-Jakob disease, Pick bodies of Pick's disease, tangles and Lewy bodies in Parkinson's disease and in a subpopulation of Lewy bodies in the diffuse Lewy body disease coexistent with Alzheimer's disease also were stained. Amyloid P was not found in the age-matched controls.

Conclusion.—Amyloid P appears to be an integral feature of most, if not all, amyloid deposits and of cerebral neurofibrillary pathology.

▶ Amyloid P is a normal α-1-glycoprotein of serum. In mice it appears to be an acute phase reactive protein, but its function in humans remains undetermined. This paper indicates that it nonspecifically involves amyloid fibrils in several neurologic diseases, and, hence, may be a nonspecific, perhaps degradative, reactive protein.—W.G. Bradley, D.M., F.R.C.P.

Cessation of Driving and Unsafe Motor Vehicle Operation by Dementia Patients
Gilley DW, Wilson RS, Bennett DA, Stebbins GT, Bernard BA, Whalen ME, Fox JH (Rush-Presbyterian-St Luke's Med Ctr, Chicago; Univ of Victoria, British Columbia)
Arch Intern Med 151:941–946, 1991   2–28

Background.—The potential effects of impaired cognition resulting from dementia on driving skills bears on public safety. In 2 previous small-scale investigations, patients who continued to drive after onset and diagnosis of Alzheimer's disease had a higher rate of motor vehicle accidents than controls; level of cognitive function was not assessed in these investigations. A retrospective survey was designed to relate degree of dementia of various causes and other factors to probability of unsafe driving behavior and duration of driving after diagnosis.

Methods.—Two hundred five patients diagnosed with probable or possible Alzheimer's disease and 138 patients with dementias of vascular or other causes, all of whom continued to drive after disease onset, were examined. Of these, 93 were still driving at the time of the survey. Degree of dementia was assessed using the mini mental state examination and the Mattis Dementia Rating Scale; driving impairment was determined from accident records and informant reports.

Reports.—Although one third of the patients still driving had been involved in some type of unsafe vehicle operation in the preceding 6 months, the likelihood of an accident could not be related to severity of dementia. However, there was a significant association of accidents with the use of sedative prescription medications by these patients and with subjective informant reports of impaired driving ability. When all 333 patients who were driving at the time of diagnosis were included in the analysis, the median time driving after diagnosis was significantly longer with Alzheimer's disease (34.4 months) than in patients without Alzheimer's disease (24.1 month).

Conclusions.—As is found in many epidemiologic investigations of drivers in automobile accidents, medications with sedative components increased the likelihood of accidents in dementia patients. Accidents were equally likely to occur at any point in the development of dementia: thus, the longer a patient continued to drive, the greater the cumulative risk of having an accident.

▶ Patients with recurrent seizures are universally prohibited from driving. The situation is less clear with dementia, although judgment plays a major role in driving safely. This study of a large number of patients with dementia demonstrates an undoubted increase in the risk of accidents for this group of patients. Further studies will be needed to determine the criteria for recommending discontinuation of driving for such patients.—W.G. Bradley, D.M., F.R.C.P.

Intramuscular Desferrioxamine in Patients With Alzheimer's Disease
Crapper McLachlan DR, Dalton AJ, Kruck TPA, Bell MY, Smith WL, Kalow W, Andrews DF (Univ of Toronto, Canada; New York State Inst for Basic Research in Developmental Disabilities, Staten Island; Behaviour Research Program, Toronto, Canada; Queen Street Mental Health Centre, Toronto)
Lancet 337:1304–1308, 1991   2–29

Background.—There is epidemiologic and biochemical evidence to suggest a causal role for aluminum in the pathogenesis of Alzheimer's disease. However, there is no evidence of a causal link for aluminum in disease progression. The results of a 2-year, single-blind clinical trial were examined to investigate whether progression of the dementia of Alzheimer's disease could be slowed by deferoxamine (DFO) mesylate. Deferoxamine is a trivalent ion chelator that was selected because of its high stability constants for iron and aluminum and because of the extensive clinical data on its use in aluminum and iron overload.

Methods.—Of 48 patients living at home with probable Alzheimer's disease, 25 were allocated randomly to DFO administered intramuscularly twice daily 5 days per week by a caregiver, and 23 received orally administered placebo or no treatment. The initial dose was 500 mg per day, but the dose was reduced to 125 mg on day 17 and was maintained at that level for the remainder of the 24-month trial. All patients underwent complete psychometric assessment at baseline. General medical and neurologic examinations were peformed at 6-month intervals. Activities of daily living also were assessed and video recorded at 6-month intervals. Caregivers maintained a daily record of medical status.

Results.—There were no significant differences between the groups in baseline measures of intelligence, memory, or speech ability. There was no difference in the rate of decline between patients treated with orally administered placebo and nontreated patients. Analysis of the videotapes revealed that DFO treatment significantly slowed the rate of decline in daily living skills. Nontreated patients declined twice as fast as DFO-treated patients. Side effects were minimal. Four patients complained of loss of appetite and 1 patient had gradual weight loss. However, these effects were reversed by temporary suspension of DFO treatments.

Conclusion.—Sustained intramuscular administration of DFO may slow the clinical progression of dementia associated with Alzheimer's disease.

▶ Crapper McLachlan has produced much evidence over the years that aluminum is closely associated with neuronal degeneration in Alzheimer's disease. An attempt to treat the disease by removing the aluminum is a natural extension of the hypothesis. This single-blind, controlled study appears to indicate an improvement with DFO therapy in Alzheimer's disease. Unfortunately, the study is somewhat flawed by the fact that the placebo group did not receive identical intramuscular injections twice daily, as did the DFO group. The placebo effect of intramuscular injections undoubtedly exceeds those of oral tablets. If true, this study is of great importance, but other studies will be necessary to confirm this finding.—W.G. Bradley, D.M., F.R.C.P.

Tacrine in Alzheimer's Disease
Eagger SA, Levy R, Sahakian BJ (Inst of Psychiatry, London)
Lancet 337:989–992, 1991   2–30

Background.—The cause of Alzheimer's disease is unknown. However, many symptoms are related to changes in neurotransmitters of the cholinergic system. Tacrine has been proposed as a possible therapeutic agent. The efficacy and safety of tacrine (tetrahydroaminoacridine) plus lecithin were assessed in a randomized, double-blind, placebo-controlled, crossover trial.

Methods.—A total of 65 patients with probable Alzheimer's disease were included. The active treatment was the maximally tolerated dose of as much as 150 mg of tacrine and 10.8 g of lecithin daily. Patients were assigned randomly to active or placebo treatment and crossed over after 13 weeks of treatment and 4 weeks of washout. The outcome was measured by the mini mental state examination, the abbreviated mental test score, and the rating by the caretaker of the activities of daily living scale.

Results.—There was a significant benefit of tacrine over placebo in the mini mental state examination and the abbreviated mental test score systems, but not in the rating of the activities of daily living. Serum liver enzymes increased with dosage, but this was reversible.

Conclusions.—There was significant symptomatic improvement in patients with Alzheimer's disease who received tacrine. The clinical relevance of this improvement is left to the individual judgment of the practitioner.

▶ There is considerable loss of nucleus basalis cells and their cholinergic transmitter function in the brain of patients with Alzheimer's disease. Many studies have attempted to correct the cholinergic deficit. There has been considerable controversy about tacrine. This randomized, double-blind, placebo-controlled crossover study showed a definite benefit in patients with probable Alzheimer's disease. It should be noted that lecithin also was used in the experimental group.—W.G. Bradley, D.M., F.R.C.P.

Frontal Lobe Degeneration: Clinical, Neuropsychological, and SPECT Characteristics
Miller BL, Cummings JL, Villanueva-Meyer J, Boone K, Mehringer CM, Lesser IM, Mena I (Harbor–Univ of California, Los Angeles Med Center, Torrance, Calif)
Neurology 41:1374–1382, 1991   2–31

Background.—Research on degenerative dementias that primarily affect the frontal lobes has expanded in recent years. However, many unresolved issues still exist on the clinical and blood flow characteristics of frontal lobe degeneration (FLD). Magnetic resonance imaging single photon emission CT (SPECT), and neuropsychological tests were used to assess the characteristics of 8 patients with FLD.

Patients.—The earliest and most common clinical presentations were social withdrawal and behavioral disinhibition. Psychiatric symptoms typically preceded the onset of dementia by several years. Neuropsychological assessment demonstrated selective impairment of frontal and memory tasks. There was relative sparing of attention, language, and visuospatial skills. Examination with SPECT revealed frontal and temporal hypoperfusion, with relative sparing of parietal and occipital blood flow.

Conclusions.—The most severe abnormality in patients with FLD is hypoperfusion in the prefrontal cortex. These disorders result in profound impairment of performance on neuropsychological tests and in behavioral disturbances characterized by apathy, social disinhibition, poor judgment, and depression. Although global regional cerebral blood flow (rCBF) is lessened, the parietal lobes are spared selectively, resulting in relative preservation of tasks such as constructions and calculations.

Although hexamethyl propyleneamine oxime SPECT seems to be diagnostic in the early phases of this syndrome, it is not know whether rCBF changes occur before clinical changes.

▶ The present findings should be contrasted with those of the typical patient with senile dementia of the Alzheimer type, particularly with relatively early onset type, who instead shows significant parietal and temporal dysfunction characterized by memory, language, and visuospatial deficits without frontal lobe abnormalities. On the other hand, many of the metabolic dementias, which are potentially reversible with prompt treatment, present with apathy and other frontal lobe signs.—A.M. Galaburda, M.D.

Treating Organic Abulia With Bromocriptine and Lisuride: Four Case Studies
Barrett K (School of Postgraduate Medicine and Biological Science, Stoke on Trent, England)
J Neurol Neurosurg Psychiatry 54:718–721, 1991   2–32

Background.—Abulia, an inability to perform acts voluntarily or make decisions, is used to describe problems of drive and volition as a result of brain damage. Bromocriptin, a dopamine agonist with predominantly postsynaptic action, has been used successfully to treat akinetic mutism, the most severe form of abulia. Bromocriptine was used to treat abulia of varying severity.

Patients.—In the 4 patients included, abulia was caused by brain damage from alcohol in 2 patients, by Wilson's disease in 1 patient, and by basal ganglia infarct in 1 patient. All the disorders affected the basal ganglia or diencephalon, or both. Bromocriptine dosage varied from 25 to 70 mg.

Results.—All of the patients improved considerably while receiving bromocriptine, and 3 deteriorated when the dose was reduced or withdrawn. In 1 patient, bromocriptine was replaced by lisuride with good effects after a depressive disorder developed.

Conclusions.—These findings are encouraging and indicate the need for a placebo-controlled trial of bromocriptine.

▶ Patients with various forms of brain damage may suffer the syndromes of abulia, akinetic mutism, and persistent vegetative state. The 4 patients described here were affected with moderate severity and showed a degree of response to postsynaptic dopaminergic agonists that appeared comparable to the response seen in the movie "Awakenings." Some patients also improve with therapy with amphetamine or methylphenidate.—W.G. Bradley, D.M., F.R.C.P.

Some Cytoarchitectural Abnormalities of the Entorhinal Cortex in Schizophrenia

Arnold SE, Hyman BT, Van Hoesen GW, Damasio AR (Univ of Iowa)
Arch Gen Psychiatry 48:625–632, 1991   2–33

Background.—There is evidence to suggest that patients with schizophrenia may have abnormalities in temporal-lobe structure and function. The entorhinal cortex plays a role in normal neuropsychological function and is vital for neural systems that mediate corticohippocampal interactions. The entorhinal cortex in schizophrenic patients was examined to determine whether structural abnormalities in this region could account for some of the psychological abnormalities of schizophrenia.

Methods.—The cytoarchitecture of entorhinal cortex was examined in 6 schizophrenic patients aged 23–80 years at the time of death and in 16 controls aged 33–80 years at the time of death. All 6 schizophrenic patients had undergone long-term institutionalizations. Four patients had undergone prefrontal lobotomies, and 2 had leukotomies.

Results.—Each of the schizophrenic brains had abnormal structural patterns in the rostral and intermediate portions of the entorhinal cortex. The abnormalities included bilateral deep invaginations of the normally smooth middle of the entorhinal cortex surface, disruption of cortical layers around the invaginations, heterotopic displacement of neurons, and poorly developed superficial lamination with a paucity of neurons in the superficial layers. In the deeper layers, some of the pyramidal cells were abnormally oriented. The changes observed, particularly the heterotopic and laminar invaginations, are static abnormalities of the entorhinal cortex that are likely to be of developmental origin.

Conclusion.—Although the neuropathologic abnormalities observed in entorhinal the cortex cannot account for the array of findings in schizophrenia by themselves, it is likely that these changes are incompatible with normal neuropsychologic processes and, thus, may have a role in the symptomatology of schizophrenia.

▶ As the authors caution, it is difficult to be certain about the anatomical findings in this set of observations. However, other observations recently published implicate other portions of the temporal lobe, particularly the superior temporal gyrus, in some schizophrenics. Taken together, it is possible that a trend is developing that involves the temporal lobes in the anatomical basis of schizophrenia.—A.M. Galaburda, M.D.

3 Epilepsy and EEG

The Risk of Seizure Recurrence Following A First Unprovoked Seizure: A Quantitative Review
Berg AT, Shinnar S (Yale Univ; Albert Einstein College of Medicine, NY)
Neurology 41:965–972, 1991   3–1

Background.—There is still controversy concerning whether a patient should be treated after a first unprovoked seizure. A meta-analysis of 16 previously published reports was undertaken to evaluate factors that may account for the variability in results and to determine factors that would identify individuals at risk for recurrent seizure.

Findings.—For the 16 investigations, the estimated risks of recurrent seizures ranged from 23% to 71%. Three factors accounted for much of the variation in results: the inclusion criteria that determined whether patients were enrolled only at the time of their first seizure or whether patients with previous seizures were included; retrospective prospective ascertainment of patients; and the interval between the first seizure and the time at which risk was assessed. The average overall pooled estimate of recurrence risk was 51%. When only reports that used first-seizure patients were considered, the risk was 40% in prospective analyses and 52% in retrospective analyses, whereas the risk was 67% in non–first seizure reports. At or near 2 years after the first seizure, the risk of recurrence was 36% in prospective analyses and 47% in retrospective analyses. The cause of seizures and EEG were the strongest predictors of recurrence. The risk was lowest (24%) in the idiopathic group with normal EEGs and highest (65%) in the remote symptomatic group with normal EEGs. Despite some inconsistencies, partial seizures also were associated with increased recurrence risk, particularly among patients with remote symptomatic first seizures.

Conclusions.—There is considerable agreement among the published reports concerning the overall risk of recurrence after a first unprovoked seizure. Differences in investigation methods and distributions of important prognostic factors may account for the differences among results. The cause of seizures and EEG are strong predictors of recurrence, with patients having idiopathic seizures and normal EEGs exhibiting the lowest risk.

▶ This article addresses one of the most important issues in epilepsy: What is the risk for recurrence and should the first seizure be treated? The reported risk of a second seizure has been wide ranging, leading to considerable disagreement on treatment approaches. Two findings of note are reported. First, the outcome is different between prospective and retrospective studies. Retrospective studies are more likely to have incomplete data and have biased study populations. Second, recurrence was much lower with an idiopathic single seizure. This article should help guide us in identifying patients with low risk of recurrence so that we do not start them on anticonvulsant medications.—E. Ramsay, M.D.

Randomised Study of Antiepileptic Drug Withdrawal in Patients in Remission
Medical Research Council Antiepileptic Drug Withdrawal Study Group
Lancet 337:1175–1180, 1991   3–2

Background.—Withdrawal of antiepileptic drug therapy and the associated seizure recurrence have important consequences. Consensus is lacking on the success of drug withdrawal policies, and the advice given to patients therefore varies considerably. A multicenter, randomized, clinical trial was done to compare seizure control under a policy of slow antiepileptic drug withdrawal with routine maintenance of therapy.

Methods.—Clinicians in 40 British and 5 other European centers participated. Randomization was done in 1,013 patients who had been seizure free for at least 2 years. An additional 776 patients were eligible, but they were not randomized. Patients in the slow withdrawal group had decrements in their dosage every 4 weeks, with the decreases depending on the drug being taken and whether the patient was an adult or a child. Follow-up was conducted at 3 months, 6 months, 1 year, and yearly thereafter.

Results.—Two years after randomization, 78% of patients who continued treatment were seizure free, compared with 59% of those in whom treatment was withdrawn; however, the difference between the groups declined thereafter. Hazard ratio peaked about 9 months after entry. Only a small proportion of seizure risk in the patients in the continued treatment group resulted from noncompliance. The most important factor in reducing the risk of seizure was longer seizure-free periods. The most important factors in increasing the risk of seizure were taking more than 1 antiepileptic drug and a history of tonic-clonic seizures. Smaller effects were noted for other factors, such as history of neonatal seizures and specific EEG features, but confidence intervals for these observations were wide. Comparison with eligible but nonrandomized patients suggested that the results could be applied to a wider patient population.

Conclusions.—Relative risks of seizure recurrence for patients who elect to withdraw from antiepileptic drug treatment after a period of seizure remission are reported. A statistical model to predict relapse may be developed by the stratified proportional hazards model. Patient counseling may be assisted by validation in this population.

▶ What should one do with an epileptic patient who has been seizure free on medication for more than 2 years? This multicenter study indicated that withdrawal of medication was associated with a higher frequency of seizures than in the control group that continued anticonvulsant therapy. This important paper should be read in full.—W.G. Bradley, D.M., F.R.C.P.

Benign Familial Neonatal Convulsions: Evidence for Clinical and Genetic Heterogeneity

Ryan SG, Wiznitzer M, Hollman C, Torres MC, Szekeresova M, Schneider S
(Univ of Texas, San Antonio; Case Western Reserve Univ)
Ann Neurol 29:469–473, 1991   3–3

Background.—Most primary epilepsies probably have a multifactorial origin, and the role of genetic factors in these disorders has not been defined. The syndrome of benign familial neonatal convulsions (BFNC) is a rare, transient, primary epilepsy of infancy with unequivocally autosomal dominant inheritance. Recently, the gene for BFNC was assigned to chromosome 20q. To determine whether BFNC is genetically heterogeneous, linkage analysis was performed in 2 previously unreported BFNC pedigrees whose clinical features suggested that the disorder is heterogeneous.

Patients.—The proband of the first family was a healthy, term neonate of Mexican-American ancestry. On the ninth day of life, she had 4 clonic convulsions. The infant was treated with phenobarbital, which was discontinued 1 month later. At 9 months of age the patient was developmentally normal and had no recurrence of seizures. Thirteen relatives of the proband also had neonatal seizures, but none had seizures after the age of 2 months. All family members had normal intellectual development. The proband of the second family was a healthy, term neonate of European ancestry. On the second day of life, she had 11 partial clonic seizures. At least 2 additional seizures occurred during the next 3 weeks (despite administration of phenobarbital), but no other seizures occurred thereafter. Twelve relatives of the proband had a clear history of idiopathic neonatal convulsions, and seizures often did not remit until they were 6–24 old months. Two relatives had febrile convulsions, and 4 had apparent audiogenic seizures. There were also 2 obligate carriers. One relative continued to have frequent convulsions until late adolescence. All family members appeared intellectually normal.

Findings.—Linkage studies performed in both families with chromosome 20 markers D20S19 and D20S20 favored linkage of the disease and marker loci in the second family by a maximum odds ratio of 45:1 at 6% recombination. However, in the first family, the odds were greater than 20,000:1 against linkage at 10% recombination or less.

Conclusions.—The syndrome of BFNC is clinically and genetically heterogeneous. Further investigations will have to be performed to clarify the relationship between phenotype and genotype in this disorder.

▶ It is not surprising to find genetic heterogeneity for a syndrome as clinically diverse as BFNC. However, it is encouraging that new families are being identified in which the abnormality can be assigned to chromosome 20q. Identification of the abnormal gene product in just one familial epilepsy should have considerable impact on our understanding of genetic epilepsies and on the development of new anticonvulsant drugs.—G.M. Fenichel, M.D.

Theophylline and Status Epilepticus in Children
Dunn DW, Parekh HU (Indiana Univ)
Neuropediatrics 22:24–26, 1991   3–4

Background.—Theophylline is known to trigger seizures, but its effect on outcome of seizures is unknown. The effect of theophylline on the occurrence and outcome of status epilepticus was evaluated in children.

Patients.—Of 114 episodes of status epilepticus occurring in 97 children during a 2-year period, 16 occurred in children receiving theophylline within 24 hours before the seizure. Serum theophylline levels were obtained within several hours for all 16 patients. In 8 patients, the serum theophylline concentration appeared to be greater than 20 µg/mL at the onset of status epilepticus; in the other group of 8, the theophylline level was either therapeutic or low.

Findings.—In the group with high theophylline levels, 5 of the children had possible precipitating factors. Mean duration of the episode was 1.3 hours. One child died and 3 sustained significant new neurologic damage. In the group with normal to low theophylline levels, all children were receiving chronic theophylline therapy and 6 had possible precipitating factors. Mean duration of status epilepticus was 1.75 hours. There were no deaths in this group, and only 1 child sustained a transient neurologic deficit. In the overall group of 114 episodes of status epilepticus, incidence of death or persistent neurologic deficit was 23%.

Conclusions.—At toxic levels, theophylline appears to be a significant factor in increased morbidity in children with status epilepticus. Failure to compensate for the increased cerebral metabolic rate of status epilepticus, resulting from hypoxia from the underlying respiratory disorder and the reduced cerebral blood flow that occurs with theophylline increases the risk of a poor outcome. For asthmatic children who are at risk of seizures, theophylline is not the initial drug of choice.

▶ Theophylline has long been known to cause seizures at toxic blood concentrations. It is now generally recognized that it can cause status epilepticus at therapeutic levels in children who are not epileptic. Its value in the treatment of asthma has diminished with the development of other drugs, and its use on an outpatient basis in children is being abandoned.—G.M. Fenichel, M.D.

Temporal Lobectomy for the Treatment of Intractable Complex Partial Seizures of Temporal Lobe Origin in Early Childhood
Hopkins IJ, Klug GL (Royal Children's Hosp, Melbourne)
Dev Med Child Neurol 33:26–31, 1991   3–5

Background.—Recently, there has been renewed interest in the surgical treatment of children and adolescents with intractable epilepsy. Temporal lobectomy is performed most often. The use of temporal lobectomy for intractable epilepsy was examined in 11 children in the first decade of life.

Methods.—Between 1978 and 1988, 21 children underwent temporal lobectomy for epilepsy, 11 of whom were younger than 10 years at operation. There were 8 boys and 3 girls, (mean age, 2 years at onset of epilepsy; 5 years 6 months at operation). All children had complex partial seizures diagnosed on clinical grounds. The seizure type was confirmed with ictal video/EEG monitoring in 7 patients. The frequency of seizures ranged from weekly to several daily in the 6 months before operation. All patients had been treated with a wide range of anticonvulsants. Six operations were left-sided and 5 were right-sided. Ten children had standard temporal lobectomies, leaving the superior temporal gyrus intact and limiting posterior resection to 4.5–5.5 cm from the tip of the temporal lobe. Most of the tissue was removed as a block. One patient had a more limited resection of the lateral aspect of the temporal lobe to remove a small superficial tumor, and medial temporal structures were left intact.

Results.—After a mean follow-up period of 3.6 years, 8 children were free of seizures and 2 had a reduction in seizure frequency to less than 25% of the presurgery rate. Epilepsy and general neurologic status were worse in 1 patient with progressive encephalitis. Four children have shown significantly improved behavior, and none have shown a worsening of behavior. Major surgical complications did not occur. Minor surgical complications included partial upper-quadrantic visual field defects in 2 children and very minor hemiparesis in 2 other children. Pathologic examination of the excised tissue revealed that the cause of the epilepsy was likely mesial temporal sclerosis in 4 children, glioma in 5, dysplasia in 1, and chronic progressive encephalitis in 1.

Conclusion.—The remission rate in young children who undergo temporal lobectomy for intractable epilepsy in the first decade of life is comparable to that obtained in older children and adults in recently reported series.

▶ Temporal lobectomy is an important alternative in children with intractable seizures of temporal lobe origin. The large percentage of children with glioma in this series reinforces the now accepted need for MRI rather than CT in the routine evaluation of children with intractable focal seizures.—G.M. Fenichel, M.D.

EEG Laterality in the Era of Structural Brain Imaging
Myslobodsky MS, Coppola R, Weinberger DR (Natl Inst of Mental Health, Washington, DC; Tel-Aviv Univ, Ramat-Aviv, Israel)
Brain Topogr 3:381–390, 1991   3–6

Introduction.—Although bilateral EEG recording is commonly performed when brain laterality is assessed for research purposes, there are uncertainties about its precision and validity. Structural brain imaging methods allow examination of the EEG electrode placements according to the 10-20 system and of the validity of inferences made from the data. Common sources of error in placement were reviewed, along with factors that may contribute to the EEG imbalance.

Plagiocephaly.—Subtle, normal cranial deformities may be included in laterality EEG data. Plagiocephaly (often characterized by a unilateral occipital flattening with bulging of the ipsilateral frontal region and prominence of the ipsilateral ear occurs in 10% or more of the population. Asymmetry of the cranial vault bones in the frontal and sagittal planes often violates the assumption that electrodes spaced for computing local current density are equidistant and at right angles to each other. Measurements other than a simple assessment of the hemicircumference must be considered, including skull inhomogeneity, basal angle, head shape, sulcal variance, neural packing density, irregularity of skull sutures, and asymmetries of the mastoid prominence. An intrinsic imbalance of the sternomastoid muscles may be a more subtle source of laterality errors.

Components of α Asymmetry.—In determining the magnitude of such errors by structural brain imaging, α or α afterdischarge of visual evoked potential covaries predictably with skull thickness and parenchymal brain asymmetry. The weight of the bone factor may differ depending on α amplitude. Cortical generators, if recruited in a synchronous activity, may change the cortex/scalp attenuation ratio of the EEG from trial to trial. The larger the cortical area occupied by electrical activity, the smaller the ratio between cortical vs. scalp EEG amplitude. This solid angle principle implies that the limit of the spatial distribution of α would be set by the anatomical size of the area, but this issue has remained unexplored. One explanation to the question of whether gradual buildup of EEG α is associated with generalization of rhythm is that α may occupy areas of different size as it spreads, thus changing cortex/scalp attenuation ratios on the right and left sides.

Conclusions.—With structural brain imaging, sufficient information may be obtained to warrant individualized montages, which may or may not be derived from the 10-20 system. Increasing sample size may reduce variance between individuals, but it can do little in controlling variance between the hemispheres in individuals. With full awareness of all components of EEG laterality, the faint asymmetries measured can be proved relevant.

▶ Interpretation of EEG findings involves, in addition to the presence of pathologic frequencies, the assessment of symmetry between the 2 hemispheres. Some findings, such as differences in the amplitude of occipital α, have long been identified. This article discusses other technical and anatomical factors that are important. With the growing use of topographic mapping and spatial displays of voltage and power, appreciation of nonpathologic causes of asymmetries is very important. Only when these are adequately appreciated should minor asymmetries be considered of potential clinical importance.—E. Ramsay, M.D.

4 Neuro-Imaging

Evaluation of the Extracranial Carotid Arteries: Correlation of Magnetic Resonance Angiography, Duplex Ultrasonography, and Conventional Angiography
Mattle HP, Kent KC, Edelman RR, Atkinson DJ, Skillman JJ (Beth Israel Hosp, Boston)
J Vasc Surg 13:838–845, 1991   4–1

Background.—Magnetic resonance angiography is a promising new imaging technique for the assessment of the carotid arteries. Its accuracy for detection of extracranial carotid stenoses was investigated by correlating "bright blood" and "black blood" MR images with duplex scan and conventional angiography (Fig 4–1).

Patients.—Thirty-nine arteries in 20 patients were evaluated with MR angiography, duplex scanning, and conventional angiography. Indica-

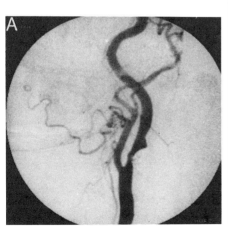
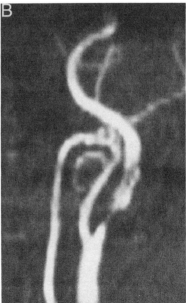

Fig 4–1.—**A,** digital subtraction angiography reveals an 80% stenosis of the internal carotid artery. **B,** bright blood MR angiography suggests a similar degree of stenosis. (Courtesy of Mattle HP, Kent KC, Edelman RR, et al: *J Vasc Surg* 13:838-845, 1991.)

tions for evaluation included stroke in 2 patients, transient ischemic attack in 2, and amaurosis fugax in 9; 7 patients were asymptomatic.

Results.—Compared with conventional angiography, duplex scanning was inaccurate in 6 instances, whereas MR angiography was inaccurate in 3. With the scanner, the degree of stenosis was overgraded in 3 and undergraded in the other 3, whereas MR angiography overgraded all 3 lesions. When a greater than 70% stenosis was defined as a positive scan, MR angiography yielded a sensitivity of 100% and a specificity of 92%, whereas duplex scanning yielded a sensitivity of 86% and a specificity of 84%. In cases where MR angiography and duplex scanning were in agreement, the correlation with conventional angiography was 100%. In differentiating preocclusive stenoses from occlusions, MR angiography accurately identified 7 of 8 lesions, whereas duplex scanning differentiated these 2 conditions in none of the arteries. Magnetic resonance angiography predicted ulceration in 9 of 13 arteries.

Conclusions.—Magnetic resonance imaging is a reliable, noninvasive technique for imaging the extracranial carotid artery. The combination of bright and black blood MR angiography allows precise delineation of the lesions, similar to that in conventional angiography. As techniques improve, MR angiography ultimately may eliminate the need for the conventional angiography in the evaluation of carotid stenoses. Its use as a screening technique is not yet economically feasible, but MR angiography is a reliable alternative to duplex scanning for noninvasive carotid imaging.

▶ A variety of new MR techniques and enhanced image quality and processing puts MR angiography in a position to challenge duplex ultrasonography successfully in the noninvasive evaluation of the extracranial carotid arteries. Time-of-flight imaging or phase imaging, combined with 2-dimensional or 3-dimensional data acquisition, increases the options available for visualizing the cervical, petrous, cavernous, and intracranial carotid artery and its branches. Time-of-flight MR angiography can yield dark or bright blood, and both may have selective uses, e.g., bright blood MR angiography instead of black blood at the skull base and black blood in areas where turbulence is a potential problem in overestimating the degree of stenosis. Magnetic resonance angiography will be able to replace routine angiography only when accurate characterization of ulcerations and precise determination of degree of vessel narrowing is forthcoming. Until that time, MR angiography of the extracranial carotid will remain an adequate, but expensive, screening examination.—R.M. Quencer, M.D.

Diagnosis of Acute Cerebral Infarction: Comparison of CT and MR Imaging

Bryan RN, Levy LM, Whitlow WD, Killian JM, Preziosi TJ, Rosario JA (Johns

Hopkins Hosp, Baltimore; Baylor College of Medicine)
AJNR 12:611–620, 1991   4–2

Background.—There is yet no imaging technique that allows precise diagnosis and delineation of acute cerebral infarction. The appearance of early stroke on MR images and CT scans was compared in a prospective trial.

Methods.—Thirty-one patients who met the standard clinical criteria for acute stroke were examined within 24 hours of the ictus. Follow-up

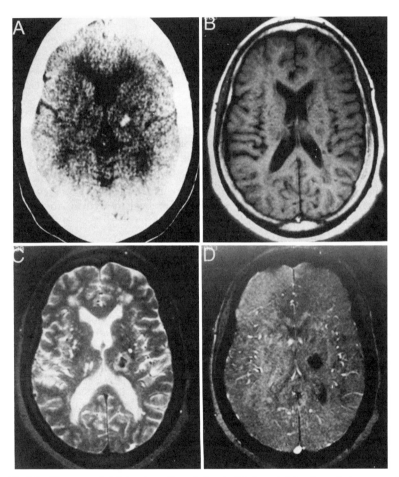

Fig 4–2.—Hematoma in left basal ganglia at 1 day. **A,** CT shows left basal ganglia hematoma. **B,** T1-weighted MRI (500/20). Hematoma is isointense. **C,** T2-weighted MRI (3,000/100) shows decreased signal intensity in center of hematoma and increased signal in periphery. **D,** GRE image (33/17/30 degrees) shows hematoma has markedly decreased signal intensity. (Courtesy of Bryan RN, Levy LM, Whitlow WD, et al: *AJNR* 12:611–620, 1991.)

examinations were performed 7–10 days later in 20 patients, and findings were correlated with the initial studies.

Findings.—For the diagnosis of acute stroke, MRI was significantly more sensitive than CT (82% vs. 58%). On the initial MR scans, increased signal intensity from acute infarcts was visible on proton density- or T2-weighted images, but changes on proton density-weighted images were more conspicuous, especially for portions of strokes involving peripheral gray matter. In addition, proton density-weighted images showed better anatomical delineation when the internal and external capsules, thalamus, and basal ganglia were involved. On follow-up examinations, MRI identified 95%, and CT identified 82% of the stroke regions. Of these, 54% were larger or better defined than on initial studies. The 2 studies were comparable in delineating acute hemorrhage. Two basal ganglia hematomas were detected, as reflected by decreased signal intensity on T2-weighted images and gradient echo images (Fig 4–2) and increased density on CT. In another acute hemorrhage in the basal ganglia, increased signal intensity on T1-weighted images was evident. This latter hemorrhagic pattern differed from that of the usual hematoma and reflected ischemic lesions with damaged capillary endothelium through which there was leakage into the surrounding parenchyma (ischemic petechial infraction). On follow-up studies, MRI detected more cases with evidence of hemorrhage than did CT.

Conclusions.—Magnetic resonance imaging appears to be more sensitive than CT in the diagnosis of acute cerebral infarction. In addition, MRI allows differentiation of any associated hemorrhage.

▶ As in most cases of intracranial pathology, MRI is more sensitive than CT in detecting the presence of an acute cerebral infarction. It is crucial, however, that if intraparenchymal hemorrhage is present, it is equally visible on MR images as on CT, because treatment often is based on whether the infarct is bland or hemorrhagic. Whereas the authors do show that hemorrhagic infarcts can be identified on MRI (see Fig 4–2) and CT, it is possible that, in a larger series of patients, smaller peripheral acute bleeds may not be as easily detected or confidently diagnosed with MRI as with CT. This, of course, would have an impact on which single imaging study should be ordered in cases of acute stroke. Furthermore, another question needs to be answered in a separate clinical study: Does the improved detection by MRI of early stroke have an impact on patient treatment and prognosis?—R.M. Quencer, M.D.

Clinical Correlates of White-Matter Changes on Magnetic Resonance Imaging Scans of the Brain

Mirsen TR, Lee DH, Wong CJ, Diaz JF, Fox AJ, Hachinski VC, Merskey H

(Univ of Western Ontario; John P Robarts Research Inst, London, Canada)
Arch Neurol 48:1015–1021, 1991   4–3

Background.—Magnetic resonance imaging allows identification of white matter changes. A high prevalence of white matter changes has been found on T2-weighted images, especially in persons with cerebrovascular disease. The differences between periventricular hyperintensity (PVH) and changes distant from the ventricles, or leukoaraiosis (L-A) were investigated.

Methods.—Ninety-four patients were enrolled prospectively. Thirty had Alzheimer's disease, 9 had mixed dementia, and 4 had multi-infarct dementia; 50 healthy persons served as controls. In addition, 1 man suspected of having encephalitis was included. The clinical and radiologic correlates of changes in cerebral white matter were noted.

Findings.—Periventricular hyperintensity was seen twice as frequently in patients with Alzheimer's disease as in healthy controls. In controls, the presence of PVH was correlated significantly with 1 measure of cerebral atrophy and the presence of changes in the adjoining deep white matter. Leukoaraiosis on MRI was not related to cognitive decline or to the presence of focal abnormalities on neurologic assessment.

Conclusions.—Patients with Alzheimer's disease had PVH twice as often as did healthy persons. The significance of white matter changes in L-A, however, remains unsettled.

▶ Attempts to relate cognitive decline and dementia to various findings on MRI have included determination of enlargement of CSF spaces, changes in ventricular size, abnormal signals from brain parenchyma, and selective areas of brain tissue loss. Although all white matter changes may seem similar, clinical correlates can be proposed if the images are analyzed closely. Distinguishing between PVHs and deep white matter hyperintensities could be useful, but a suggestion to rely on proton density images for PVH is made. Masking of PVH by the normally hyperintense CSF is possible if only T2-weighted images are obtained. Close evaluation of the temporal lobes on coronal MRI might be even more helpful than attempts to distinguish between various types of white matter involvement because, in Alzheimer's Disease, selective loss of temporal gray matter and associated temporal horn and choroidal fissure enlargement have been noted.—R.M. Quencer, M.D.

The Morphologic Correlate of Incidental Punctate White Matter Hyperintensities on MR Images

Fazekas F, Kleinert R, Offenbacher H, Payer F, Schmidt R, Kleinert G, Radner H, Lechner H (Karl-Franzens Univ, Graz, Austria)
AJNR 12:915–921, 1991   4–4

Background.—Incidental punctate white matter hyperintensities (WMHs) are sometimes seen on MRI studies of elderly patients shortly before death. Autopsies were performed on the brains of such patients to define the morphological correlate of WMH.

Methods.—Six patients aged 52–63 years at death were included. In 2 patients, the WMH was the only abnormal finding and appeared to be unrelated to brain tumor in 4. Brains were removed after death and fixed for at least 3 weeks; 4 brains were rescanned with MRI. Identification of the lesions was optimized by cutting the specimens parallel to the MRI plane and examining whole-hemisphere microscopic sections.

Results.—Most of the WMHs could be seen on postmortem scans, but few would have been identified without knowledge of the MR findings. Histologic examination revealed areas of reduced myelination, atrophy of the neuropil around fibrohyalinotic arteries, and different stages of perivenous damage. The most extensive form of perivenous damage was large areas with marked refraction of myelinated fibers. In 1 patient, edematous glial swelling in foci of ganglion cell heterotopia caused subcortical WMH.

Conclusions.—The morphological substrate of WMH is probably minor perivascular damage without infarction. Analysis of such small lesions will require histologic correlations with MRI scans of living patients or studies of unfixed material.

▶ The ubiquity of punctate WMHs identified on proton density- and T2-weighted MR images makes it necessary to understand pathologic correlates of these findings. The small WMHs are frequently multiple, are not periventricular in location, and, as this and other articles have shown, do not represent white matter infarctions. Rather, nonspecific demyelination and loss of cerebral tissue commonly in deep perivascular regions underlie these MR abnormalities. This stresses the importance of not attaching undue significance to these findings, which are frequently seen in older patients. Furthermore, it is noteworthy that in vivo MR is more sensitive in detecting the white matter lesions than either pathologic examination of the brain or postmortem brain MR, facts to remember when performing imaging–pathologic correlative studies.—R.M. Quencer, M.D.

Magnetic Resonance Imaging of Central Nervous System Lesions in Patients With Lupus Erythematosus: Correlation With Clinical Remission and Antineurofilament and Anticardiolipin Antibody Titers

Bell CL, Partington C, Robbins M, Graziano F, Turski P, Kornguth S (Univ of Wisconsin, Madison)

Arthritis Rheum 34:432–441, 1991   4–5

Background.—The CNS is involved in as many as 70% of patients with systemic lupus erythematosus. Involvement may be either focal or diffuse, and it is characterized by intermittent remission.

Methods.—To determine whether patients with focal and diffuse clinical manifestations have corresponding focal and diffuse anatomical changes, MRI of the brain and serologic studies were performed in 11 patients with diffuse CNS involvement and in 8 with focal CNS involvement. All 19 patients underwent MRI, neurofilament antibody determination by Western blot, and anticardiolipin antibody determination.

Results.—In 17 patients the MRI findings were abnormal, and in 2, the findings were normal. Abnormalities were most often seen in occipital, parietal, and frontal lobes. In patients with diffuse CNS lupus, changes did not correspond to the territory of any major cerebral vessel. In patients with diffuse disease, there were minimal changes in periventricular white matter, a feature important in differentiating patients with lupus from those with multiple sclerosis. Patients with diffuse disease had symmetrically distributed areas of increased signal intensity in subcortical white matter. After treatment with high-dose methylprednisolone, these areas resolved. Sera from patients with diffuse disease contained increased levels of antineurofilament antibodies. In contrast, patients with focal CNS lupus had areas of increased signal intensity and atrophic changes in regions corresponding to major cerebral vessels. There was no positive response to treatment with high-dose steroids. Sera of patients with focal disease had normal levels of antineurofilament antibody but increased levels of cardiolipin and lupus anticoagulant.

Conclusions.—Patients with diffuse CNS lupus apparently respond to high-dose steroid thereapy, whereas those with focal disease do not. Hence, results of combined MRI, clinical, and serologic evaluation may be used to determine which patients with CNS lupus may benefit from such treatment.

▶ Because of the frequency of white matter abnormalities and the long differential diagnosis associated with such lesions, it is important to characterize the pattern of distribution as well as possible. Although multiple sclerosis is most commonly thought of when presented with white matter lesions in patients of the age group described in this article, other causes, (e.g., dysmyelination vascular disease (including vasculities); infectious, postinfectious, and posttreatment white matter disease) must be considered. The pattern of white matter lesions described in this article, although not incompatible with multiple sclerosis, certainly deviates from the classic periventricular, irregularly marginated lesions of multiple sclerosis, and it should force one to consider a primary vascular cause for these findings. The observation that high-dose steroids may reverse the diffuse signal abnormalities in systemic lupus erythematosus indicates that, in this stage of the disease, an ischemic process associated with edema may be present. This might help separate this type of vasculitis from long-standing chronic multiple sclerosis, in which a similar reversal of white matter lesions would not be expected.—R.M. Quencer, M.D.

SPECT and MR Imaging in Herpes Simplex Encephalitis
Schmidbauer M, Podreka I, Wimberger D, Oder W, Koch G, Wenger S, Goldenberg G, Asenbaum S, Deecke L (Univ of Vienna, Austria)
J Comput Assist Tomogr 15:811–815, 1991   4–6

Background.—Herpes simplex virus is the most common cause of acute necrotizing encephalities in humans. Early diagnosis is vital for successful antiviral treatment. An investigation was undertaken to correlate findings in neuro-imaging with the clinical course of acute necrotizing encephalities.

Case Report.—Woman, 60, showed decreased mental functioning after 2 days of malaise and vomiting. Two days later, paresis of the right forearm occurred and she lost consciousness. Computed tomography scans obtained on days 4 and 17 after onset were normal. Acyclovir therapy was started. The patient regained consciousness 28 days after onset. The cell count in CSF increased to $156/mm^3$, with lymphocytes predominating. The protein content in CSF reached 110 mg%. Single photon emission CT (SPECT) with ^{99m}Tc-hexamethyl-propyleneamineoxime (HMPAO) as the tracer showed markedly increased HMPAO accumulation in the left mesiobasal temporal cortex and in the left anterior basal ganglia. Magnetic resonance imaging performed 1 week after SPECT revealed a hyperintense lesion along the hippocampus that extended to the left insula and gyrus rectus. The second SPECT study performed 48 days after onset revealed the same HMPAO distribution, but focal tracer uptake had decreased. Because there was no further clinical improvement and CSF pleocytosis persisted, a second course of antiviral treatment was administered. The final MRI examination showed widening of the left temporal horn and decreased Gd-diethylenetriaminepentaacetic acid enhancement. The final SPECT examination showed decreased HMPAO deposition in the left inferior temporal lobe.

Conclusions.—Both SPECT and MR examinations peformed over the course of acute encephalitis can provide valuable information for the differential diagnosis of acute necrotizing encephalitis. In such patients, increased HMPAO uptake in the limbic temporal lobe and anterior basal ganglia on SPECT and a high content of mobile protons on MRI reflect the distinct pathomorphologic features of acute necrotizing encephalitis. Delay of clinical improvement with persistently high HMPAO uptake in the lesion may reflect protracted acuity of inflammation. In the postinflammatory state, SPECT can delineate areas with decreased metabolic activity.

▶ This paper describes 2 adult patients with herpes simplex encephalitis, and the history of 1 of the 2 is detailed in this abstract. Establishing the diagnosis of herpes simplex encephalitis early in the clinical course is important to the prompt commencement of acyclovir therapy. Unfortunately, early in the course, the diagnosis with CT may be difficult to establish, particularly if hemorrhage is not present or if a bilateral temporal process is not identified, or both. Magnetic resonance substantially improves the detection of herpes simplex encephalitis and, therefore, MR should be ordered whenever herpes simplex encephalitis is suspected. Furthermore, functional imaging here presented as SPECT with Tc-HMPAO can give insights into disease progression and activity, which is not accomplished nearly as well with CT or MR.—R.M. Quencer, M.D.

Magnetic Resonance Imaging of Limbic Encephalitis
Kodama T, Numaguchi Y, Gellad FE, Dwyer BA, Kristt DA (Univ of Maryland, Baltimore)
Neuroradiology 33:520–523, 1991   4–7

Background.—Limbic encephalitis is a rare disorder most often associated with lung cancer, especially small cell carcinoma. It is marked by affective symptoms and striking memory impairment and, less often, by hallucinations and overt psychosis. Lymphocytic pleocytosis and elevated protein often are found in CSF. Generally, this diagnosis has not been based on neuroimaging because CT studies usually are normal or show only mild ventricular dilatation. Only 6 patients with limbic encephalitis examined with MRI have been described previously. Two patients with serial MR images were described.

Case 1.—Woman, 34, with dysphagia, lethargy, diplopia, impaired memory, and disorientation had normal head CT scans and CSF showing mild lymphocytic pleocytosis. Initial T2-weighted spin echo MRI showed abnormal high signal intensity along the orbital suface of the left frontal lobe but no temporal lobe abnormalities. The patient was given a diagnosis of malignant thymoma, which was partially resected. After surgery, her memory was severely impaired. A second T2-weighted MR scan done 2 weeks after the first showed abnormal increased signal in the hippocampal formations, but no abnormal enhancement with gadopentetate dimeglumine. The previous abnormal signal intensity in the left frontal lobe had almost resolved. Open biopsy showed a mild mononuclear infiltration of the subarachnoid space of the right hippocampus, with scattered reactive astrocytes and occasional rod cells in the subjacent cortex. Two weeks after the biopsy, MRI showed marked reduction of the high-intensity lesions in the hippocampal formations.

Case 2. Woman, 55, had temporal lobe seizures and altered mental status. She had a mastectomy 15 years previously without recurrence or metastasis. Her memory was impaired, but she had no abnormal neurologic signs. Mild lymphocytic pleocytosis and slightly elevated protein were seen in CSF. Initially CT and MR studies showed normal temporal lobes, but a small enhancing lesion, compatible with a meningioma, was attached to the faix. Sixteen days later, a second

MR study showed abnormal high signal in the right hippocampal formation. Five days after that coronal MR showed high signal in both hippocampal formations. Meningoencephalitis histopathologically similar to that of case 1 was seen in open biopsy of the right hippocampal formation. The patient was discharged, being free from seizures. Three months later only subtle high signal was found in the right hippocampal formation.

Conclusions.—Clinical symptoms of limbic encephalitis can occur when inflammatory changes are too mild to be reflected by abnormal signals in MR images. These inflammations can occur in portions of the brain, and they can resolve without residual radiologically detectable abnormalities. Because bilateral temporal lobe involvement may occur in viral encephalitis and other conditions, differential diagnosis of limbic encephalitis may be difficult based on MR images alone.

▶ The high degree of sensitivity of MRI in demonstrating intracerebral abnormalities heretofore undetectable by other imaging studies is exemplified by this report of limbic encephalitis. With this predominately non–mass-producing medial temporal lobe lesion (unilateral or bilateral) on T2-weighted images, our differential diagnosis is widened beyond those entities one would normally consider in a patient with increasing dementia—namely, a viral encephalitis, gliomatosis cerebri, or an underlying vascular disease. The lack of contrast enhancement and the value of a changing picture on follow-up MR studies may assist in arriving at a proper diagnosis, thus eliminating the need for biopsy as was done in these two cases. Although limbic encephalitis is rare, one should be aware of the MR findings, particularly in the setting of an underlying malignancy.—R.M. Quencer, M.D.

Prominent Dural Enhancement Adjacent to Nonmeningiomatous Malignant Lesions on Contrast-Enhanced MR Images
Wilms G, Lammens M, Marchal G, Demaerel P, Verplancke J, Van Calenbergh F, Goffin J, Plets C, Baert AL (Univ Hosps KU Leuven, Belgium)
AJNR 12:761–764, 1991   4–8

Background.—Prominent dural enhancement on contrast-enhanced MR images has been considered a highly specific feature of meningioma and has been described in as many as 60% of cranial meningiomas.

Methods.—A retrospective of 306 malignant intracranial tumors was conducted to examine prominent dural enhancement adjacent to nonmeningiomatous malignant lesions studied by contrast-enhanced MRI.

Findings.—There were 6 glioblastomas, 3 parenchymal metastases, and 1 dural metastasis, accounting for 3% of all malignant intracranial tumors and 16% of 61 superficial malignant intracranial tumors seen during a 2-year period. In 5 patients, the dural enhancement resembled the dural tail seen in meningiomas. Seven patients underwent surgery. In 2 patients, the dura appeared normal, and there was no leptomeningeal

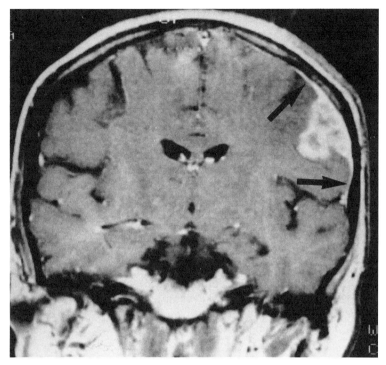

Fig 4–3.—Metastasis from mediastinal adenocarcinoma. A coronal T1-weighted (600/15) image shows inhomogeneous enhancement of lesion. Notice a dural tail on both sides of the lesion *(arrows)*. Although there was no surgical confirmation, this was assumed to be a metastasis, because a lesion was not visible on CT or MRI 6 months later. (Courtesy of Wilms G, Lammens M, Marchal G, et al: *AJNR* 12:761-764, 1991.)

tumoral invasion. Four others showed extensive invasion of the lepto-meninges. In 2 of these patients, the lesion was firmly attached to the dura, but no dural invasion was evident despite extensive external carotid artery supply to the tumor in 1. In the patient with dural metastasis, huge nodular lesions were present along the inner aspect of the dura with tail-like extension to the surrounding dura. In none of the patients did the dura in the vicinity of the tumor show any sign of tumoral invasion or extension to the dura. In 3 patients without surgical confirmation, the clinical course of the disease proved the malignant nature of the lesion. In 1 patient with metastasis, the absence of a lesion on MRI performed 6 months earlier provided additional proof of the nonmeningiomatous nature of the lesion (Fig 4–3).

Conclusion.—Prominent dural enhancement on contrast-enhanced MRI appears to be less frequent in malignant tumors than in meningioma and appears to represent reactive changes of the dura rather than tumoral invasion.

▶ Imaging signs that can impart a degree of specificity to certain abnormalities are constantly being sought, and this applies particularly to intracranial masses where many peripherally based masses (primary tumors, metastases, meningiomas, etc.) may have a similar MRI appearance. The presence of enhancement along the outer meningeal surface ("tail-sign") was originally felt to be a strong indicator of a meningioma because of associated dural invasion. However, as this "sign" is more closely scrutinized, it is clear that other lesions may have a similar appearance (see Fig 4–3). Invasion of the leptomeninges by malignant cells in nonmeningioma masses, the secondary reactive changes in the overlying dura, and the subsequent enhancement with Gd explains the imaging similarity to the dura enhancement in meningiomas. The unjustified reliance on a single radiologic sign in establishing a diagnosis is emphasized by this paper.—R.M. Quencer, M.D.

Marked Cerebrospinal Fluid Void: Indicator of Successful Shunt in Patients With Suspected Normal-Pressure Hydrocephalus
Bradley WG Jr, Whittemore AR, Kortman KE, Watanabe AS, Homyak M, Teresi LM, Davis SJ (Huntington Med Research Insts; Huntington Mem Hosp, Pasadena, Calif)
Radiology 178:459–466, 1991   4–9

Background.—Patients with normal-pressure hydrocephalus (NPH) usually have gait apraxia, dementia, and incontinence. Creation of a ventriculoperitoneal shunt benefits some, but for others who undergo the risk of surgery it is unsuccessful. A method of preselection for shunt surgery would be beneficial. The criteria of prominent CSF flow void in the cerebral aqueduct to determine candidates for shunt surgery were evaluated.

Methods.—The MRI images of 20 patients who had undergone creation of ventriculoperitoneal shunts were blindly reviewed for CSF flow void and presence of deep white matter infarction (Figs 4–4 and 4–5). Imaging was performed before shunt creation in 9 patients, after in 7, and both before and after in 4.

Results.—There was a significant association between CSF flow void (based on extent rather than degree of signal loss) and a good-to-excellent surgical response rate. The presence of deep white matter infarction on MRI was not associated with a poor surgical response.

Conclusions.—The CSF flow void should be considered along with other determining factors in choosing patients for shunt creation. The presence of mild-to-moderate deep white-matter infarction, previously considered a contraindication for shunting, should not discourage surgery.

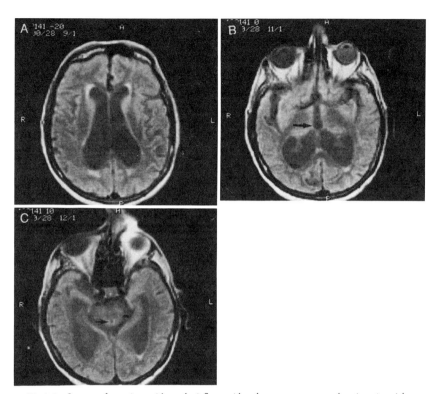

Fig 4–4.—Images of a patient with grade 1 flow void and poor response to shunting. **A,** axial sections through the lateral ventricles indicates ventricular enlargement out of proportion to minimally enlarged cortical sulci. **B,** axial section through the midbrain demonstrates mild enlargement *(arrow)* (SE 2,000/28). **C,** axial section through the midbrain demonstrates a "normal" CSF flow void in the aqueduct *(arrow)* (SE 2,000/28). **D** and **E,** axial sections through the pons demonstrate no evidence of CSF signal loss in the fourth ventricle *(arrow)* (SE 2,000/28). (Courtesy of Bradley WG Jr, Whittemore AR, Korman KE, et al: *Radiology* 178:459–466, 1991.)

▶ Publications covering new techniques and observations concerning NPH command our attention because the diagnosis, both clinically and radiographically, is often elusive. Magnetic resonance can detect the effects of fluid motion by showing signal loss in flow-sensitive spin-echo images, so it is natural that attempts be made to relate such signal loss to a number of conditions including NPH. In this paper, a greater-than-normal CSF flow-related signal loss was present in patients who were found to respond well to ventriculoperitoneal shunt, a fact that may be independent of whether ischemia/ infarction is present in the deep cerebral white matter. However, others have observed a similar extensive CSF flow void in cases of marked atrophy and ventriculomegaly; therefore, some caution in overreliance on this sign is suggested. Calculated CSF velocities (phase MR) in various areas of the ventricular system (third ventricle, aqueduct, fourth ventricle) might give us more insights into CSF flow alterations and eventually be most useful in diagnosing NPH.—R.M. Quencer, M.D.

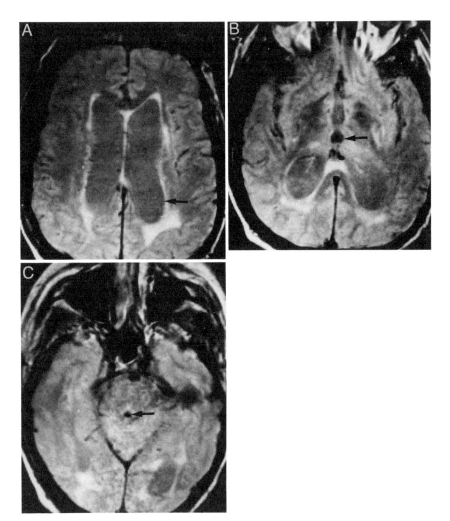

Fig 4–5.—Normal pressure hydrocephalus. Man, 76, who was seen with gait apraxia, mild dementia, and occasional incontinence underwent successful creation of a shunt, with resolution of symptoms, after this examination. **A–C,** transverse axial sections obtained without flow compensation (SE 3,000/25). **A,** section through the lateral ventricles demonstrates enlargement (*solid arrow*) and periventricular hyperintensity characteristic of deep white matter infarction (*open arrow*). **B,** section through the third ventricle demonstrates marked cerebrospinal fluid flow void (*arrow*) in the posterior third ventricle. **C,** section through the pontine isthmus demonstrates mildly enlarged aqueduct with marked cerebrospinal fluid flow void (*arrow*). (Courtesy of Bradley WG Jr, Whittemore AR, Kortman KE, et al: *Radiology* 178:459–466, 1991.)

Acute Spinal Cord Injury: Magnetic Resonance Imaging Correlated With Myelopathy

Yamashita Y, Takahashi M, Matsuno Y, Kojima R, Sakamoto Y, Oguni T, Sakae T, Kim EE (Kumamoto Univ; Kumamoto Orthopaedic Hosp, Japan;

Univ of Texas, Houston)
Br J Radiol 64:201–209, 1991   4–10

Background.—Magnetic resonance imaging visualizes a number of pathologic changes in the traumatized spinal cord that are not demonstrated by traditional imaging methods. The MR findings in acute spinal cord injury were correlated with functional outcome to evaluate the prognostic usefulness of MRI in this setting.

Patients.—Thirty-one patients aged 13–87 years with acute spinal cord injury were examined. Magnetic resonance imaging was performed within 24 hours after injury in 13 patients, within 7 days after injury in 13, and 7–14 days after injury in 5. Thirteen patients underwent surgical decompression; 11 underwent traction for dislocated vertebrae; and 18 were treated conservatively. One patient died 5 days after injury. Twenty-six patients with spinal cord abnormalities on initial imaging had follow-up MRI. Clinical follow-up ranged from 6 to 20 months.

Findings in Acute Injury.—Vertebral body fractures, subluxations, and ligament tears were often observed in patients with severe cord dysfunction. A majority of the 12 patients lacking skeletal and ligament injuries had ossification of the posterior longitudinal ligament. Changes of cord compression were seen in 23 patients and were severe in 11 of them; the commonest cause was vertebral subluxation. Cord compression was present in 20 of 26 patients with abnormal signal intensities from the cord. Central cord syndrome often was noted in patients lacking fracture or subluxation.

Prognosis.—Patients whose recovery was poor tended to have marked cord compression, swelling of the cord, and abnormal intensity on T_1- and T_2-weighted images. The degree of cord compression was the most useful prognostic indicator, followed by abnormal intensity on T_1-weighted images. Patients in whom hyperintensity on T_2-weighted images persisted or worsened tended to have a poor outcome. Two patients had extensive and irregular intensity on both T_1 and T_2 images after cervical traction.

Conclusion.—Magnetic resonance imaging is useful for the assessment of acute spinal cord injury and for predicting the prognosis and planning treatment in these patients.

▶ The use of MR in acute spinal cord injury has become an important part of these patients' overall evaluation, not so much for determining prognosis but, rather, for identifying surgically correctable abnormalities. If an acute traumatic disk herniation with cord compression is identified, a diskectomy with anterior interbody fusion may be performed in hopes of reversing early neurologic deficits, and, if an epidural hematoma with cord compression is identified, evacuation of the hematoma may be warranted. It certainly is true, as this article points out, that MR can also be useful as a prognostic indicator of patient outcome. Edema alone (high signal on T_2-weighted images) signifies a potentially better outcome than does the presence of hemorrhagic contusion (mixed low and high signal on T_2-weighted images). Increased use of MR in patients with neurologic deficits secondary to acute spinal trauma is recommended.—R.M. Quencer, M.D.

Radiation Myelopathy: Significance of Gadolinium-DTPA Enhancement in the Diagnosis

Michikawa M, Wada Y, Sano M, Uchihara T, Furukawa T, Shibuya H, Tsukagoshi H (Tokyo Med and Dental Univ)
Neuroradiology 33:286–289, 1991   4–11

Background.—Radiation myelopathy is one of the major complications of radiation therapy. Its clinical manifestations are divided into 4 major groups, one of which is chronic progressive radiation myelopathy (CPRM). Although myelography is useful for excluding metastatic spinal compression, it is of limited value in depicting the intramedullary lesions caused by CPRM. Magnetic resonance imaging has proven useful in the diagnosis of intramedullary spinal lesions. Two patients with CPRM in whom MRI with Gd-diethylenetriaminepentaacetic acid (Gd-DTPA) enhancement clearly demonstrated the intramedullary lesions of CPRM were described.

Case Report.—Man, 65, who had undergone radical neck dissection for stage IV, T0N2M0 squamous cell carcinoma of the right cervical region 25 months earlier, had neck pain, progressive right hemiparesis, and left hemihypesthesia without facial involvement. He had undergone radiation therapy, during which the cervical spinal cord from C1 to C3 had received 40 Gy. Neurologic examination showed Brown-Séquard syndrome, suggesting a lesion in the right half of C2 level. Magnetic resonance imaging of the cervical cord showed mild but unremarkable cervical cord enlargement. With Gd-DTPA enhancement, there was a robust ring of enhancement in the region of C1 and C2 on sagittal images and in the right side of the spinal cord at C2 level on axial images. His neurologic symptoms were alleviated by treatment with 50 mg/day of prednisolone. A follow-up MRI examination performed 2 weeks after corticosteroid treatment showed a slightly atrophic cervical cord. However, the ring enhancement after Gd-DTPA injection remained unchanged. The improvement of the spinal cord edema and the protracted clinical course argued against intramedullary metastases.

Conclusion.—Magnetic resonance imaging with Gd-DTPA enhancement is an extremely useful and sensitive procedure for visualizing intramedullary spinal lesions in patients who might have CPRM.

▶ It often is difficult to separate radiation myelopathy from spinal cord tumor. Modern imaging techniques have assisted, but they are not always definitive. This paper suggests that Gd ring enhancement of the spinal cord may be a feature of radiation myelopathy. This picture is very different from that usually seen with a spinal cord extramedullary or intramedullary metastasis.—W.G. Bradley, D.M., F.R.C.P.

Subacute Necrotizing Myelopathy: MR Imaging in Four Pathologically Proved Cases

Mirich DR, Kucharczyk W, Keller MA, Deck J (Toronto Hosp)
AJNR 12:1077–1083, 1991   4–12

Background.—Magnetic resonance imaging is now widely used in the investigation of the spine, but there have been few reports of subacute necrotizing myelopathy (SNM). Clinical characteristics, MRI, other imaging studies, and pathologic findings in 4 proven cases of SNM were examined.

Findings.—The patients had gradual motor and sensory deterioration of the lower limbs, impaired function of the bowel and bladder, and, in 1 patient, a deficit in the upper limbs. The condition got acutely worse in each patient before hospitalization. None showed any signs of a spinal dural arteriovenous fistual. The initial MRI scan showed focal enlargement of the spinal cord along with nonspecific T-1 and T-2 lengthening, with rimlike enhancement in 1 patient. Steroid treatment was tried and failed in all 4 patients. On follow-up, MRI showed slight enlargement of lesions in 2 patients, a stable thoracolumbar lesion in another, and atrophy of a cervical lesion in the other. Each patient underwent open spinal cord biopsy, which showed necrotic foci and abnormal parenchymal vessels with thickened, hyalinized walls (table).

Conclusions.—If spinal dural arteriovenous fistulas are absent, imaging studies cannot differentiate SNM from tumor. Its prolonged course separates it from acute transverse myelitis. A possible distinguishing feature is rimlike as opposed to solid contrast enhancement.

▶ This paper points out the difficulty of diagnosing SNM, an entity that is associated with a dural arteriovenous fistual and consequent venous hypertension of the spinal cord. With MR, the diagnosis of a transverse myelitis or early changes of a cord tumor are suspected because the underlying flow voids associated with the arteriovenous fistual are either subtle or not visualized. When confronted with an older patient with clinical history of progressive cord dysfunction and nonspecific increased T2 relaxation time of the cord, SNM should be considered. Although a spinal MR angiogram can be attempted, the most direct approach to the diagnosis is routine angiography. This can be followed by embolotherapy of the abnormal feeding vessel or vessels.—R.M. Quencer, M.D.

Summary of 4 Pathologically Proved Cases of Subacute Necrotizing Myelopathy

Case No.	Age (yr)	Sex	Clinical Findings	CSF	Electro-myography	CT Myelography	Spinal Cord MR	Surgical Findings	Postbiopsy Course
1	58	M	Progressive P & P for 1 yr; acute paraplegia; loss of bowel & bladder function	Increased protein; lymphocytosis	Thoracic cord lesion, probably tumor	Not done	Thoracic FFE; increased T2 signal from T4 to conus; 7 mo later, slight enlargement; no spinal dural AVF	Vein adherent to enlarged spinal cord; sonography suggested foci of necrosis or small cysts; quick-section histology initially suggested low-grade astrocytoma	No change
2	62	M	Progressive P & P for 2 yr; acute paraplegia	Increased protein; lymphocytosis	Radiculopathy; disk herniation or extramedullary tumor	Enlarged conus medullaris	Conus FFE; decreased T1 signal; increased T2 signal; 1 mo later, no change; no spinal dural AVF	Vein adherent to enlarged conus; myelotomy yielded necrotic material	No improvement; bladder became atonic
3	77	F	Progressive P & P over 3 mo; acute paraplegia; loss of bowel & bladder function	Increased protein; lymphocytosis	Supported inflammatory process/myelitis	Normal	Conus FFE with increased T2 signal; 2 mo later, slight FFE, decreased T1 signal in conus; no spinal dural AVF	Enlarged conus; myelotomy yielded necrotic material	No change
4	47	F	Brown-Séquard syndrome (C4 level) developed over 3 wk; acute worsening of right-sided paresis	Increased protein; lymphocytosis	Not done	Enlarged cervical cord	Cervical FEE, right > left; increased T2 signal, rim enhancement; 4 mo later, lesion smaller & no enhancement; no spinal dural AVF	Asymmetric enlarged cervical cord; myelotomy yielded white friable material; quick-section histology initially suggested low-grade astrocytoma	No change

Abbreviations: P & P, paresis and paresthesias; FFE, focal fusiform enlargement; AVF, arteriovenous fistula.
(Courtesy of Mirich DR, Kucharczyk W, Keller MA, et al: AJNR 12:1077–1083, 1991.)

5 Neuromuscular Disease and Autonomic Nervous System

Subacute, Reversible Motor Neuron Disease
Tucker T, Layzer RB, Miller RG, Chad D (Univ of California, San Francisco; Univ of Massachusetts, Worcester)
Neurology 41:1541–1544, 1991   5–1

Introduction.—Patients with motor neuron disease (MND) rarely achieve spontaneous remission. Data were reviewed on 4 patients who achieved remission from a syndrome that was difficult to distinguish from amyotrophic lateral sclerosis (ALS).

Patients.—The 3 men and 1 woman aged 39–74 years had clinical findings of widespread lower MND, such as asymmetric weakness, visible fasciculations, and muscle atrophy. In 2 patients, there were hyperactive tendon reflexes and a positive Babinski's sign. The diagnoses were ALS in 2 patients and ALS with probable upper motor neuron signs in 2 patients. Patients had neurogenic abnormalities of varying severity, including fibrillation potentials, fasciculation potentials, reduced interference pattern, and reinnervation potentials. In 2 patients there were fibrillation potentials, positive wave forms, and fasciculation potentials in at least 3 extremities and muscles of different innervations, and in 2, there were mild neurogenic disabilities of restricted distribution. Results of cerebrospinal fluid examination were normal, and there was no paraproteinemia, heavy metal intoxication, or systemic illness. Disability progressed rapidly in all patients; however, all began to improve by 4 months and recovered completely by 5–12 months.

Conclusion.—Subacute, reversible MND progresses with striking rapidity. This condition might reflect a radiculopathy, but a CNS disorder is more likely because of the upper motor neuron signs. These conditions are very rare, but they should be considered when counseling patients in whom ALS is suspected.

▶ Neurologists seeing many patients with ALS have commented on rare remissions. Few of us, however, have described these patients in the literature.

Tucker and her colleagues have collected 4 such cases. They differ from typical ALS in being somewhat more rapid, but that has not been my experience. The underlying disease still remains to be determined, but the fact that ALS can, on rare occassions, remit should be presented to every patient who is being given a diagnosis of ALS.—W.G. Bradley, D.M., F.R.C.P.

Linkage of a Gene Causing Familial Amyotrophic Lateral Sclerosis to Chromosome 21 and Evidence of Genetic-Locus Heterogeneity

Siddique T, Figlewicz DA, Pericak-Vance MA, Haines JL, Rouleau G, Jeffers AN, Sapp P, Hung W-Y, Bebout J, McKenna-Yasek D, Deng G, Horvitz HR, Gusella JF, Brown RH Jr, Roses AD, and Collaborators (Duke Univ; McGill Univ, Montreal; Massachusetts Inst of Technology; Massachusetts Gen Hosp, Boston)
N Engl J Med 324:1381–1384, 1991   5–2

Background.—Amyotrophic lateral sclerosis (ALS) is a progressive neurologic disease that commonly leads to paralysis and death. No cause of or cure for it has been found. It is familial in some patients, inherited as an autosomal dominant trait with age-dependent penetrance. The familial form can be examined using molecular genetic techniques. Through such techniques the basic molecular defect causing motor neuron degeneration may be discovered.

Methods.—In 23 families with familial ALS, linkage of the gene causing the disease was sought in 4 DNA markers on the long arm of chromosome 21.

Results.—Multipoint linkage analyses revealed the linkage between the gene and these markers. The maximum lod score was 5.03, obtained 10 centimorgans distal to the DNA marker D21S58. The families had a significant probability of genetic-locus heterogeneity.

Conclusions.—Localizing a gene causing familial ALS offers a way to isolate this gene and study its function. The insight gained from understanding this gene's function may aid in the design of rational treatment for familial and sporadic disease forms.

▶ Searching for the cause of neurologic degenerations is like looking for a needle in a haystack. Gene linkage offers the possibility of eventually determining the abnormality in familial disease such as familial ALS. The cause in sporadic cases may be very similar. In ALS in particular, families with several living affected members are rare; they should be referred to research centers for studies such as these.—W.G. Bradley, D.M., F.R.C.P.

Motor Neuropathies, Motor Neuron Disorders, and Antiglycolipid Antibodies

Pestronk A (Washington Univ)
Muscle Nerve 14:927–936, 1991   5–3

Background.—Patients with certain forms of motor neuron disease and peripheral neuropathy have serum antibodies against GM1 ganglioside, one of a family of acidic glycolipids. High titers of anti-GM1 are found in a majority of patients with some acquired lower motor neuron (LMN) disorders and motor neuropathies. Titers may relate to clinical status in individual patients.

Antibody Estimation.—Most laboratories use an enzyme-linked immunosorbent assay (ELISA) to determine serum titers of antiglycolipid antibodies. The specificity of the ELISA for IgM is best when human rather than bovine serum albumin is used to block nonspecific binding sites.

Clinical Correlations.—The highest serum IgM anti-GM1 titers are found in LMN syndromes and multifocal motor neuropathy. Treatment of the latter cases often is more effective when anti-GM1 antibody is found in the absence of an M protein. High antibody titers are more frequent in distal than in proximal LMN syndromes. High titers are unusual in most motor and sensory neuropathies and are rare in patients having typical chronic inflammatory demyelinating polyneuropathy. Patients with amyotrophic lateral sclerosis have IgM anti-GM1 antibody more often than do normal individuals. Antibody estimates provide a useful marker of disease and may help in selecting treatment.

Pathogenetic Import.—It has been difficult to produce an experimental autoimmune neuropathy associated with anti-GM1. It is not clear whether these antibodies are in fact pathogenic, but they likely are a manifestation of ongoing autoimmune disease in patients with motor system involvement.

▶ This is a useful review of the literature relating to neurologic complications of antiglycolipid antibodies. The key question in all such patients is whether the antibodies are producing the neurologic damage, are merely epiphenomena, or are quite unrelated to the neurologic problem. General experience indicates that only a minority of patients improve with treatment that lowers the antibody titer. Nevertheless, if *any* patient improves, this is important. More research is required before the relevance of these observations will become clear.—W.G. Bradley, D.M., F.R.C.P.

Immunosuppressive Treatment in Multifocal Motor Neuropathy

Feldman EL, Bromberg MB, Albers JW, Pestronk A (Univ of Michigan; Washington Univ)
Ann Neurol 30:397–401, 1991   5–4

Background.—Multifocal motor neuropathy (MMN) is characterized by distal asymmetrical weakness and conduction block on motor, but not sensory, axons. It has been suggested that MMN may respond to immunotherapy.

Methods.—The results of immunosuppressive treatment in 13 patients with MMN were reviewed. All 13 patients had MMN and increased titers of serum antibodies to the GM1 ganglioside.

Results.—None of the patients responded to oral prednisone treatment, and there was no clinical response in 4 patients treated with plasma exchange. Cyclophosphamide was administered to 9 patients, 8 of whom showed clinical improvement, with a decrease in antibody titers. In 3 patients, the discontinuation of cyclophosphamide resulted in a clinical relapse and increase in the titers of serum anti-GM1 antibodies.

Conclusions.—Cyclophosphamide treatment may be an effective means to induce and maintain clinical remission of MMN. Eighty-eight percent of these patients improved after cyclophosphamide treatment, whereas none responded to prednisone. These findings also provide more evidence that MMN is an immune-mediated process.

▶ There has been considerable controversy over whether GM1 ganglioside antibodies are the cause of amyotrophic lateral sclerosis. However, a small group of patients with asymmetric motor neuropathy, many with evidence of multifocal block on nerve conduction studies, does have high anti-GM1 antibody titers. Although in vitro studies suggest that the antibodies can be neurotoxic, few patients have improved with plasmapheresis or prednisone therapy. This paper indicates that cyclophosphamide therapy may be effective. The dose regimen is not stated clearly, but it begins with intravenous cyclophosphamide, 3 g/m², and is followed later by oral cyclophosphamide, 2 mg/day.—W.G. Bradley, D.M., F.R.C.P.

Ubiquitin-Immunoreactive Intraneuronal Inclusions in Amyotrophic Lateral Sclerosis: Morphology, Distribution, and Specificity

Leigh PN, Whitwell H, Garofalo O, Buller J, Swash M, Martin JE, Gallo J-M, Weller RO, Anderton BH (Inst of Psychiatry, London; Midland Ctr for Neurosurgery and Neurology, Smethwick, England; Royal London Hosp; Southampton Gen Hosp, England)
Brain 114:775–788, 1991   5–5

Background.—Several types of neuronal inclusions have been described in amyotrophic lateral sclerosis (ALS). In Alzheimer's disease,

Parkinson's disease, and Pick's disease, neuronal inclusions are labeled by antibodies to ubiquitin, and this recently has been found to be the case in ALS as well. Ubiquitin antibodies were used to seek evidence of abnormal protein degradation in ALS–motor neuron disease.

Methods.—Spinal cord material from 31 patients with ALS (median age, 68 years) and from 23 neurologically normal and 22 neurologically abnormal controls was investigated. Tissue was investigated by light microscopy and various immunocytochemistry studies, including qualitative analysis for the presence of ubiquitin-immunoreactive inclusions.

Results.—Ubiquitin-immunoreactive inclusions were found in anterior horn cells of all of the patients with ALS, in 1 of the neurologically abnormal controls, and in none of the neurologically normal controls. Included among the patients with ALS were cases of both familial and sporadic disease. The ubiquitin-immunoreactive inclusions appeared as dense rounded or irregular cytoplasmic inclusions—dense bodies—or loose by arranged bundles of filamentous material—skeins. A correspondence was noted between the presence of inclusions and the selective pattern of neuronal vulnerability in ALS, although most patients did not show inclusions in pyramidal neurons of the motor cortex. Bunina bodies were found in 67% of patients and were seldom labeled by ubiquitin antibodies. Twenty-three percent of patients with ALS had intraneuronal inclusions resembling Lewy bodies, and these frequently were identified by ubiquitin antibodies.

Conclusions.—Distinctive ubiquitin-immunoreactive inclusions are found in patients with ALS in anterior horn cells, as well as in cranial nerve motor neurons and, occasionally, in cortical motor neurons. Although they may not be entirely specific, they are not readily identified by antibodies to cytoskeletal proteins. These bodies may reflect accumulations of altered or abnormal neuronal proteins that are resistant to degradation via the ubiquitin proteolytic pathway.

▶ Ubiquitin appears to be an intracellular nonlysosomal protein playing a major role in the degradation of short-lived and abnormal proteins. This paper indicates that ubiquitin-mediated degeneration of proteins may play a role in ALS, as it does in other specific neuronal degenerations. This is probably a secondary phenomenon, but it offers an insight into the intracellular pathology in neurons in these diseases.—W.G. Bradley, D.M., F.R.C.P.

Treatment Related Fluctuations in Guillain-Barré Syndrome After High-Dose Immunoglobulins or Plasma-Exchange
Kleyweg RP, van der Meché FGA (Univ Hosp Dykzigt, Rotterdam, The Netherlands)
J Neurol Neurosurg Psychiatry 54:957–960, 1991   5–6

Background.—About 10% of patients managed by plasma exchange for Guillain-Barré syndrome (GBS) have treatment-related fluctuations in clinical status. These changes are taken as added evidence that plasma exchange is beneficial.

Methods.—The course of disease was reviewed in 147 patients entered into the Dutch Guillain-Barré trial, which compared high-dose intravenous immunoglobulin therapy with plasma exchange therapy.

Results.—Six of 72 patients treated by plasma exchange had treatment-related fluctuations, as did 8 of 74 receiving immunoglobulin therapy. In patients who relapsed, the decline in clinical state usually was less marked than before the initial response. One patient in the plasma exchange group and 3 of those receiving immunoglobulin therapy required several courses of treatment.

Conclusions.—These findings support the biologic effectiveness of intravenous immunoglobulin therapy for GBS. The final results are awaited, however, before recommending routine immunoglobulin therapy for patients with GBS.

▶ Several double-blind controlled studies have demonstrated that plasmapheresis improves the rate of recovery in GBS. Preliminary results are indicating a similar improvement with high-dose intravenous immunoglobulins. This paper records episodes of exacerbation following completion of plasmapheresis or immunoglobulin infusion, indicating the effectiveness of the treatments. When such patients deteriorate, they need a further course of treatment.—W.G. Bradley, D.M., F.R.C.P.

Treatment of Chronic Inflammatory Demyelinating Polyneuropathy With Intravenous Immunoglobulin

Cornblath DR, Chaudhry V, Griffin JW (Johns Hopkins Univ, Baltimore)
Ann Neurol 30:104–106, 1991   5–7

Background.—Both prednisone and plasmapheresis have been used to improve neurologic function in patients with chronic inflammatory demyelinating polyneuropathy. Intravenous human immunoglobulin also has been beneficial in several small trials.

Methods.—Fifteen patients (9 males and 6 females; age, 14–68 years) with chronic inflammatory demyelinating polyneuropathy were treated with intravenous immunoglobulin if 1 or more other therapies had failed, if there was an unsatisfactory response to current therapy, or if the patient wished to avoid another therapy because of possible side effects. Intravenous immunoglobulin was administered during a hospital stay. Five patients received a dose of .3 g/kg/day for 4 days, and the remaining 10 patients received .4 g/kg/day for 4–5 days.

Results.—These 15 patients bring the number of reported patients treated with intravenous immunoglobulin to 102. There have been clinically significant responses in 68% of patients. A multicenter, controlled trial is required assess the efficacy of intravenous immunoglobulin therapy and determine subgroups of patients who may respond to this therapy.

▶ Intravenous immunoglobin is the current "wonder" cure for many immunologic diseases, including myasthenia gravis, Guillain-Barré syndrome, and chronic inflammatory demyelinating polyneuropathy. In some patients, the response appears to be dramatic. However, this paper reports that not all patients respond and emphasizes the necessity of a double-blind, controlled trial before we can be certain of the efficacy of immunoglobulin therapy. Such a study (Abstract 5–8) recently has been published, showing that 400 mg/kg/day for 5 days is better than plasmapheresis.—W.G. Bradley, D.M., F.R.C.P.

A Randomized Trial Comparing Intravenous Immune Globulin and Plasma Exchange in Guillain-Barré Syndrome

van der Meché FGA, Schmitz PIM, and the Dutch Guillain-Barré Study Group (Academic Hosp; Daniel den Hoed Cancer Ctr, Rotterdam, The Netherlands)
N Engl J Med 325:1123–1129, 1992   5–8

Background.—Perhaps 15% of patients with Guillain-Barré syndrome (GBS), subacute inflammatory demyelinating polyneuropathy, are left with deficits, prompting a search for more specific treatment. Plasma exchange hastens improvement and limits the need for artificial ventilation. There are also indications that high-dose intravenous immune globulin may be effective. If so, immune globulin has significant practical advantages compared to plasma exchange.

Methods.—A multicenter trial was conducted to determine whether intravenous immune globulin is as effective as plasma exchange treatment. Patients ill with GBS for less than 2 weeks who were unable to walk without aid were randomized to receive either 5 plasma exchanges (200–250 mL/kg each) within 7–14 days or 5 daily doses of immune globulin (.4 g/kg daily) intravenously.

Results.—After 150 patients were admitted to the trial, muscle strength had improved significantly in one third of those receiving plasma exchange therapy and in 53% of those receiving immune globulin. Improvement occurred more rapidly in the latter patients. The mean duration of intubation was a little more than 2 weeks in patients receiving globulin therapy, and more than 3 weeks in those on plasma exchange. There were 5 complications in the course of 380 globulin infusions (hypotension in 2 patients, dyspnea in 1, fever in 1 and microscopic hematoma in 1), none requiring interruption of treatment.

Conclusion.—Immune globulin is a safe and effective treatment for GBS and has practical advantages compared to plasma exchange therapy.

▶ This important Dutch study compares standard plasmapheresis with intravenous immune globulin therapy in 150 patients with severe GBS of less than 2 weeks' duration. It demonstrates that immunoglobulin is significantly better than plasma exchange (P=.024). The outcome of the plasmapheresis series was poorer than that in the previous North American and French trials, perhaps as a result of the early inclusion of cases in the Dutch study. It looks as though immunoglobulin therapy will become the treatment of choice for this condition.—W.G. Bradley, D.M., F.R.C.P.

Two-Tiered DNA-Based Diagnosis of Transthyretin Amyloidosis Reveals Two Novel Point Mutations
Ii S, Minnerath S, Ii K, Dyck PJ, Sommer SS (Mayo Clinic and Found, Rochester, Minn)
Neurology 41:893–898, 1991   5–9

Background.—Protein deposits with abundant β-pleated sheet structure in the extracellular space result in amyloidosis. Depositions of transthyretin (TTR) or monoclonal immunoglobulin light chains are the usual cause of amyloidosis affecting nerve or muscle.

Methods.—Eleven consecutively seen unrelated patients with polyneuropathy caused by TTR amyloidosis underwent 2 tiers of genetic testing. The first step was direct genomic sequencing to determine whether any changes were present in the TTR gene. The second step was polymerase chain reaction amplification of specific alleles (PASA) to screen for previously described mutations.

Findings.—Each patient was found to be heterozygous for a mutation by direct sequencing of the promoter region, exons, and splice junctions. In 6 patients, valine 30 was substituted by methionine, the Portuguese-Japanese type; in 2, serine 77 was substituted by tyrosine, the Illinois type; and in 1, threonine 60 was substituted by alanine, the Appalachian type. Two previously undescribed mutations were found in the remaining patients, 1 in which phenylalanine 33 was substituted by leucine and another in which phenylalanine 64 was substituted by leucine. The probands of the 2 novel mutations had no pathologic findings that distinguished them from the patients with other mutations. For each of the 5 mutations described, a specific PASA assay was developed.

Conclusion.—Two novel mutations associated with amyloid polyneuropathy were identified. The PASA assays can be performed by any laboratory that can perform polymerase chain reaction. For the few samples that include an undescribed mutation, a specialty laboratory can perform direct genomic sequencing to delineate the mutation. The methods described may be used widely to diagnose genetic diseases.

▶ With the previous recognition of the molecular genetic basis of most familial types of amyloid neuropathy, the possibility of preclinical or clinical recognition and eventual treatment by genetic engineering becomes available. This paper is a step on the way to elucidating the various mutations underlying familial amyloid polyneuropathy, and it offers a new technique for recognizing the mutations.—W.G. Bradley, D.M., F.R.C.P.

Biochemical Effect of Liver Transplantation in Two Swedish Patients With Familial Amyloidotic Polyneuropathy (FAP-met[30])
Holmgren G, Steen L, Ekstedt J, Groth C-G, Ericzon B-G, Eriksson S, Andersen O, Karlberg I, Nordén G, Nakazato M, Hawkins P, Richardson S, Pepys M (Univ Hosp, Umeå, Sweden; Huddinge Hosp, Stockholm; Sahlgrenska Hosp, Gothenberg, Sweden; Miyazaki Med College, Miyazaki, Japan; Hammersmith Hosp, England)
Clin Genet 40:242–246, 1991   5–10

Background.—Patients with the autosomal dominant inherited disorder familial amyloidotic polyneuropathy (FAP) have progressive peripheral and autonomic neuropathy and neural and systemic amyloid deposits. Within these amyloid fibrils is a variant transthyretin (TTR) molecule designated TTR met 30, the principal source of which is the liver. To determine whether replacing the source of variant TTR with a source of normal TTR should reduce levels of the pathogenic mutant protein, the biochemical effects of liver transplantation in patients with FAP met 30 were evaluated.

Methods.—The 2 patients were a 52-year-old Swedish man and a 30-year-old man of Portuguese descent, both of whom had a family history of FAP. Both had progressive polyneuropathies with symptoms including intense diarrhea, general muscular atrophy, and urinary hesitancy. Both patients received successful cadaveric liver transplants and underwent radioimmunoaswsay and enzyme-linked immunosorbent assay for variant TTR, restriction fragment-length polymorphism analysis, and imaging of amyloid deposits.

Results.—Restriction fragment-length polymorphism analysis showed that both patients were heterozygous for the TTR met 30 mutation. Both had dramatic reductions in TTR met 30 levels to normal. Amyloid imaging in 1 patient showed no reduction in the quantity of amyloid at 6 months, but no further progression of the neuropathy.

Conclusion.—This treatment appears to clear variant TTR from the blood and arrested clinical progression in 1 patient. Further monitoring, including serum amyloid P scintigraphy, will determine whether elimination of the abnormal protein eventually will affect the neurologic symptoms.

▶ The mutations responsible for FAP now have been characterized in most cases. The mutated TTR is produced mainly by the liver. This is a lethal disease; hence, heroic measures such as liver transplantation may be justified. This report indicates that liver transplantation may prove to be effective for such patients. More patients will need to be studied, but this is yet another neurologic degeneration that may respond to potential treatment.—W.G. Bradley, D.M., F.R.C.P.

The Clinical Spectrum of Peripheral Neuropathies Associated With Benign Monoclonal IgM, IgG and IgA Paraproteinaemia: Comparative Clinical, Immunological and Nerve Biopsy Findings
Yeung KB, Thomas PK, King RHM, Waddy H, Will RG, Hughes RAC, Gregson NA, Leibowitz S (Royal Free Hosp School of Medicine; United Med and Dental Schools of Guy's and St Thomas's Hosps, London)
J Neurol 238:383–391, 1991   5–11

Background.—Benign monoclonal gammopathies are associated increasingly with late-onset peripheral neuropathy. Clinical, electrophysiologic, nerve biopsy, and immunologic tests were conducted in patients with peripheral neuropathy associated with benign monoclonal paraproteinemia to identify distinguishing features in the neuropathy associated with 3 different paraprotein classes and to compare them with those of chronic idiopathic demyelinating polyneuropathy.

Findings.—Of 62 patients, the paraprotein class was IgM in 46 patients, IgG in 11, and IgA in 5. Although there were variations, the clinical features were similar among those with IgM and IgG paraproteinemia. Most patients had a late-onset, slowly progressive, distal sensorimotor demyelinating polyneuropathy. Tremor and ataxia were prominent features, particularly among patients with IgM paraproteinemia. A relapsing–remitting course was observed in 3 IgM patients and 3 IgG patients. There were no distinguishing clinical and electrophysiologic features between patients with IgM and IgG paraproteinemia and those with chronic idiopathic demyelinating polyneuropathy. Of the 5 patients with IgA paraproteinemia, 4 had distal sensorimotor neuropathy and 1 had proximal demyelinating motor neuropathy. Only 1 had tremor, and none had a relapsing course. Nerve biopsy studies showed immunoglobulin deposition on myelin only in patients with IgM paraproteins, more commonly among those with a κ light chain. Immunoglobulin deposition was absent in the endoneurium but was always present in the perineurium in normal and abnormal nerves. Similarly, electron microscopic studies showed widening of the myelin periodicity in patients with IgM paraproteins, but only among those with immunoglobulin deposition on myelin. The response to treatment could not be evaluated systematically, but, in general, patients with neuropathy associated with IgG and IgA paraproteins showed more satisfactory response to corticosteroids and plasma exchange than did patients with IgM paraproteins.

Conclusions.—Neuropathies associated with IgM paraproteins with anti–myelin-associated glycoprotein are characterized by immunoglobulin deposition on myelin and by widely spaced myelin but usually also with poor response to therapy. In neuropathies associated with IgG and IgA paraproteins, immunoglobulin deposition is rare but is more likely to respond to treatment.

▶ An idiopathic gammopathy occurs in a significant number of elderly individuals, and the chance association with some other disease such as chronic peripheral neuropathy is not expected. Koch's postulutes demand that the abnormal protein be demonstrated to be neurotoxic and that removal of the protein cure the condition. In few instances has Koch been satisfied! Nevertheless, the similar clinical picture in these patients strongly suggests that, in many, the gammopathy may be the cause of the neuropathy. This large and excellent review provides evidence that many of the patients improved with immunosuppressant therapy.—W.G. Bradley, D.M., F.R.C.P.

Neuropathy Associated With Monoclonal Gammopathies of Undetermined Significance
Gosselin S, Kyle RA, Dyck PJ (Mayo Clin and Mayo Found, Rochester, Minn)
Ann Neurol 30:54–61, 1991   5–12

Background.—Monoclonal proteins in the serum or urine of patients with undiagnosed peripheral neuropathy may provide a marker for primary amyloidosis, myeloma, lymphoma, leukemia, Waldenstroëm's macroglobulinemia, or monoclonal gammopathy of undetermined significance (MGUS). The natural history and neurophysiologic characteristics of neuropathies associated with MGUS were reviewed to assess further the linkage between monoclonal proteins and peripheral neuropathy.

Patients.—The clinical characteristics, course, and electromyographic features of 31 patients with monoclonal IgM-MGUS, of 24 patients with IgG-MGUS, and of 10 patients with IgA-MGUS were reviewed retrospectively.

Findings.—There were 4 statistically significant differences that distinguished IgM-MGUS neuropathies from IgG-MGUS and IgA-MGUS neuropathies: higher frequency of sensory loss and ataxia; higher frequency of nerve-conduction abnormality (i.e., 10 attributes of nerve conduction were significantly worse but none were significantly better); higher frequency of dispersion of the compound muscle action potential; and higher frequency of IgM-MGUS in the MGUS neuropathy cohort when compared with all patients with MGUS. None of these differences could be attributed to selection or severity biases. However, the severity of neuropathy was not associated with the amount of IgM or the estimated size of the monoclonal peak. The type and severity of IgM-MGUS neuropathy were not related to the presence or absence of anti–myelin-associated glycoprotein antibody activity.

Conclusions.—These findings leave undecided the direct mechanistic linkage between monoclonal proteins and the presence of neuropathy. It appears that a simple relationship between the presence and amount of IgM-MGUS or the anti–myelin-associated glycoproteins antibody actvity and neuropathy does not exist.

▶ This is an important series that is subject to the bias of selective referral of patients to Gosselin and colleagues at the Mayo Clinic. However, it does support previous reports that the neuropathy associated with IgM gammopathies is more frequent and somewhat different from neuropathies with IgA or IgG gammopathies. The underlying mechanism still needs to be elucidated.—W.G. Bradley, D.M., F.R.C.P.

Phenelzine Associated Peripheral Neuropathy: Clinical and Electrophysiologic Findings
Goodheart RS, Dunne JW, Edis RH (Royal Perth Hosp, Australia)
Aust N Z J Med 21:339–340, 1991   5–13

Introduction.—Phenelzine sulfate is a monoamine oxidase inhibitor commonly used to treat depression. It may produce orthostatic hypotension, drowsiness, and weakness as well as peripheral paresthesia. Two patients who had a generalized sensorimotor neuropathy in clear relation to phenelzine treatment were examined.

Case 1.—Man, 43, previously had progressive numbness and dysesthesia in his feet and, more recently, in his fingertips as well as mild foot weakness. He had been depressed for 8 years; and for 2 years, he had received 30 mg of phenelzine sulfate twice daily. Sensation was impaired to the elbows and knees; reflexes were reduced or absent; and the foot muscles were mildly weakened. Nerve conduction studies showed absent sensory responses and reduced or absent lower-limb compound muscle action potentials. Fibrillation potentials were recorded from distal lower extremity muscles. Both clinical and electrophysiologic improvement ensued when phenelzine was withdrawn.

Case 2.—Man, 46, received phenelzine for major depression and anxiety for 2 years. He had progressive sensory symptoms in his legs and feet; both sensation and muscle power were objectively affected. Needle examination showed fibrillation potentials in the foot muscles. Sensory symptoms improved when phenelzine was stopped, and limb power recovered nearly completely within 6 weeks. Numbness reappeared when phenelzine was resumed and resolved only partly when treatment was again withdrawn. The patient had consumed alcohol excessively in the past but had been abstinent for 10 years.

Conclusions.—The electrophysiologic abnormalities in these patients are consistent with an axonal process. Both patients had normal pyridoxine levels.

▶ Many reports of drug-related peripheral neuropathies are suspect, with little certainty with regard to cause and effect. However, these two cases very strongly suggest that phenelzine can cause a peripheral neuropathy. In one case, improvement occurred with withdrawal of the medication, and the neuropathy returned with rechallenge. The mechanism of the neuropathy still needs to be determined.—W.G. Bradley, D.M., F.R.C.P.

Treatment of Painful Diabetic Neuropathy With Capsaicin 0.075%
Scheffler NM, Sheitel PL, Lipton MN (American Ctr for Foot Health Research, Baltimore)
J Am Podiatr Med Assoc 81:288–293, 1991   5–14

Background.—The most common diabetic neuropathy is symmetric sensory neuropathy. The foot usually is involved first, and the chief complaint is pain with nocturnal exacerbations of symptoms. A variety of treatments have been used to reduce the severity of symptoms. A double-blind, placebo-controlled trial was done to evaluate the effectiveness of topical capsaicin .075% cream.

Methods.—Fifty-four patients with type I or II diabetes mellitus who were unresponsive or intolerant to conventional therapy for diabetic neuropathy were included. All had moderate to very severe pain that interfered with sleep or activities on an everyday basis. Patients were assigned randomly to receive a group receiving capsaicin or a group receiving vehicle cream, which they were instructed to apply 4 times a day to the affected area. Pain was assessed by the investigator and patient before, during, and after 8 weeks of treatment.

Results.—At 2 weeks, improvement was seen in 58.3% of the capsaicin group and 48% of the vehicle group. By week 8, 89.5% of the capsaicin group had improved, compared with 50% of the vehicle group. Mean decreases in pain intensity were 49.1% in the capsaicin group and 16.5% in the vehicle group. Patients in the capsaicin group also had significantly more improvement in sleeping at week 8 and in walking at week 6. There were no serious adverse effects in either group.

Conclusions.—Topical capsaicin .075% cream appears to be a safe and effective technique of managing painful diabetic neuropathy. Improvements in pain and daily activities is achieved in most patients. Capsaicin cream should be considered as an early therapeutic choice for patients with this condition.

▶ Burning feet and other painful distal neuropathies commonly are caused by diabetes. This is 1 of a series of recent papers demonstrating that topical capsaicin cream can produce significant relief of the pain. The higher concentration cream (.075%) appears to be more effective than the lower concentration (.025%). However, some patients cannot tolerate the transiently increased burning produced by the higher concentration capsaicin. Nevertheless, this is clearly a therapeutic advance.—W.G. Bradley, D.M., F.R.C.P.

The Natural History of Diabetic Femoral Neuropathy
Coppack SW, Watkins PJ (King's College Hosp, London)
Q J Med 79:307–313, 1991   5–15

Background.—Diabetic femoral neuropathy is an infrequent but occasionally disabling disorder characterized by pain, weakness, muscle wasting, and reflex abnormalities. There is little objective sensory change. Pain typically is neuropathic in nature and is present in the anterior thigh above the knee. There may be weakness of knee extension or quadriceps wasting, and the knee jerk may be decreased or absent.

Clinical.—Eight of 27 patients with diabetic femoral neuropathy were symptomatic at the time diabetes was diagnosed. Cutaneous hyperesthesias were frequent and tended to be worse in bed or at night. Several patients also described numbness or hypoesthesia in the thigh. All patients but 6 had noted weakness.

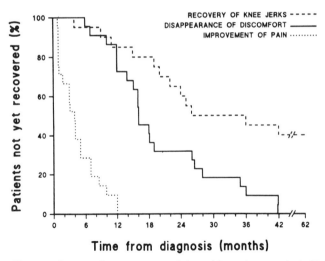

Time from diagnosis (months)

Fig 5–1.—The rates of recovery from symptoms and signs of femoral neuropathy in 27 diabetic patients. The "improvement of pain" line is the time until the first report of improvement in sensory symptoms, from 22 patients. The "disappearance of discomfort" line is the time until complete resolution of sensory symptoms, in 23 patients. The "recovery of knee jerks" is time course of return to normal of the abnormalities of patella tendon reflexes in 20 patients. No recovery was observed later than 42 months after diagnosis, and follow-up was for a median of 62 months. (Courtesy of Coppack SW, Watkins PJ: *Q J Med* 79:307–313, 1991.)

Course.—Eighteen patients were reassessed after an average of 4 years. Only 2 patients had severe relapses. Recovery usually was noted within 3 months and was complete by 18 months (Fig 5–1). None of the patients had persistent disability, although half had some residual symptoms or signs. Residual features included both sensory symptoms, such as exercise-related pain, and weakness of the legs.

Conclusions.—Diabetic femoral neuropathy tends to resolve gradually, leaving nondisabling deficits in many patients. The prognosis for resolution of pain and weakness is good.

▶ Patients with lumbosacral plexopathy frequently have diabetes as the underlying cause. In most cases, the femoral nerve bears the major brunt of the damage. This paper reviews a classic series of 27 patients and emphasizes the pain and muscle wasting. The relatively good prognosis has been suspected for some time but is clearly illustrated here. The rate of recovery is similar to that of idiopathic brachial plexopathy. The underlying pathology of the latter may also be a vasculopathic process.—W.G. Bradley, D.M., F.R.C.P.

The Appearance of the Piriformis Muscle Syndrome in Computed Tomography and Magnetic Resonance Imaging: A Case Report and Review of the Literature
Jankiewicz JJ, Hennrikus WL, Houkom JA (Naval Hosp, San Diego, Calif)
Clin Orthop 262:205–209, 1991   5–16

Introduction.—The piriformis syndrome (PS) is a controversial cause of hip pain because of the lack of objective findings. Magnetic resonance imaging is becoming increasingly valuable in the diagnosis of musculoskeletal disorders and may prove useful in the evaluation of patients with suspected PS.

Case Report.—Woman, 27, had chronic aching pain in the right buttock that was aggravated by walking, squatting, and sexual intercourse. Freiberg's, Pace's, and Lasègue's signs were positive. Pelvic and rectal examination revealed severe tenderness and a sausage-shaped fullness, with reproduction of pain by digital pressure over the soft tissues on the posterolateral pelvic wall—just proximal to the ischial spine and superior to the spinococcygeal ligament. An enlarged mass anterior to the right piriformis muscle was demonstrated by CT, correlating with the finding of sausage-shaped fullness on clinical examination. The mass was further defined by MRI as an enlarged piriformis muscle with normal and homogeneous muscle signal intensity. Injection of the right piriformis muscle trigger point with local anesthetic and a corticosteroid produced immediate pain relief.

Discussion.—The PS has been considered an entrapment neuropathy caused by pressure of the sciatic nerve by an enlarged or inflamed piriformis muscle. The sciatic nerve usually passes between the piriformis muscle above and the gemellus muscle below. In about 20% of the population the piriformis muscle is split, and 1 or both parts of the sciatic nerve pass through the muscle belly. In another 10%, the tibial and peroneal portions of the sciatic nerve are not enclosed in a common sheath, and 1 portion may pierce the muscle. If the piriformis muscle and fascia become inflamed, usually as a result of trauma, the sciatic nerve can become compressed between the swollen muscle and bony pelvis, causing an entrapment neuropathy. It also is proposed that focal hyperirritability of the piriformis muscle, usually caused by trauma, may result in a trigger-point syndrome. Both CT and MRI are valuable noninvasive procedures that can provide support for the existence of this syndrome.

▶ Sciatica without a lumbar disk lesion is a common problem. A few of these patients may have PS. This has always been difficult to diagnose, but this paper suggests that imaging studies may be of help.—W.G. Bradley, D.M., F.R.C.P.

Ischemic Injury to the Spinal Cord or Lumbosacral Plexus After Aorto-Iliac Reconstruction

Gloviczki P, Cross SA, Stanson AW, Carmichael SW, Bower TC, Pairolero PC, Hallett JW Jr, Toomey BJ, Cherry KJ Jr (Mayo Clinic and Found, Rochester, Minn)
Am J Surg 162:131–136, 1991   5–17

Background.—Paraplegia is a rare but severe and unpredictable complication after aortoiliac reconstruction. The clinical manifestations and mechanisms of neurologic injury after aortoiliac reconstruction were evaluated retrospectively.

Methods.—Between 1980 and 1989, 9 patients had ischemic injury to the spinal cord and lumbosacral roots or plexus after 3,320 aorto-iliac reconstructions, for an overall incidence of .3%. Neurologic injury occurred in 2 of 1,901 elective and 3 of 210 emergency abdominal aortic aneurysm repairs, and in 4 of 1,209 repairs for occlusive disease, 3 of whom had clinical evidence of distal embolization preoperatively. Treatment included placement of a bifurcated graft in 8 patients, extra-anatomical revascularization in 1, supraceliac aortic cross-clamping in 2, and exclusion of both internal iliac arteries in 1.

Results.—Neurologic deficits were observed immediately after surgery in 4 patients and after 24–72 hours in 5. The extent and type of injury correlated with long-term outcome. Only 1 of 3 patients with infarctions of the thoracolumbar cord and the conus had modest recovery. One of 2 patients with anterior spinal artery syndrome showed some recovery. All 3 patients with bilateral root lesions and mild patchy spinal cord ischemia with relative preservation of cord functions showed marked recovery. One patient with unilateral lumbar plexopathy had moderate recovery. The early mortality rate was 22%. Severe perioperative

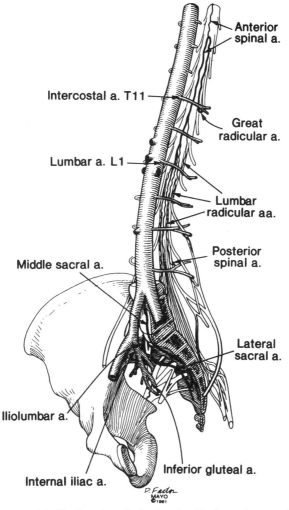

Fig 5–2.—Anatomy of the blood supply to the distal cord and lumbosacral roots and plexus. (Courtesy of Gloviczki P, Cross SA, Stanson AW, et al: *Am J Surg* 162:131–136, 1991.)

complications occurred in 7 patients, mostly because of associated visceral and somatic ischemia and sepsis.

Discussion.—Interruption of the pelvic circulation is a major causal factor in the development of ischemic injury after aortoiliac reconstruction. Occlusion of the great radicular artery, which supplies the anterior spinal artery in the thoracolumbar segment, commonly has been implicated (Fig 5-2). If this artery is chronically occluded or stenosed, the lower lumbar or sacral radicular arteries, which originate from the internal iliac artery, may contribute significantly to the blood supply of the

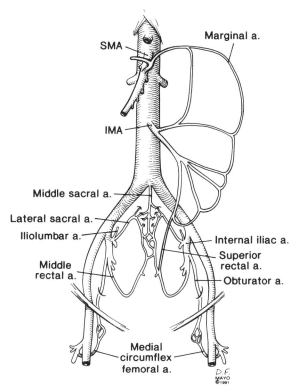

SMA

Marginal a.

IMA

Middle sacral a.

Lateral sacral a.

Iliolumbar a.

Internal iliac a.

Superior rectal a.

Middle rectal a.

Obturator a.

Medial circumflex femoral a.

D.F.
MAYO
©1991

Fig 5–3.—Primary and collateral circulation to the pelvis. (Courtesy of Gloviczki P, Cross SA, Stanson AW, et al: *Am J Surg* 162:131–136, 1991.)

terminal cord (Fig 5–3). If the internal iliac artery is diseased, collaterals from the middle sacral, contralateral internal iliac, mesenteric, or deep femoral arteries may become important.

Conclusion.—Prevention of spinal cord injury during aortoiliac reconstruction currently is not possible. However, the incidence of this complication may be reduced by recognizing high-risk patients, including those with ruptured abdominal aortic aneurysm and shaggy aorta syndrome, and by paying attention to certain guidelines such as avoidance of hypotension and prolonged supraceliac cross-clamping, use of gentle technique to prevent embolization, revascularization of at least 1 internal iliac artery, and use of heparin. Patients with ischemic injury of the lumbosacral roots or plexus have better recovery that those with cord injury.

▶ Ischemic injury of the spinal cord and lumbosacral plexus in aortoiliac reconstruction is a known complication. this excellent review helps to define frequency, prognosis, and ways of limiting the incidence of this problem.—W.G. Bradley, D.M., F.R.C.P.

Unexplained Syncope Evaluated by Electrophysiologic Studies and Head-Up Tilt Testing

Sra JS, Anderson AJ, Sheikh SH, Avitall B, Tchou PJ, Troup PJ, Gilbert CJ, Akhtar M, Jazayeri MR (Sinai Samaritan Med Ctr, Milwaukee; Milwaukee Cardiovascular Data Registry; Sandaha Home, Lahore, Pakistan; Presbyterian Univ Hosp, Pittsburgh)

Ann Intern Med 114:1013–1019, 1991   5–18

Background.—Despite thorough investigation, the cause of syncope remains unexplained in many patients. Electrophysiologic testing may be helpful but often is not. A retrospective analysis was done to characterize patients with unexplained syncope and to evaluate the roles of electrophysiologic examination and head-up tilt testing.

Methods.—The investigation included 86 patients referred for evaluation of unexplained syncope during a 2-year period, including 50 men and 36 women (mean age, 56 years). Physical examination, neurologic evaluation, surface ECG, and 24-hour ambulatory monitoring all failed to identify the cause of their syncope. All patients underwent electrophysiologic testing, and those with a negative result were administered head-up tilt testing. If the baseline test was negative, it was repeated after intravenous infusion of isoproterenol, 1 μg/min. Substantial arterial hypotension in association with presyncope or syncope was considered a positive response.

Results.—Electrophysiologic testing gave abnormal results in 34% of patients (group 1). Sustained monomorphic ventricular tachycardia was induced in 72% of these patients, and supraventricular tachycardia was induced in 17%. Syncope was provoked by head-up tilt testing in 40% of patients (group 2). Of these, 65% had an abnormal response on the first examination, and 35% had an abnormal result after infusion of isoproterenol; in every case, the symptoms were similar to those experienced spontaneously. Significant bradycardia developed in 9 of these patients. The cause of syncope remained unexplained in 26% of patients (group 3). Seventy-six percent of group 1 had structural heart disease, compared with 6% of group 2 and 30% of group 3. Therapy was based on electrophysiologic studies in group 1. In group 2, all patients had a negative results on head-up tilt test while receiving either β blockers or disopyramide. No specific treatment was administered to group 3. Syncope recurred in 10% of patients over a median follow-up of 18.5 months.

Conclusions.—The underlying cause of syncope can be identified in most patients with the combination of electrophysiologic evaluation and head-up tilt testing. Further episodes of syncope can be prevented by therapeutic strategies based on the results of these tests. Cardiovascular abnormalities appear to be the most common cause of syncope in the sample reported.

▶ Unexplained syncope frequently presents to the neurologist. Patients may have neurologic, cardiologic, or autonomic problems. This paper emphasizes the autonomic and cardiologic abnormalities and the methods of detection.—W.G. Bradley, D.M., F.R.C.P.

Factors Influencing Outcome of Prednisone Dose Reduction in Myasthenia Gravis
Miano MA, Bosley TM, Heiman-Patterson TD, Reed J, Sergott RC, Savino PJ, Schatz NJ (Wills Eye Hosp; Thomas Jefferson Univ Hosp, Philadelphia; Lehigh Valley Hosp Ctr, Allentown, Pa)
Neurology 41:919–921, 1991   5–19

Background.—Prednisone is a mainstay in the treatment of patients with myasthenia gravis. However, long-term immunosuppression often is needed because myasthenic symptoms recur as prednisone doses are decreased.

Methods.—Factors affecting the outcome of 114 prednisone dose reductions in 63 patients with generalized and ocular myasthenia gravis were reviewed. A successful dose reduction was defined as a patient remaining asymptomatic for longer than 1 year without prednisone or while taking a stable low dose of prednisone. In 37 patients, there was 1 dose reduction attempt, and in 26 patients there were 2–6 attempts. Thymectomy had been performed on 22 patients, and 17 patients received azathioprine, 2–3 mg/kg/day, along with prednisone for at least 6 months before the attempted reduction in prednisone dose.

Results.—The average starting dose of prednisone for successful attempts was 46.6 mg; for relapses, 41.4 mg. Factors that had no significant influence on outcome included age at onset, disease duration, sex, race, and type of myasthenia. Thymectomy, with or without thymoma, also had no effect on prednisone withdrawal outcome. However, azathioprine significantly improved the outcome of prednisone dose reduction. Reduction was successful in 13 of 17 patients treated with azathioprine. A slower rate of prednisone dose reduction and higher ending doses also improved the chances of success.

Conclusion.—Azathioprine adjuvant treatment should be considered for patients with generalized myasthenia gravis and no contraindications. The rate of prednisone dose reduction should be monitored closely, as overall rates of reduction of greater than 5 mg per month may jeopardize successful attempts. When a dose reduction attempt fails, further attempts should be made with slower dose reduction rates and increased ending doses.

▶ The importance of prednisone in the treatment of myasthenia gravis is undoubted, but its reduction and withdrawal continues to be a part of the "art" of management. This paper provides a careful review of the authors' experience. The use of azathioprine as an important adjuvant is, perhaps, the most significant finding. Prednisone dose reduction should be no more than 5 mg per month and should be very carefully monitored.—W.G. Bradley, D.M., F.R.C.P.

Treatment of Myasthenia Gravis With High-Dose Intravenous Immunoglobulin
Cosi V, Lombardi M, Piccolo G, Erbetta A (Univ of Pavia, Italy)
Acta Neurol Scand 84:81–84, 1991   5–20

Background.—High-dose intravenous immunoglobulin has produced promising results in patients with myasthenia gravis, including patients in the acute phase of the disease and those whose disease remained stationary despite long-standing immunosuppressive treatment. The results in 37 patients with myasthenia gravis treated with high-dose intravenous immunoglobulin were evaluated.

Methods.—Included were 33 female and 4 male patients (mean age, 39 years). Mean duration of disease was 99 months. Thymectomy had been done in 79% of patients. Eleven patients were treated in an acute onset or acute-relapsing phase because plasma exchange was not effective or was contraindicated. The remaining 26 patients had been in a stationary phase lasting at least 6 months, and 22 of them had received immunosuppressive treatment. The patients received intravenously administered immunoglobulin, .4 mg/kg/day, for 5 consecutive days.

Results.—In 70% there was a 1-degree improvement in the Oosterhuis Global Clinical Classification of Myasthenic Severity or disappearance of bulbar involvement, or both, 12 days after the beginning of treatment. This improvement was sustained for as long as 60 days in 59% of patients. A 2-degree improvement was seen in 54% of patients and sustained for 60 days in 38%. There was no difference in the percentage of improvement among patients treated in a stationary or an acute phase, and there were no side effects.

Conclusions.—High-dose intravenous immunoglobulin is an interesting therapeutic choice for patients with myasthenia gravis. It is virtually risk-free, which allows planning of a controlled trial comparing it with plasma exchange.

▶ A double-blind clinical trial of intravenous immunoglobulin would be helpful in myasthenia gravis. This study strongly suggests that intravenous immunoglobulin can be at least as beneficial as plasmapheresis in an acute relapse.—W.G. Bradley, D.M., F.R.C.P.

The Frequency of Patients With Dystrophin Abnormalities in a Limb-Girdle Patient Population

Arikawa E, Hoffman EP, Kaido M, Nonaka I, Sugita H, Arahata K (Natl Inst of Neuroscience, Tokyo; Univ of Pittsburgh)
Neurology 41:1491–1496, 1991   5–21

Background.—Limb-girdle muscular dystrophy (LGD) is a diagnostic term covering a genetically heterogeneous group of disorders. It is difficult to differentiate LGD from Becker's dystrophy and female manifesting carriers of Duchenne type muscular dystrophy. The dystrophin protein in patients with a clinical diagnosis of LGD was examined.

Methods.—From 1979 to 1990, 3,048 diagnostic muscle biopsy specimens were processed by the National Institute of Neuroscience in Tokyo. Forty-one patients had a clinical diagnosis of LGD. Dystrophin content in all patients was analyzed using both immunofluorescence and immunoblot methods.

Findings.—Five male patients with an abnormal dystrophin pattern diagnostic of Becker's muscular dystrophy were identified. There also were 2 female patients with dystrophin patterns consistent with a diagnosis of manifesting carrier of Duchenne type muscular dystrophy. In all, 17% of the patients had a dystrophinopathy, indicating that they had a disorder related to Duchenne type or Becker's muscular dystrophy. Misclassification occurred in 31% of the male patients and in 13% of female patients with isolated LGD. Through multiplex polymerase chain reaction analysis of small amounts of DNA gathered by muscle biopsy, a dystrophin gene deletion was confirmed in all 5 male patients with Becker's dystrophy.

Conclusions.—In about 40% of patients with isolated LGD or Becker's dystrophy, differential diagnosis cannot be made on the basis of histopathologic and clinical criteria. Accurate diagnosis in these patients must rely on dystrophin protein and gene studies. Without correct diagnosis, patients and their families will not receive proper genetic counseling.

▶ This paper demonstrates that, in cases previously diagnosed as having LGD on clinical grounds, almost 1 in 5 either have Becker's muscular dystrophy or are manifesting female carriers of Duchenne type musclar dystrophy. It should be noted that all such cases lacked a clean-cut autosomal recessive inheritance.—W.G. Bradley, D.M., F.R.C.P.

Limb-Girdle Syndrome: A Genetic Study of 22 Large Brazilian Families: Comparison With X-Linked Duchenne and Becker Dystrophies

Passos-Bueno MR, Vainzof M, Pavanello RCM, Pavanello-Filho I, Lima MABO,

Zatz M (Universidade de São Paulo, Brazil)
J Neurol Sci 103:65–75, 1991

5–22

Background.—Distinguishing between the X-linked muscular dystrophies and autosomal recessive limb-girdle muscular dystrophy (LGD) is very important in genetic counseling and often is very difficult. The clinical and laboratory findings in 62 patients from 22 large families with autosomal recessive inheritance were evaluated to improve characterization of LGD compared with the X-linked forms.

Methods.—All patients had a previous diagnosis of LGD. Data on age of onset and of confinement to a wheelchair were analyzed. Reproductive performance, serum enzymes, and muscle dystrophin also were assessed. Immunohistochemistry and Western blot were used.

Results.—Muscle biopsies from the majority of the families were examined, and dystrophin was normal in all. The patients in 19 families had a milder clinical course than those in the remaining 3, in which disease progression was continuous and clinically similar to X-linked Duchenne type muscular dystrophy. The parents of the affected patients had a consanguinity rate of 77%. There were no major clinical differences between the autosomal recessive and X-linked forms. Affected men had significantly higher reproductive performance than affected women. Surprisingly, estimated fitness was significantly greater for male patients with LGD than for patients of comparable age with Becker's disease.

Conclusions.—The clinical similarity of the LGD forms and the X-linked muscular dystropies suggests that the sequence of part of the dystrophin gene mapped at 6q24 may be a candidate for the cause of LGD. However, research does not support this hypothesis. Identifying the gene responsible for autosomal recessive LGD is very important both for clinical purposes and for increasing understanding of the dystrophin function and of how different genes are responsible for similar phenotypes.

▶ It is always difficult to separate the male patients with a late-onset muscular dystrophy into those with Becker's muscular dystrophy and those with LGD. There has also been a lot of argument about the existence of LGD. This paper uses the modern techniques of dystrophin analysis to separate autosomal recessive families that are dystrophin positive, showing phenotypic similarity to X-linked muscular dystrophy families. Those interested in neuromuscular disease should read this paper carefully.—W.G. Bradley, D.M., F.R.C.P.

Occidental Type Cerebromuscular Dystrophy: A Report of Eleven Cases

Topaloğlu H, Yalaz K, Renda Y, Çağlar M, Göğüs S, Kale G, Gücüyener K, Nurlu G (Hacettepe Univ, Ankara, Turkey)
J Neurol Neurosurg Psychiatry 54:226–229, 1991   5–23

Background.—Congenital muscular dystrophy (CMD) is probably an autosomal recessive disorder; it is characterized by hypotonia of early onset, joint contractures, and dystrophic changes in muscles that progress slowly. An intermediate form between classic occidental CMD and Fukuyama's CMD has been termed occidental type cerebromuscular dystrophy (OCMD). Mental development is normal, but CT shows leukodystrophic changes.

Clinical Findings.—Eleven of 23 Turkish patients seen in a 16-month period with CMD received a diagnosis of OCMD. Parental consanguinity was discovered in 8 patients. All the patients were hypotonic at birth and had delayed motor development, stiffness of several joints, and proximal muscle weakness. Seven of the 11 patients were areflexic. Facial muscle involvement was a consistent finding. The electromyogram was myopathic in most patients. Cranial CT scans showed marked white matter hyperlucency with or without ventricular dilatation. All the patients were mentally normal.

Muscle Biopsy.—Most biopsy specimens showed markedly varying fiber sizes and endomysial fibrosis. Mild necrosis of fibers with regeneration was a frequent finding. Two biopsy specimens showed mild, focal inflammation. There was no evidence of type grouping or group atrophy.

Conclusions.—These patients may well form a subgroup within CMD, but they should be considered as having a distinct disorder. The fact that some patients have normal CT findings stresses the marked heterogeneity of CMD.

Congenital Muscular Dystrophy: Brain Alterations in an Unselected Series of Western Patients

Trevisan CP, Carollo C, Segalla P, Angelini C, Drigo P, Giordano R (Università degli Studi di Padova, Padua, Italy)
J Neurol Neurosurg Psychiatry 54:330–334, 1991   5–24

Background.—Although the Japanese form of congenital muscular dystrophy (CMD) generally differs from Western cases because of changes in the CNS, brain involvement occasionally is described in non-Japanese children with CMD. An unselected group of 12 Italian children with CMD was examined clinically and radiologically.

Patients.—The 8 female and 4 male patients had a mean age of 7 years 8 months. The onset was always neonatal, with muscular hypotonia and weakness and muscle biopsy evidence of dystrophic change.

Clinical.—Five patients had evidence of mental retardation. Six patients eventually were able to walk and climb stairs, but the others could only sit. The muscular deficit improved progressively in 6 children. The single death was the result of an epidural hematoma after accidental head trauma.

Neuroradiology.—Computed tomography scanning demonstrated varying degrees of ventricular dilatation, with moderate cortical atrophy in 3 patients. Eight patients had diffuse white matter hypodensity supratentorially, also of varying degree. In 5 patients the CT abnormalities correlated with clinical CNS involvement. Autopsy of the child who died showed pachygyric change with small heterotopic areas in the white matter and disorganized cytoarchitecture. Laminar areas of demyelination also were noted.

Conclusions.—Subclinical CNS abnormalities frequently are observed in children with typical Western CMD. This disorder, like its Japanese counterpart, should be considered a type of myoencephalopathy.

▶ These 2 papers (Abstracts 5–23 and 5–24) describe a series of non-Oriental patients with CMD. In the Turkish series of Topaloğlu et al., mental development tests were normal, whereas half of the Italian patients of Trevisan et al., had mental retardation. In both series, most had evidence on CT scanning of diffuse white matter changes. The classification of cerebromuscular dystrophy still remains to be clarified.—W.G. Bradley, D.M., F.R.C.P.

A Met-to-Val Mutation in the Skeletal Muscle Na⁺ Channel α-Subunit in Hyperkalaemic Periodic Paralysis

Rojas CV, Wang J, Schwartz LS, Hoffman EP, Powell BR, Brown RH Jr (Univ of Pittsburgh; Oregon Health Sciences Univ, Portland; Massachusetts Gen Hosp, Charlestown)
Nature 354:387–389, 1991   5–25

Background.—Patients with the autosomal dominant condition hyperkalaemic periodic paralysis (HYPP) have episodes of electric inexcitability and skeletal muscle paralysis. Tetrodotoxin-sensitive sodium channels from these patients' muscle cells show abnormal inactivation. The disease appears to be caused by mutations of the skeletal muscle sodium channel α-subunit gene on chromosome 17q. Sequencing data on the α-subunit coding region was examined.

Findings.—Muscle biopsy specimens from patients with familial HYPP and controls were analyzed by cross-species polymerase chain reaction-mediated complementary DNA cloning. Two nucleotide changes in the complementary DNA of affected patients could not be explained by *Taq* polymerase errors: a G-to-T substitution resulting in a Glu-to-Asp change, and an A-to-G substitution resulting in a Met-to-Val change. The Met-to-Val substitution appeared to be the causative mutation of HYPP because it was also found in a sporadic case of HYPP as a new mutation. No further mutations were found in this region. The mutations occurred in a proposed S_6 transmembrane segment of domain IV; the affected amino acid was conserved between all previously examined sodium channels.

Conclusions.—A voltage-gated Met-to-Val mutation was responsible for HYPP. It is unknown whether this substitution affects inactivation directly or indirectly. This mutation is not found in all families with HYPP; thus different mutations could cause the same disease.

▶ Hyperkalemic periodic paralysis appears to be caused in all cases by abnormalities of the sarcolemmal sodium channels. Research is now progressing to identify the details of the mutations. This paper reports the finding of a methionine to valine substitution in the α subunit of the sodium channel in 9 familial and 1 sporadic case. However, this mutation is not present in other cases. This genetic hydrogenate may well prove to be the basis for subtle differences in the clinical picture among different families.—W.G. Bradley, D.M., F.R.C.P.

6 Movement Disorders

Immunohistochemical Studies on Complexes I, II, III, and IV of Mitochondria in Parkinson's Disease

Hattori N, Tanaka M, Ozawa T, Mizuno Y (Juntendo Univ, Tokyo; Univ of Nagoya, Japan)

Ann Neurol 30:563–571, 1991   6–1

Background.—Why nigral neurons die in patients with Parkinson's disease remains unclear. In the 1-methyl-4-phenyl-1,2,3,6-tetrahydropyridine (MPTP) model of parkinsonism, the toxic metabolite 1-methyl-4-phenylpyridinium (MPP^+) inhibits both mitochondrial NADH-ubiquinone reductase and the α-ketoglutarate dehydrogenase complex, thereby producing an energy crisis from inhibition of mitochondrial respiration.

Methods.—Immunohistochemical studies were carried out on the substantia nigra in 8 patients with Parkinson's disease and 7 controls using antisera against complexes I through IV of the mitochondrial electron transport system. All the patients with Parkinson's disease had nigral degeneration with Lewy bodies in residual neurons.

Findings.—In patients with Parkinson's disease, 13% to 74% of melanized nigral neurons had reduced staining against complex I antibody. The proportion of neurons affected in controls was significantly smaller. Staining for complexes III and IV appeared normal, but 3 patients with Parkinson's disease had reduced staining for complex II. The intensity of immunostaining did not correlate with the severity of neuronal degeneration in the substantia nigra.

Conclusion.—These findings suggest that mitochondrial complex I is abnormal in Parkinson's disease, but it is not certain whether this is a fundamental defect or is secondary to other changes.

▶ The role of abnormalities of mitochondria in the cause of Parkinson's disease is receiving increasing attention. Any degenerating cell has abnormal intracellular organelles; hence, abnormalities of mitochondria could be secondary. However, intrinsic mitochondrial deficiency could make dopaminergic neurons more sensitive to endogenous or environmental toxins. This paper, which reports decreased complex I in nigral neurons, is an important addition to the literature.—W.G. Bradley, D.M., F.R.C.P.

Preproenkephalin Messenger RNA-Containing Neurons in Striatum of Patients With Symptomatic and Presymptomatic Huntington's Disease: An In Situ Hybridization Study

Albin RL, Qin Y, Young AB, Penney JB, Chesselet M-F (Univ of Michigan; Univ of Pennsylvania)

Ann Neurol 30:542–549, 1991 6–2

Background.—Patients with Huntington's disease have striatal atrophy, although neurons containing somatostatin, neuropeptide Y, and NADPH-diaphorase are spared in comparison to other subpopulations of neurons. Striatal projection neurons may be differentially affected, as those projecting to the external globus pallidus contain mainly enkephalin. Histochemical studies were performed to determine whether the perikarya of striatal enkephalinergic neurons are affected early in the course of Huntington's disease.

Methods.—Specimens from 6 patients with verified Huntington's disease, 7 normal controls, and 2 asymptomatic suspected carriers of the Huntington's disease allele were examined. Patients' average age was 58 years; there were 3 grade 2, 2 grade 3, and 1 grade 4 specimens. Brain tissue for these studies was obtained at autopsy. In situ hybridization histochemistry was performed using a radiolabeled RNA probe complementary to preproenkephalin messenger RNA (mRNA).

Results.—In the patients with symptomatic Huntington's disease, areal density of striatal neurons expressing preproenkephalin mRNA was considerably reduced. However, in the remaining cells, the level of labeling was the same as in the controls. The presymptomatic particpants had no reduction in areal density of preproenkephalin mRNA-containing neurons in the striatum. This was so even though loss of enkephalin immunoreactivity in the external globus pallidus had been shown previously in the same brains.

Conclusions.—Like previous immunohistochemical studies, in situ hybridization shows loss of striatal enkephalinergic neurons in patients with Huntington's disease. The decrease in enkephalin immunoreactivity probably results from decreased number and density of perikarya expressing preproenkephalin mRNA in patients with symptomatic Huntington's disease. The striatal neurons probably pass though a phase in which neurotransmitter, axonal transport, or terminal structure abnormalities occur before cell death.

▶ Loss of enkephalin in the globus pallidus is an early event in Huntington's disease, being seen even in presymptomatic brains. At that stage enkephalin-containing neurons in the stratum are not reduced, although such cell bodies are lost in symptomatic cases of Huntington's disease. This suggests a (dying back) type of degeneration in the presymptomatic phase of the disease.—W.G. Bradley, D.M., F.R.C.P.

Clozapine Is Beneficial for Psychosis in Parkinson's Disease
Kahn N, Freeman A, Juncos JL, Manning D, Watts RL (Emory Univ)
Neurology 41:1699–1700, 1991   6–3

Background.—Psychotic symptoms, including paranoia and hallucinations, may occur in patients with Parkinson's disease. Reducing dopaminomimetic treatment or administering neuroleptics may help, but at the cost of worsening extrapyramidal symptoms.

Methods.—Clozapine, a neuroleptic with minimal effects on the extrapyramidal motor system, was evaluated in an open-label trial in 11 patients who had Parkinson's disease complicated by psychosis. Most of the patients had hallucinations, delusions, or recurring confusion. Clozapine was started at a low dosage such as 25 mg daily, and increased until symptoms lessened or side effects became intolerable.

Results.—Of the 11 patients, 8 improved substantially with respect to their psychotic features. Two others had some improvement, whereas 1 became more confused and was withdrawn from the trial. Motor function was not affected by clozapine administration. The final mean dose was 56 mg. Two patients tolerated other antiparkinsonian drugs for the first time and had a modest improvement in motor function.

Conclusion.—Clozapine apparently is able to control psychotic features in many patients with Parkinson's disease without making motor disability worse and does not often produce extrapyramidal side effects such as acute dystonia or parkinsonism.

▶ This open-label study supports other such studies that suggest that clozapine may be useful in treating psychosis in Parkinson's disease whether or not dementia is present. If this finding can be confirmed, it will be an advance in the treatment of patients with Parkinson's disease. It is unfortunate that the administration of clozapine did not permit any significant increase in the amount of dopamimetic medication that could be coadministered to these patients. Only 1 patient in 11 experienced severe adverse effects necessitating withdrawal from the study. In my experience, more demented patients with Parkinson's disease do not tolerate even small amounts of clozapine because of excessive sedation and hypersalivation.—W.J. Weiner, M.D.

Is Essential Tremor Benign?
Busenbark KL, Nash J, Nash S, Hubble JP, Koller WC (Univ of Kansas)
Neurology 41:1982–1983, 1991   6–4

Objective.—Essential tremor (ET) is considered a benign condition; it does not affect life expectancy, and some patients have minimal disability. However, other patients believe ET is handicapping and socially embarrassing. A standardized assessment tool, the Sickness Impact Profile, was used to examine the disability caused by ET.

Methods.—A Sickness Impact Profile questionnaire was mailed to a group of 5,700 members of the International Tremor Foundation. A group of 87 controls from the general population (mean age, 62.7 years) and a group of 145 with Parkinson's disease (mean age, 70.1 years) also were included.

Findings.—Responses were analyzed from 753 patients with ET (average age, 64.6 years). Their mean age at disease onset was 44.5 years. Propranolol was being taken by 32.3%, and primidone was being taken by 14.5%. There was a family history of ET in 61% and reduction of tremor with alcohol in 45.3%. The hands were most commonly affected (86.2%), followed by the head (42%), voice (23.1%), legs (18.9%), chin (10.1%), trunk (8%), and tongue (7.3%). All Sickness Impact Profile categories except eating showed significant differences between the ET and the general population group, with the greatest differences in communication, emotional behavior, and recreation and pastimes. The patients with ET showed no significant correlations between Sickness Impact Profile scores and tremor duration, age, drug treatment, response to alcohol, family history, or affected body parts.

Conclusions.—Some patients with ET find their condition disabling; as a group, they differ from age-matched controls on a measure of sickness-related dysfunction. Psychosocial limitations may result from the visible and audible, socially apparent nature of the condition—physicians must not ignore this effect.

▶ This study presents useful information regarding the impact of ET on the lives of patients with this disorder. This study confirms that a significant number of patients with ET find their motor disability embarrassing and disabling and certainly do not believe that their condition is benign. The study also confirms what many clinicians have long suspected, that for some patients with ET, the psychosocial limitations related to their motor disability are out of proportion to their actual degree of motor dysfunction.—W.J. Weiner, M.D.

The Hyperekplexias and Their Relationship to the Normal Startle Reflex
Brown P, Rothwell JC, Thompson PD, Britton TC, Day BL, Marsden CD (Inst of Neurology, London)
Brain 114:1903–1928, 1991   6–5

Background.—The startle syndrome, or hyperekplexia, is characterized by an exaggerated motor response to stimuli—especially auditory, but also somatoesthetic and visual. The pathophysiology is controversial, especially because uncertainty remains as to the genesis and pattern of the normal startle reflex. Patients with hereditary or symptomatic hyperekplexia were evaluated using neurophysiologic and electromyographic studies.

Patients.—Four of 8 patients were from 2 families with hereditary hyperekplexia, and 4 patients were sporadic, with the patients having presumed multiple sclerosis, sarcoidosis, presumed encephalomyelitis, and anoxic brain damage. All patients had the same pathophysiology of noise-induced startles, and 7 had abnormal jerks to somatoesthetic stimuli.

Findings.—The hyperekplexia was resistant to habituation and showed an exaggerated motor response. A normal early blink response was seen with both noise and taps to the face, separate from the subsequent true startle reflex. After the blink, electromyographic activity was first seen in the sternocleidomastoid, followed by the masseter and trunk and limb muscles. This electromyographic pattern suggested a brain stem origin for the abnormal responses. Latencies to the intrinsic hand and foot muscles were disproportionately long, and recruitment of caudal muscles was relatively slow. This was the pattern in all patients, regardless of the absolute latency of the response or the auditory or somatoesthetic nature of the stimulus. This suggested that afferents were converging on a common brain stem efferent system that formed the final pathway for all abnormal responses.

Conclusions.—The brain stem efferent system in these patients is different than that in brain stem reticular reflex myoclonus but similar to those in the normal auditory startle reflex. Thus, both abnormal and normal startle reflexes may reflect pathologic and physiologic activity of the same efferent system.

▶ The startle syndrome can be caused by a variety of etiologies, including hereditary hyperekplexia and symptomatic hyperekplexia. Although this syndrome is rare, it does produce a very characteristic clinical response with the patient's "jumping" in response to loud unexpected noises, taps to the body, or visual stimuli. The "jump" usually consists of a blink, contortion of the face, flexion of the neck and trunk, and abduction and flexion of the arms. Some patients, if standing when they "jump," may fall and injure themselves. This study demonstrates that certain forms of the startle syndrome (hereditary hyperekplexia and some examples of symptomatic sporadic hyperekplexia) are mediated by the same physiologic systems that mediate the normal startle reflex.—W.J. Weiner, M.D.

Sudden Death and Paroxysmal Autonomic Dysfunction in Stiff-Man Syndrome
Mitsumoto H, Schwartzman MJ, Estes ML, Chou SM, LaFranchise EF, De Camilli P, Solimena M (Cleveland Clinic Found; Yale Univ)
J Neurol 238:91–96, 1991   6–6

Background.—The rare disease known as stiff-man syndrome is seen with progressive and fluctuating muscle rigidity and superimposed painful spasms. Previous reports have not focused on the potential for death associated with stiff-man syndrome. Two patients with typical and stiff-man syndrome autoantibodies against γ-aminobutyricacid (GABA)-ergic neurons who died suddenly were described.

Patients.—Both patients were women in their forties, 1 with poorly controlled insulin-dependent diabetes mellitus who had increasingly severe paroxysmal attacks of muscle spasms with severe paroxysmal autonomic dysfunctions. Among these manifestations were transient hyperpyrexia, diaphoresis, tachypnea, tachycardia, pupillary dilation, and arterial hypertension. In both patients, antibodies to GABA-ergic neurons were identified in serum; in 1 patient, antibodies were identified in the CSF. Spasms continued in both patients, despite treatment including diazepam, sometimes accompanied by apnea or transient loss of consciousness. Both died suddenly and unexpectedly after 26 and 54 days of hospitalization. Cause of death could not be identified by general autopsy. Perivascular gliosis was found in the spinal cord and brain stem of 1 patient, and lymphocytic perivascular infiltration of the spinal cord, brain stem, and basal ganglia was found in the other.

Immunologic Studies.—Immunoperoxidase staining of rat brain showed GABA-ergic antibodies in patient sera at dilutions of 1:2 and 1:50. By immunoblot of total homogenate proteins of rat brain, a band with the electrophoretic mobility of glutamic acid decarboxylase was recognized in both serum and CSF of 1 patient. No band was found in the other case.

Conclusions.—In stiff-man syndrome, some autoimmune disease against GABA-ergic neurons may play a role. Stiff-man syndrome is associated with severe functional impairment and possibly sudden and unexpected death. Autoimmunity against GABA-ergic neurons may cause both overactivity of muscle and autonomic dysfunctions.

▶ There has been some controversy with regard to the role of antibodies directed against glutamic acid decarboxylase in the stiff-man syndrome. However, reports of their presence have greatly stimulated research into this rare disease. This paper describes additional clinical features of autonomic involvement and sudden death in such patients and adds support to the finding of antibodies directed against GABA-ergic neurons. The evidence is becoming increasingly strong that this is an autoimmune CNS disease.—W.G. Bradley, D.M., F.R.C.P.

Autoantibodies to GABAergic Neurons and Response to Plasmapheresis in Stiff-Man Syndrome
Brashear HR, Phillips LH II (Univ of Virginia)
Neurology 41:1588–1592, 1991   6–7

Introduction.—Stiff-man syndrome is a rare disorder of unknown cause in which progessive rigidity, spasms, and continuous motor unit activity may result from dysfunction of γ-aminobutyric acid (GABA)-ergic inhibition of α motor neurons. Some patients with this disorder have evidence of autoantibodies reactive with glutamic acid decarboxylase. A patient who had progressive stiff-man syndrome with high serum titers of glutamic acid decarboxylase-like immunoreactivity had no such finding in the CSF.

Case Report.—Woman, 32, had persistent low-back pain with progressive stiffness of gait and muscle spasms after a minor motor vehicle accident. Posttraumatic stress syndrome was diagnosed and treated with a variety of medications. She was referred to a hospital after a prolonged episode of severe lordotic spasms. Examination revealed extensive vitiligo, rigid and tender axial muscles, and marked lordosis. Her gait was rigid and slow, and she had frequent spasms of the paraspinal and limb girdle muscles. The diagnosis of stiff-man syndrome was considered. Intravenously infused diazepam, 10 mg, abolished exaggerated exteroceptive reflexes and continuous motor unit activity with no effect on mental status. The results of CSF analysis were unremarkable. The patient did not respond to a trial of clonidine, and the diazepam dosage was increased to 130 mg/day. On indirect immunofluorescent serum screening, autoantibody reactive with normal human cerebellum was seen in a pattern consistent with GABA-ergic terminals. She was admitted for a trial of plasmapheresis and possible immunosuppressive therapy. She tolerated plasmapheresis well. Her antibody titers decreased along with her exteroceptive reflex responses and motor unit activity. She also showed striking clinical improvement: her rigidity decreased, paraspinal muscles were less stiff, and she could sit up unassisted. Immunocytochemical studies were performed using the patient's serum and plasma, yielding specific labeling of human and experimental animal tissue consistent with GABA-ergic neurons and terminal fields. No such response was seen in samples from more than 200 other patients.

Conclusions.—This evidence supports the concept that stiff-man syndrome results from an autoimmune mechanism. Although plasmapheresis may result in clinical improvement, this does not prove that antibody causes the condition.

▶ The stiff-man syndrome is a rare condition. Recent studies have suggested that these patients may have autoantibodies to glutamic acid decarboxylase (1). This paper presents a further piece of evidence supporting the theory and indicates that plasmapheresis may be effective in this condition. Remaining questions include how the antibodies reach the nervous system, how long the response to plsmapheresis lasts, and whether other forms of immunosuppression are needed or are helpful.—W.G. Bradley, D.M., F.R.C.P.

Reference

1. Solimena M, et al: N *Engl J Med* 322:1555, 1990.

7 Headache and Pain

Epidemiology of Headache in a General Population: A Prevalence Study
Rasmussen BK, Jensen R, Schroll M, Olesen J (Glostrup Hosp; Gentofte Hosp, Copenhagen)
J Clin Epidemiol 44:1147–1157, 1991   7–1

Background.—The prevalence of headache has long been debated. The operational diagnostic criteria of the International Headache Society were used to examine the prevalence of specific headache entities.

Methods.—One thousand women and men (aged, 25 to 64 years) who were living in the western part of Copenhagen County were drawn randomly from the Danish National Central Person Registry. All were invited to a general health examination focusing on headache. The examination included a self-administered questionnaire on sociodemographic variables, a structured headache interview, and a general physical and neurologic assessment. Seventy-six percent of those invited participated.

Findings.—The lifetime prevalences of headache, including anyone with any kind of headache, were 93% for men and 99% for women. Lifetime prevalences of migraine were 8% for men and 25% for women. Tension-type headaches had a prevalence of 69% in men and 88% in women. The point prevalence of headache was 11% and 22% in men and women, respectively. Six percent of men and 15% of women had migraine in the previous year. The corresponding prevalences of tension-type headache were 63% and 86%. Gender differences were significant. The male to female ratio for migraine was 1:3, and for tension-type headaches, 4:5. The prevalence of tension-type headache declined with age. Migraine was not correlated with age within the age interval examined.

Conclusions.—Headache disorders are an important health problem in the general population. These data can serve as a basis for future studies of headache in selected groups with the purpose of revealing possible risk factors.

▶ Many of our present conceptions of the different types of headache and their relationships to other neurologic and medical afflictions are based on epidemiologic data. But epidemiologic investigation of headache has been impeded by methodologic obstacles such as lack of universally accepted definitions, objective pathology, and diagnostic tests. In 1988, the Headache Classification Committee of the International Headache Society attempted to remedy some of these deficiencies and published an extensive document that offers a classification scheme with precise definitions of various head-ache migraine syndromes (1). The scheme stipulates that a certain *aggregate* of charactreristic features must be present to establish a diagnosis of a spe-cific type of headache. The classification represented an important advance toward making headache diagnosis more objective. The present paper is the first to use these criteria to establish the prevalence of specific headache en-tities. The data represent a major step in epidemiologic investigations of headache.—R.A. Davidoff, M.D.

Reference

1. Headache Classification Committee of the International Headache Society: *Cephalalgia* 8, 7 (Suppl):1, 1988.

The Impact of Recurrent Headaches on Behavior Lifestyle and Health
Lacroix R, Barbaree HE (McGill Univ, Montreal; Queen's Univ, Kingston, On-tario)
Behav Res Ther 28:235–242, 1990   7–2

Background.—Some authors have proposed that behavioral avoidance is an important contributor to chronic headache pain, and others argue that avoidance behavior is a natural outcome of headache intensity. The behavioral changes of headache sufferers as they attempted to cope with recurring pain were examined.

Methods.—One hundred fifty participants completed the Comprehen-sive Pain Questionnaire (CPQ), which elicited retrospective accounts of headache-associated changes. Forty-six persons were referred by a neu-rologist, 68 were recruited through newspapers and television, and 36 volunteered from introductory psychology classes.

Results.—Participants with headaches reported marked changes in sev-eral domains of behavior and overall lifestyle. Sixty-five percent said that headaches affected their ability to work. Thirty-two percent reported de-creased satisfaction with their work, and 20% said that headaches inter-fered with their ability to get along with co-workers. Seventeen percent said a job change was necessary because of the pain. Twenty percent be-lieved their pain prevented them from taking salaried jobs. Sixteen per-cent felt that headaches prevented them from earning adequate incomes and that as a result they were in financial need. Twenty-one percent had discontinued specific leisure activities because of headache. Twenty-six percent had made changes in their social life, 15% with friends and 12% with family. About half the sample had changes in sleep habits since headache onset. Twenty percent reported taking a long time to fall asleep, and 25% woke in the night. Fifteen percent woke too early. Six percent said they did not feel refreshed in the morning.

Conclusions.—Several domains of behavior and overall lifestyle are affected by headache. These changes appeared to be persistent, even in pain-free states.

▶ Many physicians who do not suffer from recurrent headaches fail to realize the significant changes in "lifestyle" that such headaches may engender. The authors have convincingly shown that a large proportion of chronic headache sufferers significantly limit their behavior in ways that may produce economic problems and social isolation. These changes may be pervasive, disruptive, and long-lasting. Chronic headache sufferers may develop behaviors that result less from severe and continued head pain that as a result of attrempts to avoid headaches by curtailing exposure to environmental stresses.—R.A. Davidoff, M.D.

The Impact of Cigarette Smoking on Headache Activity in Headache Patients
Payne TJ, Stetson B, Stevens VM, Johnson CA, Penzien DB, Van Dorsten B (VA and Univ of Mississippi Med Ctrs, Jackson; Illinois Institute of Technology; Oklahoma State Univ; Univ of Colorado, Denver)
Headache 31:329–332, 1991   7–3

Background.—Research suggests that about one third of patients believe that cigarette smoking precipitates or aggravates headache symptoms. Health care professionals routinely recommend quitting smoking to headache sufferers. However, there is little direct evidence for a relationship between cigarette smoking and headache.

Methods.—A group of 189 patients with headache seen at an outpatient headache clinic were enrolled in an investigation of the relationship between headache and cigarette smoking. The patients completed various self-report measures and monitored their headache activity 4 times a day for 4 weeks.

Results.—Smokers had greater weekly peak headache intensity than nonsmokers. Smokers also reported higher levels of depression and general physical symptoms. Nicotine content of the preferred brand was directly associated with mean headache index, weekly headache-free days, and depression and anxiety scores. Daily smoking rate and pack-year history were related only to smokers' level of general physical symptoms.

Conclusions.—Both smoking status and cigarette nicotine content appear to affect headache activity adversely. In addition, smokers who are more anxious or depressed may exacerbate their headache activity by smoking cigarettes with a higher nicotine content.

▶ Hard data are surprisingly limited concerning the relationship between smoking and migraine. Available information is variable with regard to both the frequency of smoking by migraineurs and the effect of smoking on the underlying headache problem. At least one previous study showed that, for one third of patients, smoking (as opposed to smelling the smoke of others) activates or exacerbates their headache symptoms (1). The present study by Payne and his co-workers clearly state that smokers have more severe weekly headache pain than nonsmokers. It provides a substantial basis for recommending that migraine sufferers who smoke should discontinue their habit.—R.A. Davidoff, M.D.

Reference

1. Volans GN, Castleden CM: *Postgrad Med J* 52:80, 1976.

Benign Vascular Sexual Headache and Exertional Headache: Interrelationships and Long Term Prognosis
Silbert PL, Edis RH, Stewart-Wynne EG, Gubbay SS (Royal Perth Hosp, Australia)
J Neurol Neurosurg Psychiatry 54:417–421, 1991   7–4

Background.—The relationship of benign vascular sexual headache to benign exertional headache was examined in a series of patients reporting sexual headache. Benign vascular sexual headache was defined as a sudden constant or throbbing pain occurring at or about the time of orgasm. Masturbatory cephalagia was excluded.

Findings.—Of 45 patients, 60% had sexual headache alone, and 40% also had benign exertional headache, a sudden generalized pain occurring during any form of exertion. A majority of patients with sexual headache alone identified stress or fatigue as a contributing factor at follow up. Seven of 17 patients had recurrences, 2 of them in distinct clusters. β Blockade usually was effective. Some of the patients with both types of headache reported having episodes within 72 hours of each another. Several of these patients had exertional headache while performing isometric exercise,f including screaming and singing.

Conclusions.—In many resepcts, benign vascular sexual headache and benign exertional headache mimic a small subarachnoid hemorrhage. The paroxysmal nature of sexual headache extends beyond its association with stress and fatigue. Many patients have responded to reassurance alone, and others to a brief course of β blockade.

▶ Exertional headaches, vascular headaches, sexual headaches, and headaches produced by mild blows to the head are all thought to be related to migraine. However, in the individual attack, the severity of the headache and its precipitation can simulate a subarachnoid hemorrhage. This review of 45 patients provides information that will be helpful for the management of individual patients, and that emphasizes the benign nature of the disorder.—W.G. Bradley, D.M., F.R.C.P.

Abrupt Outpatient Withdrawal of Medication in Analgesic-Abusing Migraineurs

Hering R, Steiner TJ (Charing Cross Hosp, London)
Lancet 337:1442–1443, 1991   7–5

Background.—Analgesic-induced headaches, a common phenomenon, recently have been called an unrecognized epidemic. Physicians generally agree that withdrawal from the offending drug is possible on an outpatient basis, but most patients are admitted to the hospital for 8–15 days during withdrawal. A group of outpatients with migraine with medication abuse were examined after abrupt withdrawal.

Methods.—Forty-six migraineurs with secondary chronic daily headache were treated for medication abuse by abrupt withdrawal on an outpatient basis. Patients received an explanation of their disorder, regular follow-up, 10 mg of amitriptyline at night, and 500 mg of naproxen for headache relief.

Results.—At 6 months' follow-up, 37 patients had relief from chronic headaches. Analgesic intake was intermittent and appropriate to the original occasional migraine episodes. Six patients markedly reduced their analgesic intake, but their headache severity was unchanged. Two patients had not reduced their intake and had unchanged headache. One patient dropped out of the trial.

Conclusions.—Drug withdrawal in migraineurs who abuse analgesics and ergotamine can be done successfully on an outpatient basis. In addition, the drugs need not be withdrawn gradually. Abrupt withdrawal is well tolerated with adequate support and explanation of the disorder are given.

▶ Approximately one half of patients with acute attacks of migraine also have frequent or daily mild-to-moderate headaches in between major attacks of head pain. Many patients who have this problem use excessive amounts of over-the-counter prescribed analgesics, narcotic medications, or ergots. A number of these patients practice self-medication, but for most patients these medications are prescribed by well-meaning but naive physicians who are unaware of the dangers of worsening migraine through medication overuse. It is now believed that the daily use of these medications worsens and maintains head pain playing an important role in the transformation of episodic headache to daily headache. Eliminating the medication abuse is difficult and usually is believed to require prolonged hospitalization. The authors are to be congratulated for showing that abrupt discontinuation of medications on an outpatient basis can be accomplished successfully. Obviously, such treatment requires explanation and support from physicians, but the potential benefits are enormous.—R.A. Davidoff, M.D.

EEG and Topographic Frequency Analysis in Common and Classic Migraine

Neufeld MY, Treves TA, Korczyn AD (Tel-Aviv Univ, Israel)
Headache 31:232–236, 1991
7–6

Background.—Some reports indicate that patients with migraine have a significantly higher frequency of abnormal EEG recordings during and between attacks, the prevalence ranging from 30% to 60%. Others indicate that EEG in migraine patients is usually normal or no more abnormal than that in patients with psychogenic or tension headache. Findings on EEG were analyzed in patients with common and classic migraine.

Methods.—Twenty-two patients with common migraine, 20 with classic migraine, and 20 age-matched controls aged 18–28 years were examined. The patients were symptom free, otherwise healthy, and unmedicated during EEG recordings.

Results.—Routine EEG showed mild, nonspecific slowing in 9% of those with common migraine, 15% of those with classic migraine, and 10% of controls. Topographic EEG mapping and frequency analysis were done simultaneously in 13 patients with common migraine, 10 with classic migraine, and 11 controls. Minimal regional differences were noted on EEG mapping, with lower power in the α range in patients with eyes closed. Peak α power and its reactivity were lower in patients than in controls. This difference was significant only between patients with classic migraine and controls in the left occipital area. Peak α frequency also was slightly faster in patients. There was no frank right-left asymmetry in the peak α power in patients or controls.

Conclusions.—There may be some difference in the electrophysiologic background of migraine patients and healthy persons, but the variables examined are not useful for clinically differentiating between patients with and without migraine.

▶ Considering the modest value of the EEG in the diagnosis and management of most patients with migraine, it has been the focus of an extraordinary amount of attention. Neufeld and his colleagues have shown that the EEG abnormalities seen in young migraineurs are minimal-to-mild nonspecific, slowing, and infrequent. This paper provides evidence for the feeling that altogether too many EEGs are performed in patients with migraine. It would be fair to say that, at the present time, the major indication for performing an EEG in a migraineur would be to decide whether a change of consciousness occurring in association with a migrainous headache is possibly epileptic in nature.—R.A. Davidoff, M.D.

5-Hydroxtryptamine$_{1D}$ Receptor Agonism Predicts Antimigraine Efficacy

Deliganis AV, Peroutka SJ (Stanford Univ; Palo Alto VA Hosp, Calif)
Headache 31:228–231, 1991   7–7

Background.—Sumatriptan has been found to be an extremely effective abortive migraine agent with minimal side effects. Both sumatriptan and ergots such as dihydroergotamine (DHE) have high, similar affinity for 5-hydroxytryamine 5-HT$_{1D}$ receptor binding sites in brain membranes The hypothesis that abortive migraine efficacy derives from the ability to stimulate 5-HT$_{1D}$ receptors was tested.

Methods.—The interactions of 4 abortive antimigraine agents and 4 prophylactic antimigraine agents with 5-HT$_{1D}$ receptors were analyzed in bovine brain tissue. Radioligand binding methods and adenylate cyclase assays were used.

Results.—The affinities of 5-HT ergotamine, DHE, and sumatriptan for 5-HT$_{1D}$ receptors in bovine caudate ranged from 4–34 nM. The affinities of the prophylactic antimigraine agents methysergide, amitriptyline, (−)propranolol, and verapamil ranged from 46–11,000 nM. In adenylate cyclase studies in bovine substantia nigra, the 4 abortive antimigraine drugs inhibited forskolin-stimulated adenylate cyclase activity in a dose-dependent manner. None of the 4 prophylactic antimigraine agents had agonist effect on cyclase activity.

Conclusions.—Clinically effective abortive migraine agents inhibit adenylate cyclase activity in bovine substantia nigra. This agonist effect is mediated through an activation of 5-HT$_{1D}$ receptors. Prophylactic antimigraine agents, by contrast, do not have agonist activity at 5-HT$_{1D}$ receptors in the bovine model examined.

▶ Drs. Deliganis and Peroutka have shown that drugs that activate 5-HT$_{1D}$ receptors abort migraine attacks. Substantial biochemical and physiological evidence has shown the existence of multiple 5-HT receptor subtypes. Although the current nomenclature is confusing, recent studies based on the displacement of selective radioligands from homogenates of brain tissue have revealed that the 5-HT$_1$ category is heterogeneous and appears to comprise at least four pharmacologically distinct subtypes designated 5-HT$_{1A}$, 5-HT$_{1B}$, 5-HT$_{1C}$, and 5-HT$_{1D}$. the 5-HT$_{1D}$ subtype appears to be present in arteries and may function to reduce the release of neuropeptides from the nociceptive craniovascular nerve endings, a process that initiates the neurogenic inflammation (vasodilatation and extravasation of plasma proteins) presumed responsible for migraine pain (1). We may now have an explanation for the ability of sumatriptan and ergots to abort bouts of migraine.—R.A. Davidoff, M.D.

Reference

1. Moskowitz MA, Buzzi MG: *J Neurol* 238:518, 1991.

A Randomized, Double-Blind Comparison of Sumatriptan and Cafergot in the Acute Treatment of Migraine

The Multinational Oral Sumatriptan and Cafergot Comparative Study Group (Glaxo Group Research, Greenford, England)
Eur Neurol 31:314–322, 1991   7–8

Background.—There have been many reports on the use of ergotamine for migraine but few placebo-controlled studies, and the results of treatment vary with the route of administration. The selective 5-hydroxytryptamine receptor agonist sumatriptan also is an effective and well-tolerated acute treatment for migraine. A randomized, double-blind trial was performed to compare these 2 agents in the acute treatment of migraine.

Methods.—Included were 580 patients at 47 centers in 9 Europena countries. Patients were randomized in to a group receiving orally administered sumatriptan as a 100 mg dispersible tablet into a group receiving orally administered cafergot, containing 2 mg of ergotaimine tartrate and 200 mg of caffeine. After a baseline examination and practice recording of at least 1 migraine attack on a diary card, patients received their assigned medication and were asked to treat a total of 3 attacks or remain in the trial for 12 weeks.

Results.—Of patients in the sumatriptan group, 66% had reduction in headache intensity from severe or moderate, to mild or none within 2 hours compared with 48% of patients in the cafergot group. Headaches tended to resolve more quickly with sumatriptan, but the rate of recurrence within 48 hours was lower with cafergot. Two hours after the medication was taken, sumatriptan was significantly better at reducing the incidence of nausea, vomiting, and photophobia or phonophobia. Twenty-four percent of the sumatriptan group required further medication after 2 hours compared with 44% of the cafergot group. There was no significant difference in the number of patients with adverse effects—45% with sumatriptan and 39% with cafergot. The most common adverse effects of sumatriptan were malaise or fatigue and bad taste, usually mild and transient. More patients in the cafergot group had nausea or vomiting, or both, abdominal discomfort, and dizziness or vertigo.

Conclusions.—In the acute treatment of migraine, orally administered sumatriptan is well tolerated and is more effective than cafergot. More patients respond to sumatriptan and are completely free of pain at 2 hours. Sumatriptan may be effective even when taken as long as 4 hours after the onset of the attack. Its adverse effects usually are transient.

▶ Sumatriptan will be available shortly for the treatment of migraine attacks in the United States. Ergots previously have been the mainstay of treatment, but a surprisingly large number of patients cannot tolerate the medication or have so many side effects that they are unable to function even if the headache is aborted. Many patients require additional medications such as antiemetics and sedatives to control symptoms. In addition, ergots are surprisingly addictive in patients with frequent, recurring headaches. The Study Group's data indicate that sumatriptan is better tolerated and more efficacious than cafergot. Sumatriptan promises to be a major therapeutic addition to the present abortive treatment of migraine.—R.A. Davidoff, M.D.

Efficacy of Danazol in the Control of Hormonal Migraine
Lichten EM, Bennett RS, Whitty AJ, Daoud Y (Sinai Hosp of Detroit)
J Reprod Med 36:419–424, 1991   7–9

Background.—Migraine occurring at the time of menses often is the most difficult to control, even with combination medical treatment. The efficacy of danazol was investigated in women whose hormonally related migraine was unresponsive to standard medication.

Methods.—A group of 131 women had migraines in the luteal phase of the cycle, typically within 7–10 days before menstruation. Most of the women had more than 1 day a month of incapacitating migraines. Initially, a strict diet excluding known food triggers of headache was used and a mild diuretic was administered. Those who continued to have migraines added danazol, 200 mg, twice daily, for 2 months. Medication began on day 3 of the menses and continued for 25 days. Only diet and the diuretic were used for 2 months more.

Results.—While using danazol, 63% of patients reported control of migraines. The effect was most marked when episodes occurred within a week before menstruation. Migraines returned when danazol was discontinued but were prevented in more than 80% of women who took danazol for 6 months. In 2 women, there were severe side effects. Of the treated patients, 40% continued to have regular, although light, menses.

Conclusions.—Migraine in women probably is a hormonal event and can be controlled effectively by danazol in many patients. A daily dose of danazol, 400mg, is well tolerated when accompanied by acetazolamide.

▶ The menstrual cycle has profound effects in determining the pattern and severity of migraine in a large proportion of female patients. As many as 60% of women migraineurs link their headaches with menstruation or indicate that many of their attacks develop with a constant temporal relationship to menstruation. However, fewer than 15% of women will have their headaches exclusively at the time of menstruation. As the authors point out, menstrual migraine frequently is difficult to treat despite the use of standard prophylactic drugs, nonsteroidal anti-inflammatory drugs, and hormonal therapy with estrogens and progestins. Danazol, an androgen derivative, suppresses the pituitary ovarian axis and prevents the increase in both estrogen and progesterone levels in the luteal phase of the menstrual cycle that presumably is responsible for producing menstrual migraine. The present studies confirm previous studies indicating that danazol is a highly successful treatment for menstrual migraine in patients unresponsive to standard medical therapy.—R.A. Davidoff, M.D.

Altered Cutaneous Sensation in Trigeminal Neuralgia
Nurmikko TJ (Univ Central Hosp, Tampere, Finland)
Arch Neurol 48:523–527, 1991   7–10

Background.—The diagnosis of idiopathic trigeminal neuralgia (ITN) is based on a history of mechanically elicited pain paroxysms and the absence of neurologic deficits on routine assessment. Any sensory abnormality should prompt careful neuroradiologic and laboratory evaluation to exclude treatable causes, such as tumors. However, many reports mention occasional sensory findings in patients with ITN. A trial was done to determine whether sensory abnormalities can be found in ITN by using systematic and quantitative somatosensory measures.

Methods.—Twenty-six patients with a history of ITN had 1 or more trigger zones in the trigeminal nerve distribution. Sensory thresholds in the affected divisions and outside the affected divisions on the painful side of the face were measured and compared with those in contralateral homologous sites.

Results.—In affected divisions, warmth and tactile thresholds were higher than those in the mirror-image divisions. In adjacent divisions, comparison with contralateral divisions showed significant increases in warmth, hot pain, and 2-point discrimination thresholds. A change of tactile threshold showed a trend for significance.

Conclusions.—Increased thresholds of sensations subserved by both large- and small-diameter fibers were found in affected and adjacent unaffected divisions. Thus, there may be combined peripheral and central pathologic conditions in ITN.

▶ Most neurologists accept the idea that there should be no objective trigeminal sensory loss in patients with ITN. Indeed, crude sensory testing of such using our usual examinations is almost always normal. This elegant investigation, which has made use of finer techniques than those usually available at the bedside, has demonstrated changes is sensation in such patients. The study is a good illustration of the crudeness of our bedside techniques. It also shows that partial deafferentation (insignificant for clinical examination) is present in such patients and presumably plays a role in the pathogenesis of the paroxysmal pain.—R.A. Davidoff, M.D.

Changes in Intracranial CSF Volume After Lumbar Puncture and Their Relationship to Post-LP Headache

Grant R, Condon B, Hart I, Teasdale GM (Southern Hosp, Glasgow, Scotland)
J Neurol Neurosurg Psychiatry 54:440–442, 1991   7–11

Background.—Postlumbar puncture headache may reflect low CSF pressure, with resultant stretching of pain-sensitive intracranial structures. Low pressure is secondary to a net loss of intracranial CSF, but until recently, it has not been possible to accurately and noninvasively measure intracranial CSF volume.

Methods.—An MRI technique was used to estimate intracranial CSF volume in 20 patients with neurologic symptoms who underwent lumbar puncture. Punctures used an 18-gauge needle with the patient in the curled lateral recumbent position. A special pulse sequence (IRCP 300/400/5,000) provided an image of the CSF only.

Findings.—Eleven of the 20 patients reported headache at the time of the second MR study. Very severe headache developed in 2; it lasted at least 3 weeks. The CSF volume had decreased in all patients but one 24 hours after lumbar puncture (Fig 7–1). Most fluid was lost from the cortical sulci. The degree of fluid volume decrease correlated with the oc-

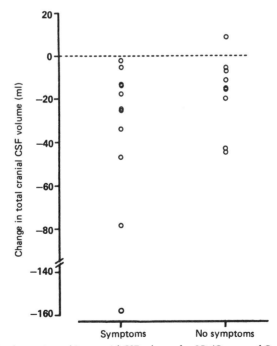

Fig 7–1.—The changes in total intracranial CSF volume after LP. (Courtesy of Grant R, Condon B, Hart I, et al: *J Neurol Neurosurg Psychiatry* 54:440–442, 1991.)

currence of post-lumbar puncture headache. There were no apparent changes in position of the intracranial structures.

Conclusion.—Changes in intracranial CSF volume are quite variable after lumbar puncture. A trend toward a relationship between CSF volume reduction and headache was evident. Estimates of cerebral blood volume might help clarify the situation.

▶ Post-lumbar puncture headache of a severe degree occurs in 5% to 15% of patients. This study provides validation for the commonly accepted view that continued leakage of fluid leads to low intracranial pressure. It will be interesting to extend this study to attempt to prove that smaller bore needles produce less decrease of intracranial CSF volume and that a "blood patch" corrects the decrease of intracranial CSF volume.—W.G. Bradley, D.M., F.R.C.P.

Disappearance of Thalamic Pain After Parietal Subcortical Stroke
Soria ED, Fine EJ (State Univ of New York; VA Med Ctr, Buffalo)
Pain 44:285–288, 1991   7–12

Background.—There have been few reports of chronic head pain disappearing after a cerebral lesion. Data were reviewed on a patient in whom thalamic pain produced by a lacunar infarct in the thalamus disappeared after a second infarct developed in the corona radiata.

Case Report.—Man, 62, had a cerebrovascular accident resulting in right hemiparesis and hemisensory syndrome. Over the next year, severe hyperpathia developed in the right half of the body, especially in the upper extremity and chest. The patient was in constant pain of varying intensity, characterized by superficial waves of ache and deep-seated burning. The pain caused severe psychologic distress and bouts of agitation, and the patient became very vigilant to fending off stimuli to the right side of his body that might set off the pain. He had athetoid posturing of the hand. Over 6 years, he received a variety of treatments, all of only marginal benefit, and he became chronically depressed. A second ictus rendered his right arm and leg powerless 7 years after the first stroke. His speech was garbled and he was unable to walk; his pain disappeared completely. On examination 5 months later, he had a right hemiparesis, most striking in the upper extremity. His hand now showed typical contractures of chronic spasticity. The sense of touch on the right side was very disturbed, including pain and temperature sense. He had no pain or hyperesthesia, and the stimuli that had formerly prompted his pain did not any longer. He reported a great improvement in his quality of life with the disappearance of his pain, despite his loss of motor function.

Conclusion.—The second event in the corona radiata interrupted the thalamoparietal interconnections and ended the pain. Stereotaxic surgery in the corona radiata has been reported by a few surgeons for rebellious chronic pain; this technique may still have value.

▶ Because we do not have a firm understanding of the pathophysiology of central pain, treatment of thalamic pain is a frustrating experience. A number of surgical procedures have been tried that include production of center median lesions, medial thalamotomy, and mesencephalic tractotomy. Some cases have had permanent relief of symptoms, but the pain is recurrent in many patients. The dorsal root entry zone technique has been used in cases accompanied by spastic hemiplegia with some success. Others have tried chronic stimulation of the internal capsule and thalamus, but the procedure has had mixed reviews. The authors of the present case report believe that stereotaxic destruction of the thalamoparietal radiations may be an efficacious treatment of the problem. This may be a reasonable approach, but, unfortunately, the results of surgical treatment are frequently contradictory; a given method may be effective in one case and fail in another, presumably identical patient.—R.A. Davidoff, M.D.

The Prognosis With Postherpetic Neuralgia
Watson CPN, Watt VR, Chipman M, Birkett N, Evans RJ (Univ of Toronto; Univ of Ottawa)
Pain 46:195–199, 1991   7–13

Background.—Postherpetic neuralgia (PHN) develops in varying proportions of patients with herpes zoster. Although PHN can last for some time, the outcome for patients initially seen at the stage of PHN is uncertain. Data on patients with moderate to severe PHN were reviewed.

Methods.—The 156 patients were observed for as long as 11 years. The patients all had PHN for at least 3 months at initial treatment.

Findings.—The patients, (median age, 71 years) had had PHN for a median time of 9 months before the initial visit. After a median follow-up of 2 years, 47% of the patients were considered to have had a good or excellent outcome, whereas 53% had a poor outcome. The outcome could not be related to age, gender, or the dermatome affected. Patients with pain for a year or longer when first seen did less well than the others. Patients having a good outcome most often used antidepressants, topical capsaican, or analagesics, but one fourth of all patients were not on treatment at the time of follow-up. Most patients with a poor outcome had pain fairly continuously despite various treatments.

Conclusions.—Nearly half of the patients with PHN in this series were doing well at final follow-up; many of them were off treatment. There appears to be a group of patients who initially do well but then deteriorate and become resistant to all treatments.

▶ A glass can be either half full or half empty depending on your view. This important long-term follow-up of patients with postherpetic neuralgia indicates that about half undergo a virtually complete remission within two years. Unfortunately, that means that half continued with their pain for many years. In most patients with continuing pain, no treatment appears to be sufficiently effective to warrant continuation. Better treatment is still needed for these patients.—W.G. Bradley, D.M., F.R.C.P.

Analgesic Effects of Vibration and Transcutaneous Electrical Nerve Stimulation Applied Separately and Simultaneously to Patients With Chronic Pain
Guieu R, Tardy-Gervet M-F, Roll J-P (Univ of Provence, Marseille, France)
Can J Neurol Sci 18:113–119, 1991   7–14

Background.—The gate-control theory for controlling chronic pain has prompted the development of various electrostimulative methods of relieving pain. Transcutaneous electrical nerve stimulation (TENS) is the most widely used modality. Vibratory stimulation (VS) also is known to have analgesic effects and can be a very efficient means of relieving pain. Both modalities chiefly activate large-diameter cutaneous afferents.

Methods.—These methods were assessed in 24 patients having chronic pain, most frequently low-back pain, which had proved resistant to medical measures. Two treatment sessions a week served to compare TENS alone, VS alone, combined treatment, and sham stimulation. Both stimuli were applied to the surface of the painful region at 100 Hz. Pain was estimated using the McGill pain questionnaire.

Findings.—Combined stimulation with VS and TENS relieved pain more frequently than either of the modalities alone and had a more marked and longer-lasting analgesic effect. Vibratory stimulation and TENS alone were much more effective than sham stimulation in terms of the number of patients relieved.

Conclusion.—Both TENS and VS are effective means of relieving chronic pain of various types, and their combination is especially effective.

▶ There is a great deal of controversy concerning the efficacy of TENS. In recent double-blind, controlled trials, TENS appeared to show no greater benefit than placebo. This study appears to be a controlled trial of TENS, vibratory stimulation, and placebo (sham stimulation). However, the sham stimulation patients received no electric sensation and were told that the current density would be very low. Moreover, the observers do not appear to have been blinded. Hence, one cannot rely on the conclusions.—W.G. Bradley, D.M., F.R.C.P.

The Effectiveness of Manual Therapy, Physiotherapy, and Treatment by the General Practitioner for Nonspecific Back and Neck Complaints: A Randomized Clinical Trial
Koes BW, Bouter LM, van Mameren H, Essers AHM, Verstegen GMJR, Hofhuizen DM, Houben JP, Knipschild PG (Univ of Limburg; Univ Hosp, Maastricht; Inst of Higher Education, Heerland, The Netherlands)
Spine 17:28–35, 1992   7–15

Background.—Although physiotherapy is widely used for back and neck complaints, its effectiveness has not been thoroughly examined in randomized clinical trials. Previous investigations of the efficacy of manipulation and mobilization of the spine for back and neck complaints were methodologically flawed, usually involved small numbers of patients, had problematic patient selection criteria, problematic operationalization of the manipulative techniques, and an absence of blinded outcome measures. The results of a randomized clinical trial attempting to avoid these flaws were reviewed.

Methods.—The efficacy of manual therapy, physiotherapy, continued treatment by general practitioner, and placebo was compared in 256 patients with nonspecific back and neck complaints of at least 6 weeks' duration. Physical therapy included exercises, massage, and electrotherapy.

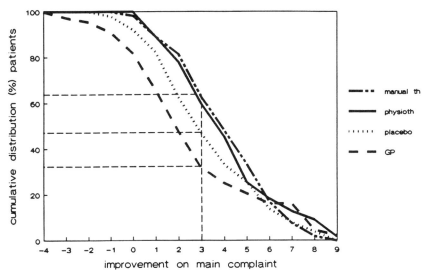

Fig 7–2.—Improvement on main complaint at 6-week follow-up (intention-to-treat analysis). (Courtesy of Koes BW, Bouter LM, van Mameren H, et al: *Spine* 17:28–35, 1992.)

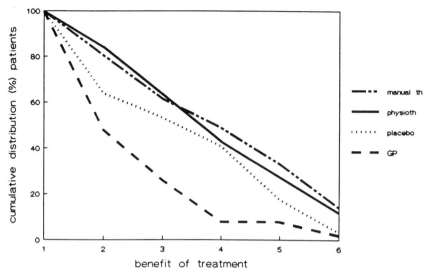

Fig 7–3.—Global perceived effect at 6-week follow-up (intention-to-treat analysis). (Courtesy of Koes BW, Bouter LM, van Mameren H, et al: *Spine* 17:28-35, 1992.)

Manual therapy was manipulation of the spine. General practitioner treatment included nonsteroid antiinflammatories, home exercise, and counseling. Main outcome measures were the severity of the main complaint, global perceived effect, pain, and functional status. Patients were assessed at 3, 6, and 12 weeks.

Results.—Both physiotherapy and manual therapy reduced the severity of complaints more than continued treatment by a general practitioner. A higher global perceived effect also was associated with these 2 treatments compared with continued treatment by general practitioner. There were no apparent differences in efficacy between physiotherapy and manual treatment. Much of their effect seemed to be related to nonspecific or placebo effects (Figs 7–2 and 7–3).

Conclusion.—Treatment with physiotherapy or manual therapy appears to be useful for patients with nonspecific back and neck complaints of at least 6 weeks' duration. Patients also responded remarkably well to the placebo therapy (detuned ultrasound and detuned short-wave diathermy) suggesting the importance of nonspecific effects.

▶ The United States loses tens of billions of dollars a year from lower back pain. The cause and the treatment of most of these cases is totally unclear. Clinical trials have shown that early mobilization after the acute injury is better than prolonged bedrest. This study demonstrates that exercises and massage had a better outcome than nonsteroidal antiinflammatories, home exercise, and general advice. More studies of this type are needed.—W.G. Bradley, D.M., F.R.C.P.

Intensive Dynamic Back Exercises for Chronic Low Back Pain: A Clinical Trial

Manniche C, Lundberg E, Christensen I, Bentzen L, Hesselsøe G (Herlev Hosp, Copenhagen)
Pain 47:53–63, 1991   7–16

Background.—Training therapy for patients with low-back pain has been a popular treatment principle for many years. However, documentation of its benefits is scanty. The effect of intensive dynamic back extensor exercises for patients with chronic low-back pain was examined in a controlled clinical trial.

Methods.—Patients with chronic low-back pain underwent a 3-month intensive training program, including a total of 30 sessions. The 105 patients were assigned randomly to 1 of 3 groups. The first group received intensive training; the second received one fifth of the first group's exercise program per session; and the third received treatment consisting of thermotherapy, massage, and mild exercise (Fig 7–4). Final assessments were done without knowledge of the patients' group assignment (Fig 7–5).

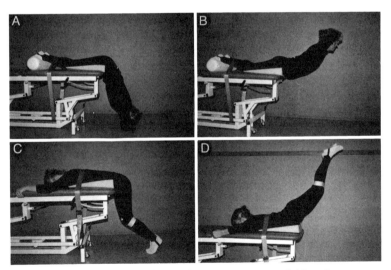

Fig 7–4.—Group C: an intensive back strengthening program. **A,** trunk lifting. Prone on a couch, hips at the edge, upper part of the body free, but supported by the hands against the floor. Strap fixation over the calves. **B,** with hands on the forehead, the trunk is lifted to the greatest possible extension in hips and spine. If necessary, starting with support from physical therapist. During pauses, the patient is supported by a chair in front of the couch. **C,** Leg lifting. Standing by the end of the couch, leaning over to a prone position with the hips against the edge in 90 degree flexion, knees at 45 degrees, and feet on the floor. Strap fixation over the chest. Strap around knees to keep legs together. **D,** both legs are straightened and lifted to the greatest possible extension in hips and spine. Again, with support from physical therapist of necessary. (Courtesy of Manniche C, Lundberg E, Christensen I, et al: *Pain* 47:53–63, 1991.)

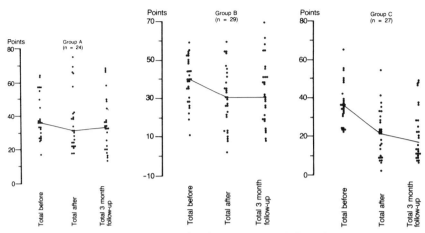

Fig 7–5.—Low back pain rating score and median. Point scoring before, after, and at 3-month follow-up. Group A: 8 patients did not participate in the 3-month follow-up. Group B: 2 patients did not participate in the 3-month follow-up. (Courtesy of Manniche C, Lundberg E, Christensen I, et al: *Pain* 47:53–63, 1991.)

Results.—Both qualitative and quantitative assessment indicated that patients in the intensive training group who completed the program at least once a week for 1 year had a significantly better back status after 1 year than at entry; those who did not continue the exercise did not show this improvement. The favorable result of intensive training occurred regardless of patient age, sex, duration and degree of back trouble severity, and preexisting sciatica or pathologic findings on spinal radiographs. Intensive training was without risk; however, patients with clinical signs of current lumbar nerve root compression or radiologic signs of spondylolysis or halisteresis of the spine were excluded.

Conclusions.—Intensive back training should be preceded by radiologic and clinical examination of the spine. One physical therapist per 2 to 3 patients should be available at the beginning of intensive training to give basic instructions and monitor for any adverse effects. Training can be done with less supervision in larger groups after a couple of months.

▶ This is a controlled clinical trial, the results of which were assessed blindly without knowledge of the treatment group. The group undertaking intensive back-strengthening exercises for 3 months showed statistically significant improvement compared with the other 2 groups, and the benefit continued if patients maintained the exercise program for up to 1 year. The studies are very convincing, but the level of exercise required is going to be difficult for many patients to achieve.—W.G. Bradley, D.M., F.R.C.P.

8 Multiple Sclerosis and Neuroimmunology

The Role of Magnetic Stimulation as a Quantifier of Motor Disability in Patients With Multiple Sclerosis

Kandler RH, Jarratt JA, Davies-Jones GAB, Gumpert EJW, Venables GS, Sagar HJ, Zeman A (Royal Hallamshire Hosp, Sheffield, England)

J Neurol Sci 106:31–34, 1991   8–1

Objective.—Magnetic stimulation has been used to estimate conduction times in central motor pathways. There is evidence from early work that central motor conduction times are prolonged in patients with multiple sclerosis (MS). Motor conduction time (MCT) values were correlated with clinical disability in 100 patients with definite MS, including 27 in relapse who were reassessed after a course of adreno corticotropic hormone or steroid. Thirty normal subjects also were examined.

Methods.—Surface recording electrodes were placed over the abductor digiti minimi, and the stimulating coil was placed in the neck near the exit foramina of the peripheral nerves. Stimulus strength was increased to produced a maximum response.

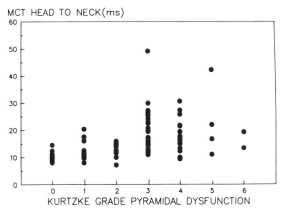

Fig 8–1.—The motor conduction times (MCT) between head and neck in clinically and laboratory-supported patients with MS with different degrees of pyramidial disability as assessed by the Kurtzke scale. Note that the total number of patients equals 100, but many of the points are overlapping. (Courtesy of Kandler RH, Jarratt JA, Davies-Jones GAB, et al: *J Neurol Sci* 106:31–34, 1991.)

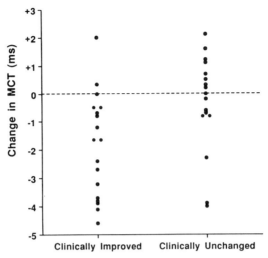

Fig 8–2.—The changes in MCT before and immediately after steroid treatment in patients with MS who showed a clinical improvement and in those who were clinically unchanged. (Courtesy of Kandler HR, Jarratt JA, Davies-Jones GAB, et al: *J Neurol Sci* 106:31-34, 1991.)

Findings.—The method proved to be highly reproducible. The MCT correlated significantly with the degree of pyramidal disability (Fig 8–1). Patients who responded to steroid treatment had a reduction in mean MCT, whereas those who failed to improve showed no significant change (Fig 8–2). An increasing MCT correlated with late relapse in patients who were followed up.

Conclusion.—Magnetic stimulation is a painless way of acquiring quantitative information on motor dysfunction in patients with MS. It should prove helpful as an objective means of monitoring treatment.

▶ The availability of some way to monitor pyramidal dysfunction in spinal cord disease is critical. The use of the magnetic stimulator to measure motor conduction time is a useful tool for prospective studies, such as those in multiple sclerosis. This may be especially important, because imaging studies of the spinal cord using MR technology are still experimental.—S. Sriram, M.D.

Cost Effectiveness of Magnetic Resonance Imaging in the Neurosciences
Szczepura AK, Fletcher J, Fitz-Patrick JD (Univ of Warwick, Coventry, England; Walsgrave Gen Hosp, Coventry, England)
BMJ 303:1435–1439, 1991   8–2

Objective.—An experience with MRI in the West Midlands region of England since 1988 was reviewed. A total of 782 patients seen at 4 neuroscience centers completed quality of life questionnaires at the time of imaging and 6 months later. Detailed cost studies also were done.

Findings.—Patient management changed after MRI in more than one fourth of cases. In another 29% of referrals, confidence in planned management increased as a result of the imaging study. In 20% of cases, the consultant's principal diagnosis changed. No improvement in quality of life was apparent at the 6-month follow-up. The cost savings from avoiding radiographic procedures were relatively small.

Conclusion.—Any diagnostic improvements achieved with MRI are gained at a higher cost. It is important to monitor the cost-effectiveness of this technology. If costs are not sufficiently reduced—even by avoiding other diagnostic procedures—and if, at the same time, patients' lives are not improved, then the benefits of MRI must be viewed very critically.

▶ As health care policymakers seek to define areas in which they control costs of the use of expensive laboratory and radiologic procedures, the use of MRI is clearly going to be scrutinized. This study from Coventry, England, shows that any diagnostic improvement is gained at a higher cost, with no significant improvement in quality of life. It does not take into account the potential risks and morbidity that were avoided, e.g., by myelogram or angiogram. Proper education of physicians in the appropriate use of the technology is likely to result in a better economic impact of MRI.—S. Sriram, M.D.

Tumor Necrosis Factor and Interleukin-1 in the CSF and Sera of Patients With Multiple Sclerosis
Tsukada N, Miyagi K, Matsuda M, Yanagisawa N, Yone K (Shinshu Univ, Matsumoto, Japan; Biotechnology Research Lab, Tokyo)
J Neurol Sci 102:230–234, 1991   8–3

Background.—The in vitro demyelinating properties of TNFα and the proinflammatory functions of interleukin (IL)-1α have suggested that these 2 cytokines may play a role in MS.

Methods.—Serum and CSF were obtained from 31 patients with MS. An enzyme-linked immunosorbent assay was used to determine the levels of TNFα and IL-1α or IL-1β.

Findings.—Tumor necrosis factor (alpha) was found in 93.5% of the CSF samples overall; TNFα was also detected in all of the CSF samples from patients with acute relapsing MS in exacerbation. Those patients had significantly higher CSF levels of TNF compared with those in remission or with controls. Increased TNF levels were also found in 35.5% of the sera, especially in sera from patients with acute relapsing MS in exacerbation. Increased levels of TNF were also common in the CSF and sera from patients with Guillain-Barré syndrome, another demyelinating disease. Neither IL-1α nor IL-1β was found in the CSF or sera of any of the patients with MS.

Conclusion.—Tumor necrosis factor levels in CSF may reflect disease activity in patients with MS. Although it is not possible to determine whether TNF is directly implicated in demyelination, it may be produced in the CNS during an acute exacerbation. It also may be involved in a number of inflammatory demyelinating disease processes.

Comparative Analysis of Cytokine Patterns in Immunological, Infectious, and Oncological Neurological Disorders

Weller M, Stevens A, Sommer N, Melms A, Dichgans J, Wiethölter (Univ of Tübingen, Germany)

J Neurol Sci 104:215–221, 1991   8–4

Background.—Cytokines are important signal transducers of the immune system. Many studies have tried to identify positive correlations between increased levels of single cytokines in serum or CSF and specific neurologic disease processes. Cytokine patterns in different immunologic, infectious, and neoplastic neurologic disorders were analyzed.

Methods.—Samples of CSF and sera were obtained from patients with relapsing-remitting and chronic multiple sclerosis (MS), Guillain-Barré syndrome, chronic inflammatory demyelinating polyradiculoneuropathy, HIV infection, bacterial meningitis, viral encephalitis, meningeal carcinomatosis, hematologic meningeal malignancies, and disseminated melanoma. Interleukins (IL) 1, 2, 4, and 6, and soluble receptor (sIL-2R), interferon-gamma (IFGN-γ), and tumor necrosis factor α (TNF-α) were measured.

Results.—Monitoring disease activity in neuroimmunologic disorders using IL-1β, IL-2, sIL-2R, or IL-4 measurement does not appear to be useful. By contrast, measures of IL-6 indicated relapse in MS and active disease in Guillain-Barré syndrome and meningeal carcinomatosis. High levels of CSF TNF-α in metastatic melanoma and frequent detection in CSF of the multifunctional B-cell growth factor, IL-6, and oligoclonal immunoglobulin bands in meningeal carcinomatosis confirmed an intrathecal immune response in disseminated leptomeningeal neoplasia that could be amenable to treatment immunomodulation.

Conclusion.—Except for the possible monitoring value of IL-6 in some disorders, there currently appears to be little to learn from cytokine determinations. The levels of many cytokines increase in many inflammatory and immunologic neurologic diseases.

▶ The importance of cytokines as mediators of demyelination is becoming evident. However, there is controversy as to the specificity of either a particular cytokine such as TNF-α or a combination of cytokines in the demyelinating process. In addition, differences in the reagents used to measure TNF α and differences in their stability (with the use of protease inhibitors) may also result in the differences in observations between laboratories. For more information on this topic, please see Reference 1.—S. Sriram, M.D.

Reference

1. Sharieff MK, Hentges R: N *Engl J Med* 325:467, 1991.

Immunosuppressive Activity of 13-*cis*-Retinoic Acid and Prevention of Experimental Autoimmune Encephalomyelitis in Rats
Massacesi L, Castigli E, Vergelli M, Olivotto J, Abbamondi AL, Sarlo F, Amaducci L (Università degli Studi di Firenze, Florence, Italy, Università Cattolica, Rome)
J Clin Invest 88:1331–1337, 1991   8–5

Introduction.—Previous studies have shown that experimental autoimmune encephalomyelitis (EAE) in Lewis rats, an in vivo model of autoimmune disorders, is suppressed by administration of all-*trans*-retinoic acid (RA). Although it may have suppressive activity on immune-mediated diseases, the usefulness of RA is limited by its toxicity. Although 13-*cis*-retinoic acid (13-cRA) is better tolerated, its activity on T-cell–mediated immunity is not known.

Methods.—The effects of 13-cRA in vivo on EAE and in vitro on T-cell–mediated immunity of splenocytes were investigated.

Results.—Administration of 13-cRA at doses that are well tolerated by humans significantly suppressed both active and passive transfer of EAE, based on clinical and histopathologic signs. Discontinuation of 13-cRA resulted in a loss of protection, but prevention of passive transfer was not affected by later discontinuation of 13-cRA. No major side effects of 13-cRA were noted. In vitro experiments showed that splenocytes from treated rats had reduced proliferative responses to the T-cell mitogen concanavalin A and to the antigens myelin and myelin basic protein. Incubation in the presence of nontoxic concentrations of 13-cRA inhibited the production of interleukin 2 from splenocytes in vitro.

Conclusion.—These data indicate that 13-cRA can induce functional and reversible immunosuppression in rats. This immunosuppression seems to act on T-cell–mediated immunity, and it can be achieved at nontoxic concentrations. A phase I clinical trial of retinoids for patients with multiple sclerosis is proposed.

▶ The lack of clear evidence of an incriminating autoantigen in a number of autoimmune diseases has resulted in the use of broad-spectrum immunosuppressants to treat autoimmune diseases. Retinoic acid analogues are compounds that inhibit T-cell function in vitro and abrogate an archetypal T-cell–mediated autoimmune disease, experimental allergic encephalitis, in vivo. Although the mechanism of this disease inhibition is unknown, the well-known effect of retinoids to induce TGFβ, a naturally occurring immunoinhibitory cytokine, makes this approach novel.—S. Sriram, M.D.

A Chronic Illness Characterized by Fatigue, Neurologic and Immunologic Disorders, and Active Human Herpesvirus Type 6 Infection
Buchwald D, Cheney PR, Peterson DL, Henry B, Wormsley SB, Geiger A, Ablashi DV, Salahuddin SZ, Saxinger C, Biddle R, Kikinis R, Jolesz FA, Folks T, Balachandran N, Peter JB, Gallo RC, Komaroff AL (Harborview Med Ctr, Seattle; Charlotte, NC; Incline Village, Nev; Washoe County Sheriff's Division, Reno, Nev; San Diego; et al)
Ann Intern Med 116:103–113, 1992   8–6

Introduction.—A total of 259 patients who had a "flu-like" illness followed by protracted, disabling symptoms of chronic fatigue and cognitive impairment sought care at a single medical practice. A large majority of the patients (183) lived near the California-Nevada border (in the area of Lake Tahoe) and were seen in 1984–1987. Several groups of patients who had had frequent close contact became ill within a period of several months.

Clinical Aspects.—Symptoms usually began suddenly. Nearly one third of the patients were regularly bedridden or shut-in. Very few patients had had similar symptoms in the years before illness began. Two thirds of patients experienced depression after onset. A total of 8% had evidence of an acute neuropathic process, which included primary seizure disorder, marked ataxia, and transient paresis.

Laboratory Findings.—Approximately one fifth of the patients had atypical lymphocytosis, and nearly one fourth of those tested had an antinuclear antibody titer of 1:20. Patients had an increased CD4/CD8 ratio. Foci of high signal intensity were seen on T2-weighted MR images in nearly 80% of the patients examined and in 21% of healthy control subjects. Positive bioassay rsults for human herpesvirus type 6 (HHV-6) were obtained in 70% of patients and 20% of controls. Only 2 patients had serologic evidence of Epstein-Barr viral infection.

Conclusion.—These patients may have had a chronic immunologically mediated inflammatory disorder of the CNS. Immunologic dysfunction may lead to the reactivation of latent HHV-6 infection. It is unclear whether this lymphotropic and gliotropic virus contributes to the symptoms or neurologic dysfunction. Also, its relationship to chronic fatigue syndrome is not known.

▶ The etiology of fatigue-like illness that follows a viral syndrome has been recognized as a clinical entity for a number of years. The lack of clear clinical features has made the identification of the illness as a distinct clinical entity difficult. This study, which was initiated by 2 physicians in private practice, shows the epidimeologic rigor of the investigators in tracking it to HHV-6.

Although this study does not infer that all postviral illnesses are the result of HHV-6 infection, the causal relationship between viral infection and chronic fatigue is significant.—S. Sriram, M.D.

9 Pediatric Neurology

Clinical Survey of Ischemic Cerebrovascular Disease in Children in a District of Japan
Satoh S, Shirane R, Yoshimoto T (Tohoku Univ, Sendai, Japan)
Stroke 22:586–589, 1991   9–1

Introduction.—Ischemic cerebrovascular disease in children is relatively rare. However, there have been few studies of this condition, and little is known of its incidence and causes.

Methods.—To clarify the clinical features of childhood ischemic cerebral disorders, data on 54 children who were treated for ischemic vascular disease during a 14.5-year period were reviewed. All the patients were younger than 16 years of age and had had CT identification of ischemic cerebrovascular disease. Data on patients with moyamoya disease were excluded.

Results.—In the previous decade, the incidence of childhood cerebral disease was calculated as .2/100,00/year. Two peaks of incidence were observed, 1 occurring in early childhood and another occurring in the junior high school years. There were 38 minor strokes, 12 reversible ischemic neurologic deficits, 3 transient ischemic attacks, and 1 major stroke. Boys and girls were affected equally. Before the stroke, 10 patients had upper respiratory tract infections, 10 had minor head trauma, and 2 had heart disease. In 91% of the patients, the middle cerebral artery region including the basal ganglia was affected. Angiography was performed on 48 patients, which demonstrated several types of occlusive lesions, mainly affecting the middle cerebral artery. Hemiparesis was present in 89% of children, and it was the most common form of disability. Although the children tended to recover better than adults, permanent disabilities such as hemiparesis or mental retardation were common.

Conclusion.—Because childhood stroke occurs during a critical period of development, prevention is even more important in children than in adults. The vascular changes are reversible in some patients. Juvenile cerebrovascular disease should be studied further to prevent these strokes.

▶ The high percentage of children in this series who had no significant risk factor for stroke is surprising. It is likely that a standard evaluation to screen for underlying causes was not done on every child in this series. One wonders whether some children who have transient ischemic attacks and reversible ischemic deficits may have experienced a migraine attack, especially those in which the event occurs after trivial head injury.—G.M. Fenichel, M.D.

Antiphospholipid Antibodies and Stroke in an Infant
Roddy SM, Giang DW (Univ of Rochester, Rochester, NY)
Pediatrics 87:933–935, 1991   9–2

Introduction.—Cerebral infarction is rare in childhood. In adults, ischemic events have been related to antiphospholipid antibodies (APA), and some adolescents with APA have had ischemic complications.

Case Report.—Male infant, 8 months, was noted at age 4 months to have dolichocephaly; 3 months later he underwent repair of sagittal synostosis. A month afterward, the patient fell down 5 steps and had CT findings of a subgaleal hematoma. The fluid was tapped, but left hemiparesis developed suddenly 2½ weeks after the fall. Findings at CT were still negative for an intracerebral lesion. There was a family history of both migraine and Tourette syndrome. A left visual field defect was seen, but there was no facial asymmetry. A left Babinski sign was noted, and the patient had difficulty with left hand movements. Magnetic resonance imaging suggested previous infarction superoposterior to the body of the right lateral ventricle. An assay for anticardiolipin antibody was strongly positive for IgG antibody. The hemiparesis improved gradually with aspirin treatment, but partial seizures occurred and an electroencephalogram indicated a right central focus. Seizure activity was controlled with carbamazepine. Titers of anticardiolipin antibody remained increased after 1 year, but there were no further clinical symptoms.

Conclusion.—Antiphospholipid antibodies can cause cerebral infarction in young children. The presence of APA in a child may predict future thrombotic events. Assessment should include an activated partial thromboplastin time test, a serologic test for syphilis, and an ELISA or radioimmunoassay for anticardiolipin antibody.

▶ A cerebral infarction developed in this infant after a head injury. Evaluation revealed the presence of APA. Although there are other reports of stroke in children who have APA, it is not clear whether this is a chance association or a cause-and-effect association. Data are not available on the incidence of APA in normal infants and children.—G.M. Fenichel, M.D.

Management of Hyponatremic Seizures in Children With Hypertonic Saline: A Safe and Effective Strategy
Sarnaik AP, Meert K, Hackbarth R, Fleischmann L (Wayne State Univ, Detroit)
Crit Care Med 19:758–762, 1991   9–3

Background.—A sudden decrease in serum sodium levels can lead to extensive brain damage and death in adults and children. Although prompt correction would seem to be indicated, several investigators have suggested that rapid correction of sustained hyponatremia may be more harmful than hyponatremia itself, resulting in central pontine and extrapontine myelinolysis.

Management.—An experience with the management of hyponatremia was reviewed in 60 children treated in hospital for 69 episodes of severe hyponatremia (a serum sodium level less than 125 mol/L). Forty-one of the patients presented with seizures. A total of 25 of the children with seizures received a bolus injection of 4–6 mL of 3% saline per kg; 28 other children received a benzodiazepine and/or phenobarbital, with or without subsequent hypertonic saline.

Outcome.—Six episodes of hyponatremic seizures resolved spontaneously. Six children who initially were given phenobarbital and/or a benzodiazepine became apneic and had to be intubated. Apnea and/or seizures resolved rapidly when hypertonic saline was given. Such treatment significantly hastened the increase in serum sodium. None of the children had deteriorating CNS function or had clinical signs of osmotic demyelination syndrome develop.

Discussion.—Symptomatic hyponatremia in these children appears to be related to increased brain water; a rapid increase in serum sodium levels normalizes the brain water content. A rapid increase might, however, be hazardous when chronic asymptomatic hyponatremia is present and the CNS osmoregulatory system has restored a normal brain water content.

▶ Hyponatremia more commonly leads to seizures in children rather than in adults. In children, an acutely developing hyponatremia is more common than a chronic picture. In both adults and children, significant brain damage can occur if the condition is not recognized and treated. This study indicates that hypertonic saline is safe in childhood hyponatremia. In the adult, however, it has been clearly demonstrated that central pontine myelinolysis is a frequent disastrous result of the use of hypertonic saline.—W.G. Bradley, D.M., F.R.C.P.

The Beneficial Effects of Early Dexamethasone Administration in Infants and Children With Bacterial Meningitis

Odio CM, Faingezicht I, Paris M, Nassar M, Baltodano A, Rogers J, Sáez-Llorens X, Olsen KD, McCracken GH Jr (Natl Children's Hosp, San José, Costa Rica; Electrophysiology Labs, Dallas; Univ of Texas Southwestern Med Ctr, Dallas)
N Engl J Med 324:1525–1531, 1991   9–4

Background.—The molecular pathophysiology of bacterial meningitis has been much studied to establish the mechanisms of the inflammation and to find ways to improve outcome. Dexamethasone has reduced meningeal inflammation and improved outcome both in experimental models and in children with meningitis. A placebo-controlled, double-blind study of dexamethasone was conducted in 101 infants and children with meningitis.

Methods.—The patients were 59 boys and 42 girls ranging in age from 6 weeks to 13 years. Eighty percent were younger than 2 years of age, and 90% were younger than 5 years. All had either culture-proved bacterial meningitis or clinical signs of the disease with CSF characteristics of bacterial infection. All patients received cefotaxime, 200 mg/kg/day; 52 received dexamethasone, .6 mg/kg/day, and 49 received placebo. The first dose of dexamethasone or placebo was given 15 to 20 minutes before the first dose of antibiotic, and treatment was continued for 4 days. The 2 groups had similar demographic, clinical, and laboratory characteristics.

Results.—The mean opening cerebrospinal pressure and estimated cerebral perfusion pressure improved significantly in the dexamethasone group within 12 hours of the start of therapy. Those measures worsened in the placebo group. Meningeal inflammation and CSF concentrations of tumor necrosis factor-α and platelet-activating factor decreased in the dexamethasone group by 12 hours, whereas increased inflammation was seen in the placebo group. The dexamethasone group also had a significantly better clinical condition and mean prognostic score at 24 hours. At a mean follow-up of 15 months, 51 children in the dexamethasone group and 48 children in the placebo group were alive. Of those, 14% of the dexamethasone group had 1 or more neurologic or audiologic sequelae compared with 38% in the placebo group. The relative risk of sequelae for a child receiving placebo was 3.8.

Conclusion.—In infants and children with bacterial meningitis, dexamethasone therapy appears to improve immediate and long-term outcome when used as an adjunctive therapy. Dexamethasone was given before cefotaxime in this study.

▶ For decades, pediatricians were reluctant to use corticosteroids in children with bacterial meningitis. It is now clear from several sources that the early administration of dexamethasone improves both neurologic and audiologic outcomes. Early administration of dexamethasone is becoming a standard of care in children with bacterial meningitis.—G.M. Fenichel, M.D.

Intraspinal Epidermoid Tumors in Children: Problems in Recognition and Imaging Techniques for Diagnosis

Caro PA, Marks HG, Keret D, Kumar SJ, Guille JT (Alfred I duPont Inst, Wilmington, Del)
J Pediatr Orthop 11:288–293, 1991   9–5

Introduction.—Acquired intraspinal epidermoid tumors are considered a late complication of lumbar puncture. The clinical manifestations of this rare tumor are similar to those of other musculoskeletal childhood problems, creating a problem in diagnosis. Furthermore, because of the long interval between lumbar puncture and the development of symptomatic tumor, this relationship may be overlooked, causing a delay in diagnosis. Four children with iatrogenic intraspinal epidermoid tumors are described.

Patients.—Four children, aged 6–10 years, were seen with progressive back pain, hamstring spasm, radicular leg pain, alteration of gait pattern, or difficulty in walking. All patients had had lumbar punctures performed between the neonatal period and 2 years of age. Three patients had other conditions that had similar clinical manifestations, including flat feet and the Klippel-Feil syndrome, Ito disease, and spondylolisthesis of the L4-L5 vertebrae. None of the patients responded to conservative treatment. Because of persistent complaints and slight deterioration in neurologic findings, an intraspinal pathology was suspected. In 2 patients, metrizamide myelography identified the intraspinal tumor. In the other 2 patients, MRI showed the mass and its relationship to other dural structures. On T1-weighted images, the mass was of very low signal intensity with a thin border of intermediate intensity. Intravenous administration of gadolinium-diethylenetriaminepentaacetic acid improved the visualization and delineation of the tumor. The T1-weighted images showed faint enhancement of the periphery of the mass, suggesting capsular enhancement. All patients improved after removal of the tumor.

Conclusion.—Iatrogenic epidermoid tumor should be included in the differential diagnosis of patients who had prior lumbar punctures and who are seen with longstanding complaints of back pain, hamstring spasm, radicular pain, and gait disturbance with minimal or no neurologic deficit or no response to conservative treatment. Magnetic resonance imaging is superior to myelography for the diagnosis of this rare tumor.

► Magnetic resonance imaging has become the modality of choice for diagnosis of spinal cord disorders in children. There is little reason to delay doing MRI on children with symptoms referrable to the spinal cord. If the cord is tethered in a growing child, ischemic injuries that persist even after the tether is released can occur.—G.M. Fenichel, M.D.

Brain Growth and Cognitive Improvement in Children With Human Immunodeficiency Virus-Induced Encephalopathy After 6 Months of Continuous Infusion Zidovudine Therapy

DeCarli C, Fugate L, Falloon J, Eddy J, Katz DA, Friedland RP, Rapoport SI, Brouwers P, Pizzo PA (Natl Insts of Health, Bethesda, Md)

J Acquir Immune Defic Synd 4:585–592, 1991   9–6

Background.—In children with HIV infection, the most common neurologic sequela is progressive encephalopathy attributable to HIV itself, because viral markers are found in the CNS. Computed tomography signs of brain atrophy may be present before the loss of developmental milestones, and signs of reduced atrophy have been noted after continuous intravenous infusion zidovudine (CI-ZDV) therapy. Ventricular size was analyzed on CT images before and after 6 months of CI-ZDV therapy.

Methods.—The patients were 7 boys and 1 girl (mean age, 7.5 years) with symptomatic HIV infection. All patients underwent neuropsychologic evaluation before and 6 months after CI-ZDV. Axial CT images of the ventricular area at the level of the foramen of Monro were obtained at the same times. Therapy began with 80 mg of ZDV given by intravenous bolus, followed by CI-ZDV infusion, 360–1,300 mg/m²/day. The measurements, including the ventricular brain ratio, were done in blinded fashion from digitized images.

Results.—The initial scans all showed evidence of moderate-to-severe central atrophy. In 7 of the 8 children, the ventricular area decreased by a mean of 21.5% and the ventricular brain ratio decreased by a mean of 20%. Reduction in ventricular brain ratio was correlated with decreased CSF protein concentration, but not with T4 or T8 lyumphocyte measurements. The 7 children had a mean improvement of 17.7% in their intelligence quotients, which correlated significantly with the decreases in CSF protein concentration. There was no significant correlation between the magnitude of the change in the ventricular area and the magnitude of intelligence quotient changes.

Conclusion.—In children with HIV encephalopathy, cognitive improvement noted after 6 months of CI-ZDV is accompanied by reduced brain atrophy and decreased CSF protein. Zidovudine may thus ameliorate the pathogenesis of AIDS encephalopathy in children. Computed tomography can provide quantitative indicators of response to therapy.

▶ Studies on zidovudine (AZT) in children were delayed until its efficacy had first been shown in adults. It appears to be a very useful drug, and we should not be surprised to see it administered shortly after birth to children who are HIV positive.—G.M. Fenichel, M.D.

Chronic Inflammatory Demyelinating Polyradiculoneuropathy of Childhood: Treatment With High-Dose Intravenous Immunoglobulin
Vedanarayanan VV, Kandt RS, Lewis DV Jr, DeLong GR (Duke Univ, Durham, NC)
Neurology 41:828–830, 1991   9–7

Introduction.—Chronic inflammatory demyelinating polyradiculoneuropathy (CIDP) in children is rare. It is commonly treated with corticosteroids, immunosuppressive drugs, and plasmapheresis. High-dose intravenous immunoglobulin (IVIG) therapy has recently been used with good results in adults with CIDP. The effects of high-dose IVIG therapy were studied in children with CIDP.

Patients.—Three girls and 1 boy (age, 7–9 years) who had CIPD diagnosed were treated with high-dose IVIG during acute exacerbations. Two children had progressive muscle weakness after a bout of chickenpox, 1 had symptoms of neuropathy after a bout of viral illness, and 1 patient had a family history of Charcot-Marie-Tooth disease. Three patients underwent sural nerve biopsy, which confirmed the diagnosis. All 4 children had prevously been treated with prednisone, and 3 patients had also been treated with azathioprine and plasmapheresis. During subsequent relapses, each child was treated with IVIG, 400 mg/kg/day, given as a slow infusion for 5 days. One child is being treated with IVIG infusions in a dose of 400 mg/kg every 2–7 weeks to maintain remission. Follow-up has ranged from 38 weeks to 90 months.

Results.—All 4 children showed excellent recovery of motor strength after each IVIG-treated relapse. This therapy has been at least as effective as plasmapheresis in improving motor function in the 3 children who had both therapies. There have been no side effects of IVIG. With plasmapheresis, 2 children contracted septicemia from infections of central lines with *Staphylococcus epidermidis*. One child had profuse bleeding from accidental extrusion of a central line. A third patient had 3 episodes of major venous thrombosis related to the placement of central lines for plasmapheresis. She has had no thrombotic episodes since her relapses have been treated with high-dose IVIG.

Conclusion.—High-dose IVIG appears to be a safe and effective adjunctive therapy for children with CIPD, particularly during acute relapse.

▶ Controlled clinical trials are difficult in rare diseases, and treatment advances are often based on small clinical case series, as in this study. It seems convincing that intravenously administered immunoglobulin can be effective in childhood CIDP; however, a recent study of adults with CIDP suggests that not all patients can be expected to improve with this therapy.—W.G. Bradley, D.M., F.R.C.P.

Treatment of Antenatal Myasthenia Gravis

Carr SR, Gilchrist JM, Abuelo DN, Clark D (Brown Univ, Providence, RI)
Obstet Gynecol 78:485–489, 1991
9–8

Background.—When a pregnant woman has myasthenia gravis, the neonate may be affected with myasthenia or, sometimes, fatal congenital anomalies. Few reports have focused on modulating the effects of the disease on the developing fetus. The fetus of a myasthenic woman was tested using plasmapheresis and immunotherapy.

Case Report.—Woman, 32, had a 14-year history of myasthenia gravis. She had given birth to 2 children, but both had died of congenital anomalies. At her first prenatal examination, at 8 weeks' gestation, she was taking pyridostigmine, 360 mg/day. She had mild diplopia, dysarthria, and facial and proximal limb weakness. To further suppress production of anti-acetylcholine receptor antibodies, plasmapheresis and prednisone therapy were begun. Six plasmapheresis sessions were given from 15 to 17 weeks' gestation, each exchange consisting of approximately 3,500 mL. Prednisone was begun at 80 mg every other day and was increased to 80 mg and 40 mg on alternating days after an increase in antibody titer at 26.5 weeks' gestation. Pyridostigmine was titrated to her symptoms, with a usual dose of 30 mg/day. The treatment decreased anti-acetylcholine receptor antibody titers from 400 nmol/L to 40 nmol/L at 25 weeks. As those titers decreased, fetal breathing motion, which was inversely correlated with titers, was seen. The patient delivered a female infant by cesarean section at 35 weeks. The baby had transient myasthenia gravis and required intermittent ventilatory support and anticholinesterase medications for 5 weeks. The mother's postoperative course was unremarkable.

Conclusion.—A patient with maternal myasthenia gravis was successfully treated by serial plasmapheresis and immunotherapy. Therapy may have improved the infant's outcome, which differed from those of the patient's previous pregnancies. The effects of the maternal myasthenia were not completely eliminated, however.

▶ Neonatal myasthenia is a well-recognized risk in children born of myasthenic mothers. The possibility of in utero involvement, with the production of severe congenital anomalies by the transplacental passage of anti-acetylcholine receptor antibodies, has received little attention. This paper suggests that treatment to reduce the anti-acetylcholine receptor antibody titer can be effective in such rare cases.—W.G. Bradley, D.M., F.R.C.P.

Prevention of Neural Tube Defects: Results of the Medical Research Council Vitamin Study

Wald N, for the MRC Vitamin Study Research Group (Med College of St Bartholomew's Hosp, London)
Lancet 338:131–137, 1991   9–9

Introduction.—For many years, it has been suspected that diet has an etiologic role in neural tube defects. Previous studies have suggested that folic acid or other vitamins may decrease the recurrence rate of these defects. A multicenter, randomized, double-blind trial with a factorial design was conducted to determine whether supplementation with folic acid or other vitamins could prevent neural tube defects.

Methods.—The study, which was performed at 33 centers in 7 countries, included 1,817 women who were at high risk of having a pregnancy with a neural tube defect because of a previous affected pregnancy. The women were randomized to 1 of 4 supplementation groups: folic acid; a mixture of vitamins A, D, B_1, B_2, B_6, C, and nicotinamide; both folic acid and the other vitamins; or neither. Supplementation began around the time of conception, and patients were evaluated every 3 months until week 12 of pregnancy. Each woman remained in the trial until she had a pregnancy and until it could be determined whether a neural tube defect was present (an "informative" pregnancy), or until the end of the trial. The trial was halted after almost 8 years when sufficiently conclusive results emerged.

Results.—Of the 1,195 informative pregnancies, 27 had a neural tube defect, 6 in the groups receiving folic acid and 21 in the other 2 groups. The prevalence of neural tube defects was 1% in women who received folic acid compared with 3.5% in those who did not receive folic acid. Folic acid had a 72% protective effect; the other vitamins had no significant protective effect. Exclusion of women who reported stopping taking their capsules before their last scheduled visit yielded similar prevalence results. Folic acid supplementation appeared to cause no demonstrable harm, although the study had limited ability to detect rare or slight adverse effects.

Conclusion.—Neural tube defects can be prevented by folic acid supplementation. Folic acid, beginning before pregnancy, is recommended for all women who have had a pregnancy with a neural tube defect. Public health measures may be pursued to ensure adequate amounts of folic acid in all women who may bear children.

▶ The etiology of neural tube defects is poorly understood, but it is believed to be multifactorial—a genetic predisposition influenced by an environmental agent. Several previous studies have suggested that folic acid supplementation might prevent neural tube defects; however, this large randomized study has proven the point. Despite these results, there is no reason to believe that folic acid deficiency is an important cause of neural tube defects. I fail to understand why the MRC Vitamin Study Research Group recommends folic acid supplementation only for those women with a prior history of neural tube defects. It seems to be an inexpensive and safe recommendation for all pregnant women.—G.M. Fenichel, M.D.

Globoid Cell Leukodystrophy: A Family With Both Late-Infantile and Adult Type

Verdru P, Lammens M, Dom R, Van Elsen A, Carton H (Universitaire Ziekenhuizen, Leuven, Belgium; Universiteit Antwerpen, Belgium)
Neurology 41:1382–1384, 1991   9–10

Background.—The rare autosomal recessive disorder globid cell leukodystrophy (GBL) causes accumulation of galactosylsphingosine, which is neurotoxic. The disease usually has its onset in the first 6 months and progresses rapidly. A patient with adult-onset GBL from a family with a history of both late-infantile and adult disease was studied.

Case Report.—Woman, 19, the daughter of consanguineous parents, was seen with postural tremor of the upper limb, pyramidal paresis of the left lower limb, and bilateral extensor plantar responses. Magnetic resonance imaging revealed diffuse symmetric occipital white matter and posterior corpus callosum hyperintensity. Cerebrospinal fluid protein content was increased, and brain stem auditory-evoked potentials showed prolonged interpeak latencies. The patient was admitted 9 months later, when she showed evidence of peripheral nerve involvement. Electromyography showed demyelinating sensorimotor neuropathy; electron microscopic examination of a sural nerve biopsy specimen showed inclusions in Schwann's cells consisting of aspecific lipid material, curved and rectilinear geometric formations, and small spiculae. Galactosylceramide β-galactosidase activity in the leukocytes was less than 2% of the normal mean. The patient had a brother who had seizures and who died with no diagnosis at 4 years of age.

Conclusion.—The molecular nature of GBL may be different in these patients than it is in those with classical GBL. The clinical course in 1 sibling does not predict benefit in a second sibling. No treatment, including bone marrow transplantation, appears to be effective.

▶ Several inborn errors of metabolism, which once were thought to be exclusively disorders of children, are now recognized in adults as well. These disorders are rarely considered in the differential diagnosis of adults with degenerative neurologic disorders—unless there is an affected child in the kindred. Infantile and adult forms are often caused by similar enzyme deficiencies, and variation in age at onset is not fully explained. Leukodystrophies should be considered in patients of all ages in whom features of progressive neurologic deterioration develop in both the central and peripheral nervous systems.—G.M. Fenichel, M.D.

Neurological Findings in the Carbohydrate-Deficient Glycoprotein Syndrome

Blennow G, Jaeken J, Wiklund LM (Univ Hosp, Lund, Sweden; Univ Hosp Gasthuisberg, Leuven, Belgium; Univ of Gothenburg, Gothenburg, Sweden)
Acta Paediatr Scand Suppl 375:14–20, 1991   9–11

Background.—A new syndrome—the carbohydrate deficient glycoprotein syndrome—was recently studied. It manifests mainly as a nervous system disorder that is already apparent in infancy. Other organ systems are also involved, (e.g., the liver, kidneys, subcutaneous adipose tissue, skeletal system, and pericardium). The primary neurologic characteristics are retarded psychomotor development, muscular weakness and hypotonia, areflexia, ataxia, strabismus, retinitis pigmentosa, seizures, and strokelike episodes. Serum glycoproteins have deficient oligosaccharide

---

Neurologic Findings at Various Ages in
the Carbohydrate-Deficient
Glycoprotein Syndrome

Neonatal and infantile stage

Hypotonia
Muscular weakness
Developmental retardation
Hyporeflexia
Alternating esotropia
Stroke-like episodes

Preschool and school stage

Ataxia
Muscular atrophy
Dysequilibrium, dyskinesia
Areflexia
Contractures, kyphoscoliosis, pigeon thorax
Walking tip-toe with support
Pinching grasp
Retinitis pigmentosa
IQ 40–60
Extrovert social behaviour
Stroke-like episodes

Puberty and adulthood stage

Increasing weakness of the lower limbs
Slowly deteriorating retinitis pigmentosa
Stable ataxia
Stable intellectual subnormality
Compressed stature

(Courtesy of Blennow G, Jaeken J, Wiklund LM: *Acta Paediatr Scand Suppl* 375:14–20, 1991.)

moieties in these patients (especially pronounced in transferrin), which can be used as a chemical marker.

Patients.—Thirteen girls and 9 boys from Swedish and Belgian families were studied. In all patients, diagnosis was confirmed by greatly increased values of carbohydrate-deficient serum transferrin. The median age at follow-up was 13 years, with a range of $2^{1}/_{2}$–48 years.

Findings.—In the neonatal and infantile period, the patients had hypotonia, muscular weakness, developmental retardation, reduced tendon reflexes, and alternating esotropia. In the preschool and early school-age period, the patients had progressive polyneuropathy with muscular weakness and contractures; extrapyramidal signs (e.g., ataxia, dyskinesia, and dysequilibrium); psychomotor retardation, with IQ levels of 40–60; transient strokelike episodes; and retinitis pigmentosa. The condition remained fairly stationary in puberty and adulthood. At best, these patients learned to walk with support, understand the spoken word well, and develop fairly good linguistic skill. The main neuroradiologic finding was pontine and cerebellar atrophy (table).

Conclusion.—Despite the well-characterized biochemical deficiency in the carbohydrate content of certain glycoproteins, the pathophysiology underlying these neurologic findings is unclear. Both photoreceptors and myelin are associated with glycoproteins, and nerve biopsy material from these patients contains inclusion bodies, suggesting abnormal myelin metabolism.

▶ Glycoprotein degradation disorders (mannosidosis, fucosidosis, and sialidosis) are rare and resemble mild forms of mucopolysaccharidoses. The initial symptoms always occur in infancy or childhood. This new disorder differs from other glycoprotein degradation disorders because of the prominent and progressive peripheral neuropathy. It is 1 of the few disorders that produces polyneuropathy in the newborn.—G.M. Fenichel, M.D.

10 Mitochondriopathies

Mitochondrial Encephalopathies: Molecular Genetic Diagnosis From Blood Samples
Hammans SR, Sweeney MG, Brockington M, Morgan-Hughes JA, Harding AE (Inst of Neurology, London)
Lancet 337:1311–1313, 1991   10–1

Background.—Patients with syndromes of myoclonic epilepsy and ragged red fibers (MERRF) and mitochondrial encephalopathy with lactic acidosis and strokelike episodes (MELAS) may have point mutations of mitochondrial DNA (mtDNA), as may patients with a variety of other neurologic conditions. Patients with various mitochondrial myopathy phenotypes, and those with progressive myoclonus and epilepsy and/or ataxia were evaluated to seek these mutations in blood and muscle mtDNA.

Results.—Neither healthy subjects nor controls with other neurologic disorders had either mutation. Members of 6 kindreds were found to have the MERRF mutation; unusual phenotypes were found in 2 of these, but all index patients had myoclonus. Seventeen patients from 16 families were found to have the MELAS mutation. This group had a wide range of clinical findings that affected the CNS, including strokelike episodes in 10 patients. Ragged red fibers on muscle biopsy, which generally are considered to be the hallmark of mitochondrial diseases, were absent in 3 patients with mtDNA mutations. The defect was easily detectable in blood as well as in muscle in all 6 patients with MERRF and in 10 of 11 patients with MELAS.

Conclusion.—Screening for mitochondrial encephalopathies may be done inexpensively and reliably by molecular genetic analysis of blood samples. For patients with young-onset stroke, these techniques could add important information for diagnosis and genetic counselling. The bp 8344 MERRF mutation is a major cause of the MERRF syndrome and is specific for this phenotype.

▶ An increasing number of diverse neurologic disorders, including encephalopathies, epilepsy, stroke, optic neuropathies, myopathies, and other neuromuscular diseases, have now been found to be caused by a wide range of mitochondrial disorders. To date, almost all the conditions that have been recognized are the result of aberrations of the mitochondrial DNA. This study demonstrates that many of these abnormalities can be detected in DNA obtained from peripheral blood cells. Specialized laboratories are required for these studies, but the techniques are becoming more widely available with time.—W.G. Bradley, D.M., F.R.C.P.

Impairment of Mitochondrial Transcription Termination by a Point Mutation Associated With the MELAS Subgroup of Mitochondrial Encephalomyopathies
Hess JF, Parisi MA, Bennett JL, Clayton DA (Stanford Univ, Stanford, Calif)
Nature 351:236–239, 1991   10–2

Introduction.—Mutations in mitochondrial DNA (mtDNA) include duplications and point mutations as well as deletions. In patients with mitochondrial myelopathy, encephalopathy, lactic acidosis, and stroke-like episodes (MELAS), there is a common A-to-G substitution in a highly conserved portion of the gene for transfer RNA$^{Leu(UUR)}$. The boundary of genes 16S rRNA and tRNA$^{Leu(UUR)}$ is the site of the human mtDNA transcription termination site (Fig 10–1). Any alternations in transcription termination ascribable to the MELAS mutation were identified.

Results.—An active fraction (mtTERM) that yielded reproducible positive results for termination activity was localized. Its most abundant species was a ~34K protein, which was assumed to represent a nuclear gene product. The MELAS mutation, although comparable to the tRNA^{Lys} gene associated with myoclonus epilepsy and ragged red fibers, was also found to be embedded in the middle of a tridecamer sequence essential for formation of the 3′ ends of 16S ribosomal RNA in vitro. Thus, the MELAS mutation was found to result in a severe impairment of the 16S rRNA transcription termination; this finding correlated with the reduced affinity of the partially purified termination protein for the MELAS template.

Conclusion.—The point mutation in MELAS results in a dramatic loss of function of the transcription termination sequence. Therefore, the molecular defect appears to be an inability to produce the correct type and quantity of rRNA compared with other mitochondrial gene products. Discovering the nature of the proteins within the 34K fraction will not only reveal the details of the termination process, but will suggest ways to investigate or treat MELAS at the molecular level.

▶ This paper may appear "too technical" for the practicing clinician, but it contains the seeds of future diagnostic tests and treatments for patients with possible MELAS. We will all have to become aware of the field of molecular genetics, which clearly plays an important role.—W.G. Bradley, D.M., F.R.C.P.

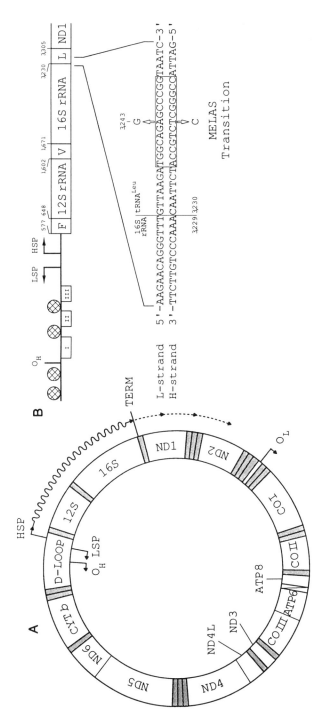

Fig 10–1.—A, representation of human mtDNA. The shaded areas represent the 22 tRNA genes. *Open regions* denote control regions, rRNA genes, and protein-coding genes. O_H and O_L demarcate the respective origins of heavy (*H*)- and light (*L*)-strand mtDNA synthesis. The abbreviations *HSP* and *LSP* mark the respective promoters for transcription from the H and L template strands. The *wavy line* originating from the HSP represents the abundant transcripts that terminate downstream of the 16S rRNA gene at a site in the gene for tRNA$^{Leu(UUR)}$, marked TERM. The *dashed lines* represent HSP transcripts passing through the site of termination. **B**, schematic of the D-loop and transcription termination region. The letters F, V, and L indicate the genes for tRNAs Phe, Val, and Leu, respectively. A portion of the gene for ND1 is shown. Boxes marked I, II and III represent conserved sequence blocks I, II and III in the D-loop region. *Cross-hatched circles* denote sites of transcription termination in vitro and potential mtTERM protein building in the D-loop region downstream of the LSP. (Courtesy of Hess JF, Parisi MA, Bennett JL, et al: *Nature* 351:236–239, 1991.)

Mitochondrial Myopathy of Childhood Associated With Depletion of Mitochrondrial DNA

Tritschler H-J, Andreetta F, Moraes CT, Bonilla E, Arnaudo E, Danon MJ, Glass S, Zelaya BM, Vamos E, Telerman-Toppet N, Shanske S, Kadenbach B, DiMauro S, Schon EA (Columbia Univ, New York; Phillips Universitat, Marburg, Germany; Univ of Illinois, Chicago; Children's Hosp Med Ctr, Seattle; Univ of North Dakota, Bismarck, et al)
Neurology 42:209–217, 1992   10–3

Background.—Cytochrome *c* oxidase (COX) deficiency of infancy manifests as mitochondrial disorders, including tissue-specific phenotypes (such as fatal infantile myopathy and a benign, spontaneously reversible myopathy) and multisystem disorders (such as Leigh's syndrome). No specific qualitative error in mitochondrial or nuclear DNA has been observed in these patients. However, a new type of mitochondrial disease of early infancy that is associated with a quantitative error in mtDNA has recently been identified in 5 children.

Patients.—The mitochondrial myopathy became evident within or soon after the first year of life. Ragged-red fibers and reduced respiratory chain activity were seen on muscle biopsy specimens. In all 5 children, the amount of muscle mitochondrial DNA (mtDNA) was severely reduced at 2% to 34% of normal. Depletion of mtDNA correlated with the absence of mtDNA-encoded translation products and the loss of cytochrome *c* oxidase enzyme activity in individual muscle fibers.

Conclusion.—Five children had mitochondrial myopathy associated with depletion of muscle mtDNA. Four had later clinical onset and slower progression than previously described cases. This mitochondrial myopathy of childhood is 1 phenotypic expression of a novel pathogenetic mechanism in mitochondrial diseases, the specific depletion of mtDNA in affected tissue.

▶ Cytochrome-*c*-oxidase (complex IV) contains 13 polypeptides; 3 large subunits are encoded by mtDNA. Deficiency of COX has been associated with fatal and benign forms of infantile myopathy, Leigh syndrome (subacute necrotizing encephalopathy), Alper syndrome (progressive infantile poliodystrophy), myoclonic encephalopathy and ragged-red fibers (MERRF), oculomyopathy, Kearns-Sayre syndrome, and Menke's disease (trichopoliodystrophy). Including those in this study, only 9 children have been reported with the specific deletion of mtDNA in affected tissue.—G.M. Fenichel, M.D.

Deletion of Mitochondrial DNA in Patients With Combined Features of Kearns-Sayre and MELAS Syndromes

Zupanc ML, Moraes CT, Shanske S, Langman CB, Ciafaloni E, DiMauro S

(Univ of Wisconsin, Madison; Columbia Presbyterian Med Ctr, New York; Northwestern Univ, Chicago)
Ann Neurol 29:680–683, 1991   10–4

Background.—There is controversy about the classification of Kearns-Sayre syndrome (KSS); mitochondrial encephalomyopathy, lactic acidosis, and stroke-like episodes (MELAS); and myoclonic epilepsy with ragged-red fibers (MERRF). Some believe it is a useful subdivision that suggests different etiologies, but others believe that all patients with mitochondrial encephalomyopathies have the same features in different proportions and combinations. Two patients with major features of both KSS and MELAS were examined.

Patients.—The patients were a 9-year-old girl and an 11-year-old boy. Both had progressive external ophthalmoplegia and pigmentary retinopathy before 20 years of age, the obligatory clinical triad of KSS. They also had ptosis and sensorineural hearing loss, along with episodes of transient hemiplegia with lactic acidosis, which is reminiscent of MELAS. The girl was found to have insulin-dependent diabetes mellitus at $3\frac{1}{2}$ years of age, and the boy was found to have hypoparathyroidism at 5 years of age. Both patients were found to have ragged-red fibers on muscle biopsy. Southern blot analysis showed distinct heteroplasmic deletion of muscle mitochondrial DNA in both patients; however, neither had evidence of the point mutation in the transfer RNA[Leu(UUR)] gene identified in MELAS.

Conclusions.—Two children had features of both KSS and MELAS. Such combinations, which suggest that mitochondrial DNA deletions can have pleomorphic clinical manifestations, should be studied in depth to help understand the pathogenesis of the differences between KSS, MERRF, and MELAS.

▶ This study is one of an increasing series that is gradually clarifying our understanding of the neurologic mitochondriopathies. These 2 patients had clinical features of both KSS and MELAS, and they had evidence of deletion of muscle mitochondrial DNA that was typical of KSS. However, the point mutation in the transfer RNA[Leu(UUR)] gene identified in MELAS was not present in these patients. The plot thickens!—W.G. Bradley, D.M., F.R.C.P.

Marked Reduction in CSF Lactate and Pyruvate Levels After CoQ Therapy in a Patient With Mitochondrial Myopathy, Encephalopathy, Lactic Acidosis and Stroke-Like Episodes (MELAS)

Abe K, Fujimura H, Nishikaway, Yorifuji S, Mezaki T, Hirono N, Nishitani N, Kameyama M (Osaka Univ; Sumitomo Hosp; Second Tanne Hosp, Osaka, Japan)
Acta Neurol Scand 83:356–359, 1991   10–5

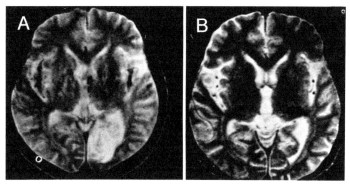

Fig 10–2.—**A** and **B**, MRI (Shimazu 1.5-tesla superconducting system; TR/TE = 2,500/120) reveals high-intensity lesions in the left occipital, but these diminish on subsequent MRI. (Courtesy of Abe K, Fujimura H, Nishikaway, et al: *Acta Neurol Scand* 83:356–359, 1991.)

Introduction.—There is no known effective treatment for mitochondrial myopathy, encephalopathy, lactic acidosis, and stroke-like episodes (MELAS), a syndrome classified as mitochondrial encephalomyopathy. A patient with MELAS in whom marked reduction in CSF lactate any pyru-

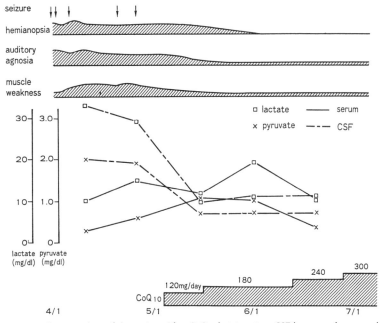

Fig 10–3.—Progress chart of the patient. After CoQ administration, CSF lactate and pyruvate levels decreased, and the clinical symptoms were improved simultaneously. (Courtesy of Abe K, Fujimura H, Nishikaway: *Acta Neurol Scand* 83:356–359, 1991.)

vate levels occurred was shown to have clinical improvement when treated with coenzyme Q (CoQ).

Case Report.—Man, 34, was admitted with untreatable seizures that had been occurring since he was 21 years of age. Magnetic resonance imaging revealed abnormal intensity lesions in the left parietal and left operculum, but they diminished in 2 months (Fig 10-2). The patient was of short stature, had a normal prenatal and perinatal history, had seizures with right hemianopia and auditory agnosia, demonstrated weak muscle strength, and had headache with nausea. Laboratory data were in the normal range, except for an abnormal increase in CSF lactate and pyruvate. The serum lactate and pyruvate levels were normal. These clinical features are compatable with a diagnosis of MELAS. To confirm the diagnosis, the patient underwent biopsy of the right quadriceps muscle, but no ragged red fibers were found. However, ragged red fibers are not always found in MELAS patients, and their absence does not exclude a diagnosis of MELAS. The patient was started on high dosage CoQ therapy. One week later, his hemianopia and state of delirium started to improve, and the doses of major tranquilizer could be tapered. A lumbar puncture performed after 3 weeks of therapy revealed markedly decreased CSF lactate and pyruvate levels. No seizures have occurred since CoQ therapy was started, and muscle weakness has gradually improved. High-dose CoQ therapy is being continued (Fig 10-3).

Conclusion.—There have been no other descriptions of CoQ efficacy in the CNS. Although exogenous CoQ is known to be unable to pass the blood-brain barrier, this patient had a broken blood-brain barrier, which allowed CoQ to pass relatively freely through it and into the brain tissue.

▶ The increasingly frequent recognition of mitochondrial abnormalities as a cause of a number of rare neurologic diseases opens up the possibility of treatment. Coenzyme Q, vitamin K, ascorbic acid and, possibly, other agents that can assist in electron transfer in defective mitochondria can now be offered to such patients. This paper reviews evidence of the effectiveness of exogenous CoQ.—W.G. Bradley, D.M., F.R.C.P.

Zidovudine Myopathy: A Distinctive Disorder Associated With Mitochondrial Dysfunction

Mhiri C, Baudrimont M, Bonne G, Geny C, Degoul F, Marsac C, Roullet E, Gherardi R (Hôpital Henri Mondor, Créteil, France; Hôpital Saint Antoine; Necker-Enfants Malades, Paris)
Ann Neurol 29:606–614, 1991   10–6

Background.—During the past 3 years, zidovudine has been implicated in the mitochondrial changes that occur in the diffuse myopathy found in HIV-infected patients. Zidovudine, a nucleoside analog that inhibits HIV replication, has been in use since 1986, with reported side effects of serious anemia and neutropenia. Because it is the sole effective therapy for AIDS, withdrawal of zidovudine as a result of reports of myopathy was considered risky. To determine the role of zidovudine in myopathy, muscle biopsy specimens from HIV-infected patients were examined.

Patients.—Muscle biopsy specimens obtained from 48 HIV-infected patients with neuromuscular symptoms were examined by conventional and electron microscopy.

Findings.—Thirteen of the patients who received long-term zidovudine therapy had a progressive, usually painful, proximal myopathy with pronounced wasting, normal to moderately elevated creatine, and a myopathic electromyographic pattern. These muscle biopsy specimens showed a characteristic structural myopathy associated with mitochondrial changes. The 13 affected patients had received a significantly higher mean cumulative dose than the other zidovudine recipients in the study. There was a decrease in respiratory chain capacity, which was demonstrated by an assay of mitochondrial enzymes, but mitochondrial DNA showed no abnormality.

Conclusion.—Long-term zidovudine therapy, especially in patients with a cumulative dose of more than 250 g, can cause severe myopathy in HIV-infected patients. The myopathy is characterized histologically by the distinctive association between structural abnormalities and mitochondrial changes. Zidovudine myopathy accounts for almost one third of the HIV-associated neuromuscular disorders evaluated since 1987, and it has been detected in 18% of patients treated for more than 200 days.

▶ This is 1 of a number of studies demonstrating the development of a mitochondrial myopathy in patients receiving zidovudine for the treatment of HIV infection. Evidence indicates that zidovudine inhibits mitochondrial DNA polymerase, hence resulting in mitochondrial dysfunction and overproduction. Although zidovudine is important in the suppression of viral replication, the myopathy can be sufficiently severe to necessitate drug withdrawal, with consequent improvement in the myopathy.—W.G. Bradley, D.M., F.R.C.P.

11 Infectious Diseases and General Medical Diseases

Subdural and Epidural Empyema: Diagnostic and Therapeutic Problems

McIntyre PB, Lavercombe PS, Kemp RJ, McCormack JG (Mater Misericordiae Hosp, South Brisbane; Royal Brisbane Hosp, Australia)

Med J Aust 154:653–657, 1991   11–1

Background.—Subdural empyema describes the presence of pus in the potential space between the dura mater and arachnoid mater. Patients may show no abnormalities on CT, and there is controversy about the need for surgical treatment. An experience with 2 such patients prompted a clinical and microbiologic review of patients with subdural and epidural empyema in Brisbane, Australia, during a 10-year period.

Patients.—The review included patients from the neurosurgical units of the Royal Brisbane Hospital, Royal Children's Hospital, Princess Alexandra Hospital, and the Mater Misericordiae Adult and Children's Hospitals. There were 10 men and 4 women. Eight cases originated in the paranasal sinuses; 3 began in the middle ear; 2 started after surgery or trauma; and 1 occurred as a complication of *Haemophilus influenzae* meningitis. Eight of the patients with community disease were younger than 20 years of age, and all of the cases of sinus origin were caused by streptococci, especially *Streptococcus milleri.* The patients were symptomatic for as long as 9 days before presentation, almost always with headache and fever. In 3 of the cases of otic origin but only 2 of the 10 sinus or posttraumatic cases, an intracranial collection was considered in the differential diagnosis within 24 hours of admission. In 8 of 13 patients, the initial diagnosis was viral or partially treated bacterial meningitis. Angiography was diagnostic in 2 patients, but the initial CT scan was not diagnostic in 3 of 11 patients. All patients required surgery, which was delayed in all 3 patients who died.

Conclusion.—Subdural and epidural empyema is an uncommon condition that remains a diagnostic challenge. Computed tomography is not a reliable diagnostic tool, although diagnosis is improved by use of intravenously administered contrast and more modern scanners. To avoid morbidity and mortality, the condition must be treated by surgical drainage and early, aggressive antimicrobial therapy.

▶ Intracranial subdural and epidural empyemata are rare disorders and, as this paper illustrates, they must be treated with urgency if a good outcome is to be obtained. Because of this, it is important that we continually review their clinical presentation and investigation. Computed tomography is not universally successful in imaging the empyema, and it will be important to investigate the success of MRI.—W.G. Bradley, D.M., F.R.C.P.

Brain Biopsy in the Management of Focal Encephalitis
Anderson NE, Willoughby EW, Synek BJL, Croxson MC, Glasgow GL (Auckland Hosp; Univ of Auckland, Auckland, New Zealand)
J Neurol Neurosurg Psychiatry 54:1001–1003, 1991   11–2

Objective.—The role of brain biopsy in the diagnosis and management of suspected herpes simplex encephalitis (HSE) was evaluated in 29 patients, including 16 who were studied prospectively and 13 who were studied retrospectively. Clinical examination, CT, and electroencephalography were used as guides for appropriate site of biopsy. The diagnosis of HSE was confirmed only in patients with positive biopsy cultures for herpes simplex virus (HSV).

Findings.—A diagnosis of HSE was confirmed in only 8 (28%) patients. The biopsy showed acute encephalitis in 14 patients (including 2 with inclusion bodies), but HSV was not cultured. In 4 patients, biopsy provided alternative diagnoses, such as lymphocytic meningitis and subdural empyema, for which curative alternative treatment was available. Treatment was not affected by failure to confirm a diagnosis of HSE. The complications included a fatal intracerebral and subdural hematoma in 1 patient, and a subdural hematoma in 1 other patient. Another patient had seizures 1 month later.

Conclusion.—Brain biopsy is not justified in the routine investigation of focal encephalitis. It provides a low yield of alternative diagnoses and is only marginally helpful in the management of patients with suspected HSE.

▶ There is much argument about the necessity for brain biopsy in suspected HSE. Other diagnoses with different therapy may be found, as occurred in this study. However, such cases are uncommon. Moreover, brain biopsies are not totally benign. Therefore, most experienced neurologists recommend initial treatment with acyclovir in patients suspected of having HSE; brain biopsy is reserved for those patients that do not respond.—W.G. Bradley, D.M., F.R.C.P.

Herpes Zoster Myelitis

Devinsky O, Cho E-S, Petito CK, Price RW (New York Hospital-Cornell Univ Med Ctr, New York; Univ of Medicine and Dentistry of New Jersey, Newark)
Brain 114:1181–1196, 1991   11–3

Background.—Herpes zoster (HZ) is typically benign, but neurologic complications are common. These complications range from transient pain and paraesthesiae associated with acute rash to postherpetic neuralgia, segmental sensory loss or motor paresis, encephalitis, myelitis, and cerebral vascular occlusion. Clinical myelopathy is rare, usually occurring in immunocompromised patients. The clinical and pathologic findings in a series of patients with HZ myelitis were evaluated.

Patients.—All 13 patients studied had systemic diseases associated with immunosuppression. The median time between the onset of HZ rash and myelopathic symptoms was 12 days. The subsequent median interval to maximal deficit was 10.5 days. Typically, the presenting neurologic symptoms were ipsilateral to the rash. Motor dysfunction predominated, followed by a spinothalamic and, less frequently, a posterior column sensory deficit.

Autopsy Findings in 9 Patients.—The most severe pathologic involvement occurred in the dorsal root entry zone and the posterior horn of the spinal cord segment corresponding to the involved dermatome. Spread was variable, both horizontally and vertically in the spinal cord. Direct varicella-zoster virus (VZV) infection of the neuroectodermal cells, especially the oligodendrocytes, was shown by immunostaining viral antigens and the presence of Cowdry type A intranuclear inclusions. In 6 cases, VZV infection was associated with focal demyelination. In 4 cases, VZV vasculitis was associated with leptomeningitis and hemorrhagic necrosis.

Conclusion.—Early treatment is beneficial in patients with HZ myelitis. The typical delayed development and slow evolution of HZ myelitis in most patients and the efficacy of newer antiviral drugs indicate that these drugs may prevent multiplication and spread of the virus in the CNS.

▶ Postherpetic neuralgia and myelopathy are the 2 most frequent complications of HZ. Treatment with acyclovir can be effective in ameliorating the severity of the HZ infection. This is an excellent review of the clinical and pathologic features of the myelopathy in HZ.—G. Bradley, D.M., F.R.C.P.

Sequential Cranial MR Findings of Asymptomatic and Neurologically Symptomatic HIV⁺ Subjects

Post MJD, Levin BE, Berger JR, Duncan R, Quencer RM, Calabro G (Univ of Miami)

AJNR 13:359–370, 1992   11–4

Background.—Human immunodeficiency virus (HIV-1) is known to infect neurologic tissue early in the course of infection. However, it is not known whether HIV causes significant functional or structural abnormalities during the period in which a seropositive individual is neurologically asymptomatic. The results of a prospective MR scan and the clinical reassessment of HIV-positive asymptomatic and neurologically symptomatic individuals with initially abnormal cranial studies were com-

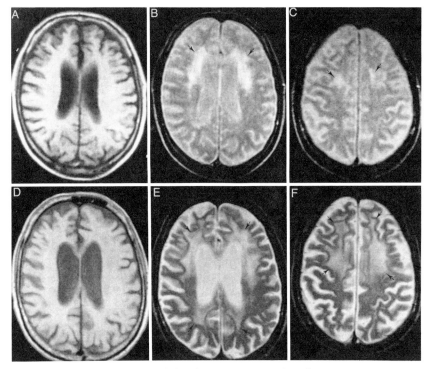

Fig 11–1.—Magnetic resonance and clinical worsening in a neurologically symptomatic HIV-positive subject, 61 years, who was mildly encephalopathic HIV positive. His neuropsychologic test battery demonstrated a subcortical dementia, and he had no hypertension and no active infection with other pathogens. His initial .5-tesla MR image on (**A**) T1W1 (700–20) showed moderate cortical and deep atrophy associated with periventricular and centrum semiovale confluent white matter lesions, the latter seen on (**B** and **C,** *arrows*) T2W1 (2,400/80). Fourteen months later, concomitant with worsening encephalopathy, the follow-up 1-tesla MR image showed on (**D**) T1W1 (850/20) an increase in the size of the sulci and ventricles and on (**E** and **F**) T2W1 (2,200/80), extension of the white matter lesions (*arrows*). (Courtesy of Post MJD, Levin BE, Berger JR, et al: AJNR 13:359–370, 1992.)

pared to determine what MR changes occur and how they correlate with serial neurologic and neuropsychologic findings.

Methods.—Twenty asymptomatic and 11 neurologically symptomatic HIV-seropositive patients were studied. The patients were prospectively reassessed by cranial MRI 1–2 years after an initial MR scan of the brain showed abnormalities.

Results.—All the patients had abnormal follow-up scans, showing atrophy and/or white matter lesions. Twenty-seven had no progression of MR abnormalities, including 18 patients with minimally abnormal scans who remained asymptomatic with improved or static neuropsychologic performance. One of 4 patients with scan changes, all of whom had clinically suspected HIV encephalopathy, showed MR, clinical, and neuropsychologic test improvement. The remaining 3 had MR, neurologic and/or neuropsychologic worsening. Autopsy in 1 of these patients confirmed the presence of HIV-1–containing multinucleated giant cells in the brain (Fig 11-1).

Conclusion.—Intracranial MR abnormality progression from HIV-1 infection appears to occur only in a minority of HIV-positive patients during a period of 1–2 years, and only in those who are neurologically symptomatic. This progression correlates with clinical deterioration. Minor cerebral MR abnormalities in HIV-positive individuals who remain neurologically asymptomatic do not change a period of 1–2 years. It is known that HIV can infect the brain early; however, in many patients, it may not significantly damage the brain anatomically early in the disease based on MR criteria.

▶ An HIV infection of the brain is likely to be an invariable consequence of AIDS. During its terminal stages, a frequent outcome of HIV infection is encephalopathy (AIDS dementia complex), which is typically characterized on MRI by cerebral atrophy and discrete or confluent white matter abnormalities. This study was designed to explore the changes in the brain as detected by sequentially performed MRIs and to establish their predictive value with respect to neurologic deterioration. The lack of a significant change in the MRIs, except in previously neurologically symptomatic individuals, suggests that it is too insensitive to discern early HIV-related changes in the brain, and that it should not be used as a screening tool.—J.R. Berger, M.D.

Neurosyphilis in Human Immunodeficiency Virus Type 1-Seropositive Individuals: A Prospective Study
Berger JR (Univ of Miami)
Arch Neurol 48:700–702, 1991   11–5

Objective.—There is increasing interest in the role of syphilis in human immunodeficiency virus type 1 (HIV-1) infection. The frequency of syphilis in asymptomatic HIV-1-seropositive (HIV+) subjects was assessed, and its contribution to the presence of neurologic disease in symptomatic subjects was determined.

Methods.—A total of 338 subjects were enrolled in a longitudinal study designed to explore the neurologic consequences of HIV-1 infection. Serologic studies of blood and CSF were performed in 235 subjects, including 166 asymptomatic HIV+ subjects, 63 neurologically symptomatic subjects, and 6 HIV-1–seronegative control subjects.

Findings.—Among HIV+ subjects, the prevalence of prior syphilis, defined by a history (40.5%) or presence of a reactive serum fluorescent treponemal antibody-absorption (FTA-ABS) test (36%), was significantly high compared with that in control subjects. Three neurologically asymptomatic HIV+ subjects and 2 neurologically symptomatic HIV+ subjects had neurosyphilis. All 5 subjects had reactive serum RPR test. All 3 asymptomatic HIV+ subjects had both a reactive CSF Venereal Disease Research Laboratory (VDRL) test and a reactive FTA-ABS test, and 2 had a history of appropriately treated syphilis. Of the 2 symptomatic HIV+ subjects with neurosyphilis, 1 had dementia, which responded to high-dose intravenous penicillin therapy; this patient also had reactive CSF VDRL and FTA-ABS tests. The other patient had penicillin-responsive myelopathy, which was accompanied by a reactive CSF FTA-ABS test and a nonreactive CSF VDRL.

Conclusion.—Unsuspected neurosyphilis is relatively common in asymptomatic HIV+ subjects, and it may account for neurologic disease in a significant minority of neurologically symptomatic HIV+ individuals. Considering the significant overlap between the spectrum of neurologic diseases caused by HIV-1 and *Treponema pallidum*, neurosyphilis should be considered in the differential diagnosis of neurologic disease in HIV+ individuals. Furthermore, the significant rate of neurosyphilis in HIV-1–infected individuals supports the liberal examination of CSF in all HIV+ individuals, especially those with a history of syphilis or serologic evidence of syphilis, regardless of prior treatment.

▶ Syphilis is "raising its ugly head" again, particularly in HIV-positive patients. It may be difficult to separate the neurologic complications of these 2 infections. Because neurosyphilis is eminently treatable, it is important that all HIV-positive patients with neurologic complications have blood and CSF syphilis serology studied.—W.G. Bradley, D.M., F.R.C.P.

Whipple's Disease Confined to the CNS Presenting With Multiple Intracerebral Mass Lesions

Wroe SJ, Pires M, Harding B, Youl BD, Shorvon S (Natl Hosp, London; Inst of Neurology, London)

J Neurol Neurosurg Psychiatry 54:989–992, 1991   11–6

Moving?

I'd like to receive my *Year Book of Neurology and Neurosurgery* without interruption.

Please note the following change of address, effective: _____

Name: _____

New Address: _____

_____

City: _____ State: _____ Zip: _____

Old Address: _____

_____

City: _____ State: _____ Zip: _____

Reservation Card

Yes, I would like my own copy of the *Year Book of Neurology and Neurosurgery*. Please begin my subscription with the current edition according to the terms described below.* I understand that I will have 30 days to examine each annual edition. If satisfied, I will pay just $59.95 plus sales tax, postage and handling (price subject to change without notice).

Name: _____

Address: _____

City: _____ State: _____ Zip: _____

Method of Payment

❏ Visa   ❏ Mastercard   ❏ AmEx   ❏ Bill me   ❏ Check (in US dollars, payable to Mosby-Year Book, Inc.)

Card number _____ Exp date _____

Signature _____

LS-0907

---

*Your *Year Book* Service Guarantee:

When you subscribe to the *Year Book*, we'll send you an advance notice of future volumes about two months before they publish. This automatic notice system is designed to take up as little of your time as possible. If you do not want the *Year Book*, the advance notice makes it quick and easy for you to let us know your decision; and you will always have at least 20 days to decide. If we don't hear from you, we'll send you the new volume as soon as it's available. And, of course, the *Year Book* is yours to examine free of charge for 30 days (postage, handling and applicable sales tax are added to each shipment).

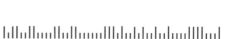

BUSINESS REPLY MAIL

FIRST CLASS MAIL   PERMIT No. 762   CHICAGO, IL

POSTAGE WILL BE PAID BY ADDRESSEE

Chris Hughes
Mosby-Year Book, Inc.
200 N. LaSalle Street
Suite 2600
Chicago, IL 60601-9981

|ıl|ıı|lıııı|lıı|lıııı||l|ıl|ılıl|ıl|ıııı|lll|ıı|

NO POSTAGE
NECESSARY
IF MAILED
IN THE
UNITED STATES

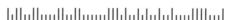

BUSINESS REPLY MAIL

FIRST CLASS MAIL   PERMIT No. 762   CHICAGO, IL

POSTAGE WILL BE PAID BY ADDRESSEE

Chris Hughes
Mosby-Year Book, Inc.
200 N. LaSalle Street
Suite 2600
Chicago, IL 60601-9981

|ıl|ıı|lıııı|lıı|lıııı||l|ıl|ılıl|ıl|ıııı|lll|ıı|

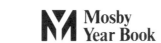

Mosby
Year Book

Dedicated to publishing excellence.

Background.—Patients with Whipple's disease may have neurologic symptoms, but they rarely have progressive cognitive decline and hypothalamic disturbance leading to death. A patient with Whipple's disease confined to the CNS, including a previously undescribed CT and MRI finding, was described.

Case Report.—Man, 32 was admitted with a 2-week history of severe morning headaches, vomiting, and drowsiness. He was drowsy and disoriented and had left upper motor neuron 7th nerve palsy, slight left-sided pyramidal weakness, and sensory inattention. Computed tomography of the head revealed several bilateral ring-enhancing mass lesions, and contrast MRI showed several high-signal mass lesions with peripheral ring enhancement. The patient had a performance IQ of 53, with impaired memory, perceptual difficulties, and frontal lobe dysfunction. The partly cystic right front lesion was partially excised. The patient received parenteral antibiotics for 2 weeks and was begun on long-term sulfamethoxazole-trimethoprim. Gastrointestinal studies were normal. The patient had improved little at 1 month; he was apathetic, docile, and did not initiate conversation. His performance IQ was 58. On MRI, the lesions were smaller, but there was considerable enlargement of the left frontal mass. After another 2 months, he had improved greatly, and MRI showed improvement or resolution of all lesions. The patient resumed limited employment 11 months after onset. Electron microscopic examination of biopsy specimens showed characteristic rod-shaped bacilliform inclusions.

Discussion.—Manifestations of Whipple's disease include signs of rapidly evolving, raised intracranial pressure and multiple ring-enhancing intracerebral mass lesions on imaging studies. Prognosis may be poor in patients with macrophage bacterial inclusion; treatment should include identification of a specific cause and long-term antibiotic treatment.

▶ Whipple's disease usually is seen as multifocal arthritis, malabsorption, and an occasional neurologic syndrome. The neurologic manifestations are legion, and they include progressive dementia, ataxia, and hypothalamic and brain stem dysfunction with ophthalmoplegia and variable basal ganglia and lung tract signs. This unusual patient presented with multiple cerebral masses containing the typical phosphatidylscrine-positive bacteria. The patient responded slowly but positively to antibiotics. It is important to keep this disease in mind in all "undiagnosable"cases.—W.G. Bradley, D.M. F.R.C.P.

Successful Treatment of Primary Amebic Meningoencephalitis
Brown RL (Wilkes-Barre Gen Hosp, Wilkes-Barre, Pa)
Arch Intern Med 151:1201–1202, 1991   11–7

Introduction.—Primary amebic meningoencephalitis, a fulminant, often rapidly fatal infection, is caused by the free-living ameba *Naegleria fowleri,* and it occurs in individuals with a recent history of swimming in warm fresh water. There are only 3 reported cases of survival in affected patients. Data were reviewed on a patient who survived without neurologic sequelae.

Case Report.—Man 32, with suspected meningitis came to the emergency department with fever, lethargy, and severe headache; he rapidly progressed to coma and was admitted to the intensive care unit. A CT scan of the brain was normal. Lumbar puncture yielded cloudy fluid with a white blood cell count of $5,356 \times 10^6/L$, a glucose level of 5.55 mmol/L, and a protein level of 6.10 g/L. In addition to routine microbiologic studies, microscopic examination for free-living amebae was performed because the patient was a summer-camp swimming instructor. It was later learned that he had been waterskiing in a small freshwater lake several days previously. High-dose penicillin was administered intravenously. At 4 hours after admission, bacterial antigen tests were negative, but 3 motile amebae were seen on light microscopic examination of the CSF. Penicillin was stopped, and amphotericin B, 75 mg/day, was administered together with rifampim, 600 mg, every 12 hours. The patient improved, and amphotericin was administered intrathecally the next day; this treatment continued for 10 days. The patient improved progressively and was asymptomatic at the end of treatment.

Conclusion.—The diagnosis of primary amebic meningoencephalitis must be considered to allow prompt, aggressive therapy. A history of swimming in warm, fresh water is crucial. Although high-dose rifampin and intrathecal amphotericin therapy may have contributed to the successful outcome in this patient, routine use of these medications is questionable.

▶ Acute amebic meningoencephalitis caused by *Naegleria fowleri* is a rapidly fatal disease, with death occurring within 2–5 days of presentation in the absence of treatment. The disease is often unsuspected and, therefore, only a handful of successfully treated patients have been reported. Clues to the diagnosis include recent contact with freshwater typically exceeding 30°C, complaints of parageusia and anosmia resulting from early involvement of the olfactory nerve and the lobes by the trophozoite, and CSF analysis revealing a neutrophilic pleocytosis, red cells, and low sugar. The organism is difficult to detect on Gram's or Wright's stain. Wet mount, as described in the case report of Dr. Brown, is the preferred technique for early detection. Although *N. fowleri* does not grow in culture media generally used for bacteria, viruses, or fungi, culture techniques are available if the organism is suspected. Amphotericin B in concentrations of less than 1 μg/mL is exquisitely amebicidal for *N. fowleri.* Intrathecal administration is recommended to supplement intravenous administration. A synergistic effect may be observed with rifampin, tetracycline or minocycline.—J.R. Berger, M.D.

Neurocysticercosis: Neurologic, Pathogenic, Diagnostic and Therapeutic Aspects

Davis LE, Kornfeld M (Univ of New Mexico, Albuquerque)
Eur Neurol 31:229–240, 1991   11–8

Introduction.—Cysticercosis is the most common parasitic infection of the central nervous system worldwide, and it is seen chiefly in developing countries. Immigration from Mexico and Latin America into the United States has increased the prevalence of neurocysticercosis, especially in the Southwest.

Pathogenesis.—A human becomes the definitive host for the tapeworm after eating inadequately cooked pork that contains viable larvae of *Taenia solium* or cysticerci. The larvae develop in the small bowel. Humans also may be intermediate hosts, like the pig, by ingesting food or water contaminated by *T. solium* ova. Cerebral edema may develop when fibroblasts form a capsulelike structure around a cyst (table). Oncospheres lodging in the meninges or choroid plexus may enter the ventricles or the subarachnoid space.

Pathology.—Giant cells often persist when inflammatory reaction to the capsule subsides. Parenchymal or meningeal ateries may be inflamed. The cerebral parenchyma may harbor single or multiple cysts, which tend to occur in the gray matter, especially the cortex. Hundreds of cysts may be present in the extreme cases. It may be difficult to determine whether a given cyst is cortical or meningeal. Diffuse meningeal thickening may make it hard to identify the parasitic membranes.

Clinical.—Symptoms may be absent for a considerable time in patients with cerebral infestation. Parenchymal cysts often present with seizures or focal neurologic signs. Hemisparesis, visual field impairment, and movement disorders are common. Cysticerci in the ventricles or meninges produce chronic meningitis. The CSF is abnormal in approximately half the patients, most often exhibiting a lymphocytic pleocytosis. Eosinophils are found in 10% to 15% of cases. The electroencephalogram often is abnormal. A CT scan may demonstrate 1 or more cystic lesions (5-20 mm in diameter) near the gray-white injunction in the cerebral cortex. Magnetic resonance imaging can demonstrate both parenchymal and ventricular cysticerci. A new immunoblot test detects both IgM and IgG antibodies to cysticerci antigens.

Management.—Active disease most often is treated with praziquantel, a well-tolerated orally active drug. Albendazole is widely used to treat neurocysticercosis in Mexico. Surgical removal of a cyst occasionally is indicated.

▶ With increased international travel and immigration, neurologists in every part of the world are seeing increasing numbers of patients with neurocysticercosis. Therefore, the clinical features, diagnosis, and treatment are of

Typical Stages of C. *cellulosae* in Brain

Stage	Time after ova ingestion	Pathology	CT scan	Common clinical features
1	weeks	larval migration	small non-contrast-enhancing edematous lesion	mainly asymptomatic occasional flu-like illness
2	weeks	early cyst formation	small homogenous contrast-enhancing lesion	mainly asymptomatic with occasional seizures, rare increased intracranial pressure in massive infection
3	2 months to 10 years	mature cyst	3–18 mm non-contrast-enhancing cyst without adjacent edema	mainly asymptomatic
4	2–10+ years	degenerating cyst with adjacent inflammation, fibrous capsule and surrounding edema	ring contrast-enhancing cyst with adjacent edema	seizures, increased intracranial pressure, focal neurologic signs
5	2–10+ years	collapsed dead fibrotic cyst that often calcifies	isodense or calcified nodule	asymptomatic or seizures

(Courtesy of Davis LE, Kornfeld M: *Eur Neurol* 31:229–240, 1991.)

great importance. This report provides an excellent review, and it should be read in its entirety.—W.G. Bradley, D.M., F.R.C.P.

Spinal Cord Schistosomiasis: A Clinical, Laboratory and Radiological Study, With a Note on Therapeutic Aspects
Haribhai HC, Bhigjee AI, Bill PLA, Pammenter MD, Modi G, Hoffmann M, Kelbe C, Becker P (Univ of Natal, Durban; Med Research Council, Durban, South Africa; Med Research Council, Hillbrow, South Africa)
Brain 114:709–726, 1991   11–9

Background.—Spinal cord disorder is the most common disease in the neurology unit at this South African Hospital that treats mostly black Zulu patients; the myelopathy remains unexplained in 10%. A protocol was established to improve diagnostic yield, and it was used for 14 patients with spinal cord schistosomiasis.

Patients.—During a 20-month period, 14 patients (12 blacks and 2 whites) received a diagnosis of of spinal cord schistosomiasis. Back pain, leg pain, weakness, sensory disturbance, and sphincter impairment were predominant. Half the patients had lesions in the conus medullaris, cauda equina, or both, as shown by clinical findings and CT myelography; the other half had clinically acute or subacute transverse myelitis with normal or equivocal CT myelographic findings. In 2 patients with conus swelling who underwent biopsy, granulomas containing bilharzial ova were found. In the other 12 patients, the diagnosis was made presumptively on the basis of clinical and laboratory findings. Bilharzial infection was found in all 13 patients tested based on blood serology and/ or detection of bilharzial ova. On CSF examination, all but 1 patient had pleocytosis, increased protein content, and low normal glucose concentration. Intrathecal IgG synthesis was shown by oligoclonal IgG bands, increased IgG index, and an increased CSF IgG synthesis rate. A CSF bilharzia enzyme-linked immunosorbent assay (ELISA) was sensitive, but it was not completely specific for the diagnosis of spinal cord schistosomiasis.

Outcome.—Improvement was rapid in 11 patients, 8 of whom received praziquantel and corticosteroids and 2 of whom had surgery; 1 patient improved spontaneously. Medical treatment resulted in significantly reduced CSF cell count, protein concentration, ELISA bilharzia titer, and intrathecal antibody production. Conus size decreased in 3 patients who had repeat CT myelography after therapy.

Conclusion.—The presumptive diagnosis of spinal cord schistosomiasis is supported by the clinical and radiologic improvement and the normalization of laboratory results after combined praziquantel and corticosteroid treatment. When the condition is diagnosed on indirect evidence, early intensive medical treatment, as opposed to surgery, is recommended. Laminectomy and biopsy are probably not necessary to make a confident diagnosis.

▶ With world travel and immigration, no physician can escape the need to know about diseases such as schistosomiasis. This excellent review of the clinical features, investigation, and management of spinal cord schistosomiasis should be carefully studied by every neurologist.—W.G. Bradley, D.M., F.R.C.P.

Does Orthotopic Liver Transplantation Heal Wilson's Disease? Clinical Follow-Up of Two Liver-Transplanted Patients

Hefter H, Rautenberg W, Kreuzpaintner G, Arendt G, Freund H-J, Pichlmayr R, Strohmeyer G (Heinrich-Heine Univ of Düsseldorf, Germany; Univ of Hannover, Germany)
Acta Neurol Scand 84:192–196, 1991   11–10

Introduction.—Because few patients with Wilson's disease have undergone liver transplantation, few data are available on the results of transplantation in this hereditary disorder. In 2 patients, there was a reversal of severe neurologic symptoms after liver transplant; these results were confirmed in 2 additional patients.

Case Report.—Woman, 19 had Wilson's disease, which was diagnosed on the basis of decreased serum copper levels, slightly decreased ceruloplasmin levels, increased urinary copper excretion, and an intense Kayser-Fleischer (KF) ring. Laparoscopy revealed cirrhosis of the liver with clear signs of portal hypertension. Because of severe hemorrhages from esophageal varices, liver transplantation was performed 3 years after the onset of symptoms. A second transplantation was required after severe rejection with the first organ. The patient was able to return to work in 4 months, and her copper metabolism returned to normal.

Results.—Both patients were well at follow-ups of 4 and 6 years. They were nearly asymptomatic clinically and had normal results on most electrophysiologic tests. Although the follow-up still is too short to exclude further copper intoxication of the liver or other organs, fading of the KF ring suggests that copper elimination is sufficient. These results are comparable with those of asymptomatic patients with Wilson's disease who were treated conventionally very early in the course of disease.

Conclusion.—This disorder may be healed by orthotopic liver transplantation, and pathogenic defect in Wilson's disease may be limited to the liver. However, liver transplantation should be used in patients at a life-threatening stage of the disease.

▶ The exact biochemical abnormality in Wilson's disease is still unknown, although the disease results from an excess deposition of copper in the brain and liver. This paper offers the hope of a cure for patients through the heroic procedure of liver transplantation. These observations suggest that a mutation in a protein produced by the liver may be the primary abnormality in Wilson's disease, and that the normal transplanted liver corrects this defect.—W.G. Bradley, D.M., F.R.C.P.

Neurological Paraneoplastic Syndromes in Patients With Small Cell Lung Cancer: A Prospective Survey of 150 Patients
Elrington GM, Murray NMF, Spiro SG, Newsom-Davis J (Natl Hosp, London)
J Neurol Neurosurg Psychiatry 54:764–767, 1991   11–11

Background.—Small-cell lung cancer (SCLC) is associated with various paraneoplastic syndromes, including the Lambert-Eaton myasthenic syndrome (LEMS), subacute sensory neuropathy (SSN), myelopathy, cerebellar degeneration, and encephalopathy. More than 1 syndrome may affect the same patient.

Series.—The study included 150 patients who were given a tissue diagnosis of SCLC, approximately one third of whom had limited disease. The mean patient age was 64 years. All patients were evaluated before receiving cytotoxic drugs.

Findings.—Two of 6 patients with suggestive clinical features proved to have electrophysiologic findings that were diagnostic of LEMS. One patient had SSN diagnosed. Twenty-four patients had sensory impairment and 15 were areflexic. Four patients had trunk and limb ataxia. The patients with LEMS and SSN had neurologic symptoms develop before other manifestations of SCLC. Four patients were seen with symptoms caused by cerebral metastasis of SCLC.

Implications.—Three of 150 patients with SCLC in this prospective series presented with neurologic paraneoplastic syndromes. Both LEMS and SSN are associated with antibody to SCLC antigen, which recognizes determinants on motor nerve terminals or dorsal root ganglia. These structures lack the blood-nerve barrier that may protect other potential neural targets.

▶ The diagnosis of paraneoplastic syndromes requires considerable acumen. There is much uncertainty about the true incidence of paraneoplastic complications. This prospective study offers information relative to this question. This incidence of Lambert-Eaton syndrome is surprisingly high, and it may be biased by the special interests of this group.—W.G. Bradley, D.M., F.R.C.P.

12 Sleep Disorders

Drivers With Untreated Sleep Apnea: A Cause of Death and Serious Injury
Findley LJ, Weiss JW, Jabour ER (Univ of Virginia, Charlottesville; Harvard Univ, Boston)
Arch Intern Med 151:1451–1452, 1991   12–1

Background.—Patients with obstructive sleep apnea have high rates of automobile accidents. The driving performance of untreated patients with this condition has been found to be worse than that of control subjects. However, there appear to be no reports of drivers with untreated sleep apnea falling asleep at the wheel and causing crashes involving serious injuries or death. Three such cases were repeated to demonstrate that individuals with untreated sleep apnea can cause serious harm to themselves and others.

Patients.—The patients were 3 men (age, 24–72 years). All were hospitalized for injuries sustained during automobile or truck accidents. All 3 had fallen asleep while driving. One hit a telephone pole, another hit a tree, and the third hit a parked truck. In the truck accident, a pedestrian was killed and the driver of the parked truck suffered severe spinal injury resulting in permanent paraplegia. Two of the patients with sleep apnea had closed head injuries, and the third had multiple facial lacerations, rib fractures, a hemothorax, and a right acromion fracture. None of the patients showed signs of alcohol or drug ingestion. Two of the patients had undergone sleep studies 2 years and 6 years, respectively, before their automobile accidents.

Conclusion.—Drivers with untreated sleep apnea may cause many preventable automobile accidents. Therefore, physicians have specific duties involving such patients. Physicians must try to identify impaired drivers with sleep apnea before they have an accident. Clinicians should routinely ask patients in at-risk groups about loud snoring and hypersomnolence. The diagnosis of sleep apnea should be considered when examining patients who fall asleep while driving. Physicians must warn patients about the risks of driving with untreated sleep apnea. Finally, clinicians must treat seriously impaired drivers and prevent them from driving until they can be treated successfully.

▶ State laws generally prohibit drivers with uncontrolled epilepsy and other causes of loss of consciousness from driving. There is increasing concern that other neurologic conditions, such as dementia, can cause serious motor-vehicle accidents. This paper highlights the risk of untreated sleep apnea and makes recommendations for physicians. We should also add alcoholism and psychiatric conditions, including depression, to the list of disorders to be considered in this context.—W.G. Bradley, D.M., F.R.C.P.

Neuronal Activity in Narcolepsy: Identification of Cataplexy-Related Cells in the Medial Medulla

Siegel JM, Nienhuis R, Fahringer HM, Paul R, Shiromani P, Dement WC, Mignot E, Chiu C (VA Med Ctr, Sepulveda, Calif; Univ of Calif, Los Angeles; San Diego Veterans Affairs Med Ctr; Univ of California, La Jolla; Stanford Univ, Palo Alto, Calif)

Science 252:1315–1318, 1991   12–2

Background.—Narcoleptic dogs exhibit most symptoms of human narcolepsy, including periods of rapid eye movement (REM) sleep just after the onset of sleep and increased sleepiness. If narcolepsy is a disease of REM sleep regulation, cataplexy and sleep paralysis presumably represent the triggering during waking of that mechanisms that ordinarily suppress muscle tone during REM sleep. This suppression of muscle tone requires an intact dorsolateral pons and medial medulla.

Methods.—Narcoleptic dogs had microwires implanted in the brain stem, and cataplexy was elicited by play and by presenting preferred foods. Physostigmine was sometimes given to increase the frequency of cataplexy.

Findings.—A group of cells in the medial medulla were active during both cataplexy and REM sleep. The cells were noncholinergic and were localized to the ventromedial and caudal regions of the magnocellular nucleus. Most of the medullary cells were inactive during cataplexy and active during REM sleep.

Discussion.—A population of cells with a common pattern of activity in cataplexy and REM sleep is present in the medullary area implicated in control of atonia, suggesting a common basis for cataplexy and REM sleep atonia. Apparently, the generalized phasic activation of brain stem neurons characterizing REM sleep does not take place in cataplexy.

▶ Narcolepsy appears to be very similar in dogs and humans. This study of narcoleptic dogs identifies a group of neurons in the brain stem that fire at high rates during an attack of cataplexy and also during REM sleep. Further study of these dogs may complete our understanding of the human condition.—W.G. Bradley, D.M., F.R.C.P.

Brain Neurotransmitter Changes in Human Narcolepsy

Kish SJ, Mamelak M, Slimovitch C, Dixon LM, Lewis A, Shannak K, DiStefano

L, Chang LJ, Hornykiewicz O (Univ of Toronto, Ont, Canada; Univ of Vienna, Austria)
Neurology 42:229–234, 1992   12–3

Introduction.—Animal and human pharmacologic studies of narcolepsy suggest that the function of several biogenic amine neurotransmitter systems may be altered. The concentrations of noradrenaline, dopamine, and serotonin—as well as their metabolites and receptor binding sites—were estimated in autopsy brain samples from 3 patients with narcolepsy.

Findings.—Compared with controls, the levels of noradrenaline and serotonin metabolites (MHPG, 5-HIAA) were markedly increased in cerebral cortical samples from the patients with narcolepsy. Two of the 3 patients had a moderate reduction in α_1-adrenoceptors, as judged from reduced levels of ^{3}H-prazosin binding. The striatal levels of dopamine and its metabolite, homovanillic acid, were normal, but dihydroxyphenylacetic acid (the second metabolite of dopamine) was reduced markedly. Binding of tritiated spiperone to the D_2 dopamine receptor was increased in the caudate and putamen.

Implications.—These findings indicate that brain monoaminergic neurotransmitter function is altered in human narcolepsy. The monoaminergic neuronal systems involved have been implicated in the regulation of sleep-wakefulness activity in humans.

▶ Dogs suffering from narcolepsy have been shown to have dysfunction of the brain stem neurons and increased levels of dopamine D_2 receptor. This autopsy study of the brains of 3 humans with narcolepsy demonstrates a somewhat similar finding. The details remain to be elucidated, but there is a clear abnormality of noradrenaline, dopamine, and serotonin metabolism, which may lead to improved understanding and treatment.—W.G. Bradley, D.M., F.R.C.P.

13 Ataxia

Cerebrotendinous Xanthomatosis
Baumgartner RW, Hauser V, Grob P, Waespe W (Universitätsspital, Zürich, Switzerland)
Schweiz med Wochenschr 121:858–864, 1991   13–1

Introduction.—Cerebrotendinous xanthomatosis (CTX) is a rare familial disorder of lipid metabolism based on an autosomal recessive defect of the liver enzyme 26-hydroxylase. The enzymal defect inhibits the biosynthesis of cholic acid and chenodeoxycholic acid, and promotes the synthesis of cholestanol and cholesterol in the liver, resulting in cholestanol and cholesterol accumulation in most tissues. The clinical manifestations of CTX are progressive neurologic deficits with intellectual deterioration, juvenile cataracts, and xanthoma of the tendons. The literature on CTX was evaluated, and 3 new cases were studied.

Patients.—Cerebrotendineous xanthomatosis was first described in 1937. Since then, more than 100 cases have been reported, including 44 in Japan, 26 in the United States, 40 in Europe, and 18 in Israel. Until the 3 patients studied were diagnosed, CTX had not previously been seen in Switzerland. All 3 patients were men aged 35–43 years at the time of diagnosis. Two of the patients were brothers. The parents of the third patient were blood relatives. All 3 patients had bilateral juvenile cataracts. Two patients underwent cataract operations on both eyes when they were in their twenties. The third patient has not yet undergone surgery. All 3 patients had spastic ataxia with severe locomotor disturbances. Two patients started to deteriorate mentally in early childhood, and both got progressively worse as they got older. Biopsy specimens of the Achilles tendon showed xanthoma formation in 2 patients. Magnetic resonance (MR) imaging of the brain showed abnormal findings in 2 patients. The third patient had normal MR scans. All 3 patients had increased urinary bile alcohol excretion.

Diagnosis.—The early diagnosis of CTX is important, because timely administration of chenodeoxycholic acid (at doses ranging from 750 to 1,000 mg daily) has been shown to reduce plasma cholestanol levels and slow cholestanol and cholesterol synthesis. Clinically, chenodeoxycholic acid therapy slows the progression of neurologic deterioration and improves the typical thought disturbances; disorientation; and spastic, ataxic, and polyneuropathologic symptoms. A decrease in tendinous xanthoma or a slowing of cataract formation have not been observed. However, chenodeoxycholic acid clearly reduces the cholestanol concentration in the plasma and CSF. and it also reduces urinary bile alcohol excretion.

Conclusion.—A diagnosis of CTX should be suspected in any patient with chronic progressive spastic-ataxic symptoms, juvenile cataracts of unclear etiology, and tendinous xanthoma in the presence of normal or slightly increased serum lipid levels.

▶ The hereditary ataxias present a difficult diagnostic problem for the clinician. A few ataxias, such as those associated with vitamin E deficiency, are treatable. Cerebrotendinous xanthomatosis is yet a further rare type of hereditary ataxia. This paper highlights some of the diagnostic pointers, such as early cataracts and mental deterioration. Detailed biochemical studies should be undertaken in such patients.—W.G. Bradley, D.M., F.R.C.P.

Treatment of Heredo-Degenerative Ataxias With Amantadine Hydrochloride
Botez MI, Young SN, Botez T, Pedraza OL (Hôtel-Dieu Hosp, Université de Montréal; McGill Univ, Montréal, Quebec, Canada)
Can J Neurol Sci 18:307–311, 1991   13–2

Background.—In a preliminary study, patients with Friedreich's ataxia (FA) and olivopontocerebellar atrophies (OPCA) were found to have low levels of the dopamine metabolite, homovanillic acid (HVA), in the cerebrospinal fluid (CSF). Because amantadine hydrochloride (AH) stimulates dopamine release, an open clinical trial was conducted to determine the therapeutic effects of AH on patients with FA and OPCA.

Treatment.—Seventeen patients with FA and 12 patients with OPCA were treated with AH, 100 mg/day, for the initial week; they were then given 200 mg/day. Therapy was continued for at least 3.5 months, with 1 exception. The mean duration of treatment was 7.9 months (range 1.5–26) for patients with FA and 8.9 months (range, 4–23) for the patients with OPCA. The visual and auditory reaction time (RT) and movement time (MT) with the right and left hand were measured before and after treatment.

Results.—For patients with OPCA, AH improved performance in 7 of 8 RT and MT measures. For patients with FA, AH improved performance on only 2 of 4 MT measures and on visual and auditory MT with the right hand; there was no improvement in RT. Patients with both OPCA and FA had low pretreatment levels of CSF HVA compared with age-matched controls, but there was no correlation between CSF HVA levels and improvement with AH. Subjective improvement was striking in patients with OPCA, but it was less evident or absent in patients with FA.

Discussion.—It appears that patients with OPCA respond better to AH than do patients with FA. Because the lesions in OPCA include cell bodies in the cerebellum, the more pronounced effect of AH in OPCA may be a result of direct interaction between damaged neurons and dopaminergic pathways. The lesions in FA are mainly spinocerebellar, and the interaction between the affected site and dopaminergic neurons is more indirect. It also has been proposed that the neuronal damage associated with neurodegenerative disorders may be related to excitation of N-methyl-D-aspartate (NMDA) receptors. The more pronounced effect of AH in patients with OPCA may be caused by the action of AH on NMDA receptors, which is also exerted strictly at the cerebellar level.

▶ This interesting open study will prompt the use of amantadine for the treatment of patients with FA and OPCA. However, as in all open studies, the placebo response may have caused the improvement, and a double-blind controlled study is essential before therapeutic benefit can be believed. We hope that the authors will undertake this next step.—W.G. Bradley, D.M., F.R.C.P.

14 Cerebral Palsy

Hemiplegic Cerebral Palsy: Correlation Between CT Morphology and Clinical Findings
Wiklund L-M, Uvebrant P (Children's Hosp, Göteborg, Sweden)
Dev Med Child Neurol 33:512–523, 1991   14–1

Introduction.—There is evidence from recent CT studies that spastic hemiplegic cerebral palsy (CP) among children born at term is mostly of prenatal origin, whereas that among children born preterm develops mainly in the perinatal period. The correlation between CT and clinical findings was analyzed in a population-based series of Swedish children with hemiplegic CP.

Study Design.—The study population consisted of 111 children (age, 5–16 years) with hemiplegic CP, of whom 28 were born preterm and 83 were born at term, and for whom at least 1 CT scan was available. The CT morphology was related to a number of clinical features, including type of hemiplegia, motor impairment, sensory impairment, other neurologic signs, growth impairment of the affected limb, additional impairments, and total handicap.

Findings.—Computed tomography was abnormal in 82 children and normal in 29. Thirteen children had bilateral lesions. Nineteen CT scans showed maldevelopment, 47 showed periventricular abnormalities, 13 had cortical/subcortical findings, and 3 had other abnormalities. All unilateral abnormal CT findings were located in the hemisphere corresponding to the hemiplegic side. There was no significant correlation between the size of the lesion and the severity of motor and other neurologic impairments within morphologic groups; however, some trends were found. Small lesions implied mild-to-moderate impairments, whereas large lesions implied moderate-to-severe impairments. Children with normal CT findings were significantly less impaired. Preterm children did not differ significantly from those born at term. Left-sided hemiplegia predominated among children born preterm (64%), whereas right-sided hemiplegia predominated among those born at term (58%). In the 13 children with bilateral lesions, the hemisphere with the dominating abnormalities correspond to the hemiplegic side. The 13 children with cortical/subcortical atrophy were more seriously impaired. Cortical lesions were associated with more severe epilepsy, arm-dominated hemiplegia, poor hand function, and facial weakness. Cortical involvement was also significantly related to low IQ. Children with normal CT findings more often had leg-dominated, modest hemiplegia; good hand function; no facial weakness; and mild motor impairment, and they only very rarely had epilepsy.

Conclusion.—The morphologic findings from CT scans of children with hemiplegic CP are useful for predicting clinical outcome, and they can be considered an important adjunct to the clinical history and clinical findings in these children.

▶ Neuroimaging has contributed much to the understanding of the mechanisms of cerebral palsy. Two groups that remain baffling are those with normal CT and those in which 1 hemisphere is generally smaller (the group categorized in this paper as cortical/subcortical atrophy). The normal group may be better defined by MRI, which is more likely to demonstrate heterotopia. No explanation is available for the group with underdevelopment of 1 hemisphere.—G.M. Fenichel, M.D.

Altered Corticospinal Projections to Lower Limb Motoneurons in Subjects With Cerebral Palsy

Brouwer B, Ashby P (Univ of Toronto; Toronto Western Hosp)
Brain 114:1395–1407, 1991   14–2

Background.—The neurophysiologic abnormalities underlying the various motor disorders of cerebral palsy (CP) have not been established. One explanation for the co-contraction of muscles during voluntary movements is that the projections of the descending pathways to the motoneurons are abnormal. This possibility was investigated.

Methods.—Twenty-two healthy individuals and 14 individuals with CP were investigated. The projections of the cortical neurons activated by

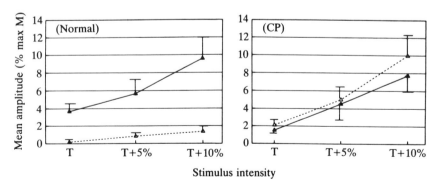

Fig 14–1.—Means of the relative amplitudes (+1 SE) of the contralateral responses recorded from TA (*filled triangles*) and SOL (*open triangles*) after magnetic stimulation (pooled data from C2-C3 and C2-C4 stimulation sites) from 10 controls and 8 patients with CP. The amplitudes of the compound muscle action potentials are expressed as a percentage of that muscle's maximum M wave (% max M). (Courtesy of Brouwer B, Ashby P: *Brain* 114:1395–1407, 1991.)

transcranial magnetic stimulation to the motoneurons of lower limb muscles were assessed.

Results.—Magnetic stimulation produced strong facilitation of tibialis anterior (TA) motoneurons in healthy individuals and little or no facilitation of the soleus (SOL) motoneurons. This differential facilitation occurred at all stimulus sites on the scalp and at all stimulus intensities at which responses were elicited. In individuals with CP, magnetic stimulation facilitated TA and SOL motoneurons almost equally, a finding that could not be explained by differences in the excitability of the respective motoneuron pools (Fig 14-1).

Conclusion.—Lesions of the immature human brain and corticospinal tract may result in altered corticospinal projections. These altered projections seem to be directed equally to the motoneurons of both agonist and antagonist ankle muscles in individuals with CP. This may explain why voluntary movements in those with CP are frequently disrupted by co-contraction of flexor and extensor muscles.

▶ One of the basic organizational arrangements of the CNS is reciprocal innervation of the muscles. During most movements and reflex activities, this ensures that, as 1 muscle contracts, the antagonist muscle relaxes. In this elegant investigation, Drs. Brouwer and Ashby have shown a breakdown of the typical reciprocal relationship between the TA and SOL muscles in patients with CP. Their data indicate that the co-contraction of muscles is caused by an abnormality of the projections from the motor cortex to the spinal motoneurons which results from the lesions of the immature nervous system responsible for CP. It is a beautiful example in the undeveloped CNS of plasticity—the reorganization of the CNS after injury.—R.A. Davidoff, M.D.

15 Chiropractic Manipulation Risks

Vertebrobasilar Ischemia After Neck Motion
Frisoni GB, Anzola GP (Università di Brescia, Brescia, Italy)
Stroke 22:1452–1460, 1991   15–1

Introduction.—Vertebrobasilar ischemic stroke can occur after chiropractic manipulation of the cervical spine, and it is seen less often after spontaneous and abrupt head movement. Three such cases were evaluated, and 36 previously reported cases were reviewed.

Clinical Aspects.—Half of the patients reviewed had head or neck pain on the side of the lesion. The symptoms frequently developed during or after the first manipulation. Five percent of the patients had an occipital lobe syndrome; 8% each had cerebellar and locked-in syndrome; 28% had Wallenberg's syndrome; and 49% had other brain stem disorders. A total of 28% of the patients died or had very severe long-term impairment.

Mechanisms.—Head rotation may lead to an asymptomatic cessation of flow in 1 or both vertebral arteries at the level of the atlantoaxial joint. Transient or intractable arterial spasm has been proposed, but it has not been proven. Vascular damage often is claimed when vertebrobasilar ischemia occurs after neck motion, but definitive evidence is not available. Progressive or delayed symptoms may develop secondary to thrombosis or a slowly progressive dissection.

Implications.—Patients at risk of vertebrobasilar ischemia following sudden neck motion cannot be identified a priori. If neurologic symptoms develop during cervical manipulation, further maneuvers are strongly contraindicated. The risks and benefits of manipulation must be carefully considered; complications probably are more frequent than generally thought.

▶ Chiropractic manipulation can be of symptomatic benefit for a good number of the pains of modern life, even though there is uncertainty about the scientific validity of many aspects of the discipline. There is, however, 1 area in which chiropractic manipulation should never be allowed—the cervical spine. This study describes 3 new cases and reviews the literature on patients who had vertebrobasilar strokes caused by chiropractic manipulation. The message of this study should be carried to the lay public and the chiropractic profession.—W.G. Bradley, D.M., F.R.C.P.

16 Normal Pressure Hydrocephalus and Pseudotumor Cerebri

Shunting Normal-Pressure Hydrocephalus: Do the Benefits Outweigh the Risks? A Multicenter Study and Literature Review
Vanneste J, Augustijn P, Dirven C, Tan WF, Goedhart ZD (St Lucasziekenhuis, Amsterdam; Free Univ of Amsterdam; Univ of Amsterdam; Municipal Hosp Slotervaart, Amsterdam)
Neurology 42:54–59, 1992   16–1

Background.—In the treatment of normal-pressure hydrocephalus (NPH), physicians must balance the possibility of missing a treatable dementia or gait disorder and the risks of ventricular drainage. To address this question, a clinical study was performed, the literature on NPH was studied, and the findings of these 2 studies were compared.

Methods.—In the clinical study, 166 consecutive patients who underwent a shunting procedure for NPH were evaluated. The patients were treated during 9½ years at 4 neurosurgical departments. Improvement was graded on a scale of 0 (no improvement) to +2 (marked improvement in gait, mental disturbances, or both). In the literature study, appropriate literature from 1966 to 1990 was examined to determine the

TABLE 1.—Multicenter Study: Improvement Depending on Etiology

Etiology of NPH	No. pts	Grades of improvement		
		None	Slight	Marked
Idiopathic	127	87	21	19 (15%)
Known etiology, communicating	11	7	0	4 (36%)
Known etiology, noncommunicating	14	3	2	9 (64%)
Total	152	97 (64%)	23 (15%)	32 (21%)

Percentages are rounded off upward or downward.
(Courtesy of Vanneste J, Augustijn P, Dirven C, et al: *Neurology* 42:54–59, 1992.)

TABLE 2.—Multicenter Study: Shunt-Related Complications and Residual Harm

Type	Total	Complications			Death	Residual harm		
		Severe	Moderate	Mild		Much worse	Worse	No
Ischemic strokes	5	1	2	2	1	—	2	2
Cerebral hemorrhages	8	4	2	2	4	1	2	1
Subdural hematomas and effusions	23	9	3	11	—	—	2	21
Intracranial infections	6	4	2	—	—	1	1	4
Epileptic seizures	5	2	2	1	—	—	—	5
Extracranial infections	>25*	4	3	>18*	4	—	1	>20*
Others	>39*	—	4	>35*	—	—	2	>39*
Total	>111* (73%)	24 (16%)	18 (12%)	>69* (45%)	9 (6%)	2 (1.3%)	10 (6.6%)	>92*

* Exact data not available.
Percentages in parentheses are rounded up or down to the unit.
(Courtesy of Vanneste J, Augustijn P, Dirven C, et al: Neurology 42:54–59, 1992.)

expected rate of improvement and complications in patients with shunted NPH.

Results.—In the clinical study, 64% of the patients failed to improve (Table 1). Improvement rates varied by etiologic group, with the largest subgroup—idiopathic NPH—having the lowest rate of marked improvement. The study area had an incidence of shunt-responsive NPH of 2.2/million/year. A total of 28% of the patients had severe or moderate shunt-related complications, and 7% died or were left with severe residual morbidity (Table 2). The ratio of substantial benefit to serious harm was only 3, and that for idiopathic NPH was only 1.7. In recent studies, the overall improvement rate increased to 74%, but the complication rate remained at 36%.

Conclusion.—Significant improvement after shunting for NPH will occur in only 15% to 20% of the patients, depending on the cause of the disorder. This is considerably lower than is commonly thought. In patients with good surgical risks, death or serious morbidity will occur in 2% to 3% of all patients with NPH and 8% to 9% of patients with idiopathic NPH.

▶ This study confirms many previous reports indicating that only a small proportion (10% to 20%) of patients with presumed NPH improve with shunting. It also emphasizes much higher morbidity and mortality rates than are generally recognized from shunting these patients; these rates are particularly high in those patients with idiopathic NPH. If there is nothing to lose by shunting, the procedure is often recommended to patients. The morbidity and mortality experience should temper this enthusiasm.—W.G. Bradley, D.M., F.R.C.P.

Fatal Tonsillar Herniation in Pseudotumor Cerebri

Sullivan HC (Case Western Reserve Univ Hosp, Cleveland)
Neurology 41:1142–1144, 1991   16–2

Background.—Pseudotumor cerebri rarely poses a threat to life. Likewise, its evaluation and treatment do not usually pose a serious risk to the patient. A young woman with pseudotumor cerebri who herniated after lumbar puncture (LP) and died was evaluated.

Case Report.—Woman, 27, was admitted in 1984 with the "worst headache of her life," which was relieved by neck hyperextension and was aggravated by neck flexion and movement. A CT scan showed no mass or hemorrhage. An LP showed an opening pressure of 350 mm H_2O, with a cell count of 0. Shortly after the LP, the patient became lethargic, had nystagmus and right-sided weakness, and went into respiratory arrest requiring intubation. Early papilledema was evident. Magnetic resonance imaging showed slightly low positioning of the cerebellar tonsils with a normal fourth ventricle. The patient improved. Four years later, she was readmitted with severe headache, productive cough, and fever. Her previous medical records were not available, and she denied any previous illness. After LP was performed, with opening pressure of 450 mm H_2O and 9 white blood cells (50% polymorphs), the patient became lethargic, had blurred disk margins, brisk symmetric reflexes, and bilateral extensor plantar responses. A second LP was performed for more spinal fluid, with opening pressure of less than 250 mm H_2O. The patient had a respiratory arrest. Although an endotracheal tube was inserted, the patient died. Autopsy showed no Arnold-Chiari malformation. The cerebellar tonsils were necrotic. The spinal cord and medulla were tumescent, which was consistent with prolonged ventilation of infarcted brain stem and spinal cord secondary to the herniation.

Conclusion.—Only 1 other case has been reported in the literature with regard to this rare complication of LP in a patient with pseudotumor cerebri. Any patient who is seen with clinical signs and symptoms of pseudotumor cerebri, which is associated with focal neurologic signs or symptoms suggestive of a posterior fossa lesion, should undergo MRI before LP. Lumbar puncture should be performed cautiously in patients in whom neuroimaging does not clearly demonstrate the presence of a craniocervical lesion but, rather, low-lying cerebellar tonsils.

▶ This case is extremely worrying for the clinician. The patient's initial presentation suggested subarachnoid hemorrhage. Relief of the headache by neck extension is usually the converse of what is expected with tonsillar herniation. Innumerable patients with pseudotumor cerebri have undergone spinal tap without complication, but this report will cause all of us to carefully evaluate the need for spinal tap in such cases.—W.G. Bradley, D.M., F.R.C.P.

17 Neuro-Ophthalmology

Isolated and Combined Pareses of Cranial Nerves III, IV and VI: A Retrospective Study of 412 Patients
Berlit P (Univ of Heidelburg, Mannheim, Germany)
J Neurol Sci 103:10–15, 1991   17–1

Background.—The prognosis is good for most ocular nerve pareses, but their diagnosis and treatment remain controversial. The value of various procedures was studied retrospectively in 412 patients with isolated ocular nerve paresis treated before the advent of MRI.

Methods.—The records of 412 patients treated between 1970 and 1985 were reviewed. The main sign in each case was ocular nerve paresis, and 52 patients had asymptomatic sensory or reflex asymmetry. The patients were treated for at least 2 weeks with anti-inflammatory drugs or measures directed to correct diabetes, hypertension, or lipid abnormalities, depending on the cause. Etiologic groups included inflammation, tumors, aneurysms, trauma, vascular origin, other causes mimicking ocular nerve palsies, and unclear origin (table).

Results.—There were 172 oculomotor nerve palsies, 165 abducens nerve palsies, and 25 trochlear nerve palsies. There were 50 cases of combined ocular nerve palsy, consisting of the third and sixth cranial nerves, in 21 cases and pareses of all 3 nerves in 17 cases. Of the 165 palsies resulting from vascular causes, 135 involved diabetes mellitus and hypertension. The most commonly affected nerve was the oculomotor, with no involvement of the pupil in 63% of cases. The abducens nerve was the most commonly affected in inflammatory disease and brain tumor, along with aneurysm of the oculomotor nerve. In 73 patients, the cause of the ophthalmoplegia was unclear. Tumors, aneurysm, and vascular processes were the most common causes of ocular nerve paralysis, which was only partial in 206 cases. Pain was present with tumor, trauma, and aneurysm, and it was much less common with trochlear palsies than with palsies of the other 2 nerves. Of the 352 patients in whom the clinical course was followed for 3 weeks, 191 had complete regression and 59 had only partial recovery. Inflammatory and vascular lesions carried the best prognosis. The outcome of vascular lesions was improved with nonsteroidal anti-inflammatory drugs.

Conclusion.—Cranial nerve pareses may result from a variety of causes. Magnetic resonance imaging may aid diagnosis when cause is not apparent. The disease can be allowed to take its course in patients with diabetes mellitus or hypertension who have ocular nerve mononeuropa-

Etiologic Factors in Isolated and Combined Pareses of Cranial Nerves III, IV, and VI

	All (n = 412)	N.III (n = 172)	N.IV (n = 25)	N.VI (n = 165)	Combined (n = 50)
Vascular lesion	40	49	56	30	36
with diabetes mellitus or hypertension	33	42	52	24	20
other causes	7	7	4	6	16
Inflammation	15	11	12	19	16
multiple sclerosis	5	3	8	7	2
infection	10	8	4	12	14
Tumor	9	7	–	11	14
Aneurysm	58	9	–	4	2
Trauma	44	6	12	3	–
Other known causes	8	8	–	4	26
Unknown	170	10	20	29	6

Note: Values are given in percent; n = 412.
(Courtesy of Berlit P: J Neurol Sci 103:10–15, 1991.)

thy, but a basic diagnosis should be made in other cases. Tumor or muscular or orbital disease must be excluded in patients with combined ocular motor nerve pareses.

▶ Extraocular nerve palsies always present a difficult diagnostic problem, and more information is always worthwhile. This study reviews the Heidelburg experience in the era before MRI scans. It contains a good deal of interesting observations.—W.G. Bradley, D.M., F.R.C.P.

18 Neuro-Otology

Benign Positional Vertigo: Incidence and Prognosis in a Population-Based Study in Olmsted County, Minnesota
Froehling DA, Silverstein MD, Mohr DN, Beatty CW, Offord KP, Ballard DJ
(Mayo Clinic, Rochester, Minn)
Mayo Clin Proc 66:596–601, 1991   18–1

Introduction.—Patients with benign positional vertigo (BPV) are generally believed to have a good prognosis, but their risk of serious CNS disorders is unknown.

Methods.—To determine the incidence, persistence, and risk of CNS disorders in patients with BPV, a population-based medical records linkage system for residents of Olmsted County, Minnesota, was reviewed to identify patients in whom BPV was newly diagnosed in 1984. Transient episodes of vertigo—with no other signs and symptoms except positional nystagmus—was the definition of BPV. Of 467 patients with vertigo, dizziness, or labyrinthitis, 195 was excluded for insufficient documentation of vertigo, 75 for continuous vertigo, 65 for absence of vertigo, 49 for previous onset of BPV, 10 each for new CNS findings and orthostatic hypotension, and 10 for various conditions or missing records. Data on 53 patients were available for analysis.

Results.—Adjusted for age and sex, the incidence of BPV was 64/100,000 population/year, and it increased by approximately 38% with each decade of life. The chief complaint was vertigo in 92% of patients, and 77% were initially examined in an internal or family medicine clinic. Only 1 patient had a stroke during follow-up; the relative risk for new stroke in these patients, compared with the expected incidence in an age- and sex-matched control population, was 1.62. Survival was not significantly different between the BPV and control groups.

Conclusion.—It appears that BPV is associated with a good prognosis. One source of bias in this study is exclusion of patients with insufficient documentation of vertigo; if these patients had the same rate of BPV as the study cohort, the incidence would have been about 107/100,000 population/year. In addition, the study does not address the risk of BPV associated with head trauma.

▶ Benign positional vertigo is a relatively common problem in practice. Perhaps half the patients have a posttraumatic syndrome, and half are idiopathic. This paper reviews the latter syndrome, which clearly has a benign prognosis and does not herald future neurologic or general disease. One drawback of the study is the large number of excluded patients for whom similar follow-up data would have been interesting.—W.G. Bradley, D.M., F.R.C.P.

Suggested Reading

Cedarbaum JM, Gandy SE, McDowell FH: "Early" initiation of levodopa treatment does not promote the development of motor response fluctuations, dyskinesias, or dementia in Parkinson's disease. *Neurology* 41:622–629, 1991.

D'Costa DF, Abbott RJ, Pye IF, et al: The apomorphine test in Parkinsonian syndromes. *J Neurol Neurosurg Psychiatry* 54:870–872, 1991.

Dexter DT, Carayon A, Javoy-Agid F, et al: Alterations in the levels of iron, ferritin and other trace metals in Parkinson's disease and other neurodegenerative diseases affecting the basal ganglia. *Brain* 114:1953–1975, 1991.

Durner M, Sander T, Greenberg DA, et al: Localization of idiopathic generalized epilepsy on chromosome 6p in families of juvenile myoclonic epilepsy patients. *Neurology* 41:1651–1655, 1991.

Fenichel GM, Florence JM, Pestronk A, et al: Long-term benefit from prednisone therapy in duchenne muscular dystrophy. *Neurology* 41:1874–1877, 1991.

Guldvog B, Loyning Y, Hauglie-Hanssen E, et al: Surgical versus medical treatment for epilepsy. I. Outcome related to survival, seizures, and neurologic deficit. *Epilepsia* 32:375–388, 1991.

Hietanen MH: Selegiline and cognitive function in Parkinson's disease. *Acta Neurol Scand* 84:407–410, 1991.

Holmberg BH, Hägg E, Hagenfeldt L: Adrenomyeloneuropathy—Report on a family. *J Intern Med* 230:535–538, 1991.

Kawabata S, Higgins GA, Gordon JW: Amyloid plaques, neurofibrillary tangles and neuronal loss in brains of transgenic mice overexpressing a c-terminal fragment of human amyloid precursor protein. *Nature* 354:476–478, 1991.

Logar C, Boswell M: The value of EEG-mapping in focal cerebral lesions. *Brain Topogr* 3:441–446, 1991.

Mash DC, Pablo J, Buck BE, et al: Distribution and number of transferrin receptors in Parkinson's disease and in MPTP-treated mice. *Exp Neurol* 114:73–81, 1991.

McDonald JW, Garofalo EA, Hood T, et al: Altered excitatory and inhibitory amino acid receptor binding in hippocampus of patients with temporal lobe epilepsy. *Ann Neurol* 29:529–541, 1991.

Meierkord H, Will B, Fish D, et al: The clinical features and prognosis of pseudoseizures diagnosed using video-EEG telemetry. *Neurology* 41:1643–1646, 1991.

Mhiri C, Baudrimont M, Bonne G, et al: Zidovudine myopathy: A distinctive disorder associated with mitochondrial dysfunction. *Ann Neurol* 29:606–614, 1991.

Murata K, Araki S: Autonomic nervous system dysfunction in workers exposed to lead, zinc, and copper in relation to peripheral nerve conduction: A study of R-R interval variability. *Am J Ind Med* 20:663–671, 1991.

Palmini A, Andermann F, Aicardi J, et al: Diffuse cortical dysplasia, or the 'double cortex' syndrome: The clinical and epileptic spectrum in 10 patients. *Neurology* 41:1656–1662, 1991.

Panayiotopoulos CP, Tahan R, Obeid T: Juvenile myoclonic epilepsy: Factors of error involved in the diagnosis and treatment. *Epilepsia* 32:672–676, 1991.

Peterson GM, Khoo BHC, von Witt RJ: Clinical response in epilepsy in relation to total and free serum levels of phenytoin. *Ther Drug Monit* 13:415–419, 1991.

Puce A, Bladin PF: Scalp and Limbic P3 event-related potentials in the assessment of patients with temporal lobe epilepsy. *Epilepsia* 32:629–634, 1991.

Roberts GW, Gentleman SM, Lynch A, et al: βA4 amyloid protein deposition in brain after head trauma. *Lancet* 338:1422–1423, 1991.

Selmaj K, Raine CS, Cross AH: Anti-tumor necrosis factor therapy abrogates autoimmune demyelination. *Ann Neurol* 30:694–700, 1991.

Semchuk KM, Love EJ, Lee RG: Parkinson's disease and exposure to rural environmental factors: A population based case-control study. *Can J Neurol Sci* 18:279–286, 1991.

Shoffner JM, Watts RL, Juncos JL, et al: Mitochondrial oxidative phosphorylation defects in Parkinson's disease. *Ann Neurol* 30:332–339, 1991.

Singer HS, Hahn I-H, Moran TH: Abnormal dopamine uptake sites in postmortem striatum from patients with Tourette's Syndrome. *Ann Neurol* 30:558–562, 1991.

Verity CM, Golding J: Risk of epilepsy after febrile convulsions: A national cohort study. *BMJ* 303:1373–1376, 1991.

Walker R, Findlay JM, Young AW, et al: Disentangling neglect and hemianopia. *Neuropsychologia* 29:1019–1027, 1991.

Wijdicks EFM, Ropper AH, Hunnicutt EJ, et al: Atrial natriuretic factor and salt wasting after aneurysmal subarachnoid hemorrhage *Stroke* 22:1519–1524, 1991.

Woods BT, Kinney DK, Yurgelum-Todd DA: Neurological "hard" signs and family history of psychosis in schizophrenia. *Biol Psychiatry* 30:806–816, 1991.

NEUROSURGERY

ROBERT M. CROWELL, M.D.

Introduction

High technology continues to generate progress in neurologic surgery. Increasingly, MRI (and its offshoot, MR angiography) have become the studies of choice for neurosurgical conditions. Remarkable improvements in diagnosis have been made in MRI with the use of contrast agents (Abstract 19-3) and spectacular 3-dimensional rendering of the cortical surface (Abstract 19-1). Magnetic resonance angiography can now depict (with rather reliable images) both the cervical vessels (Abstracts 19-4 and 19-5) and the intracranial vessels (Abstracts 19-6 and 19-8). Other diagnostic techniques that have advanced recently are SPECT (Abstract 19-9), transcranial infrared spectroscopy (Abstract 19-10), and motor evoked potentials (Abstract 19-11).

Radiosurgery has further blossomed in 1992 through the application of high technology methods. Rather impressive results for invasive pituitary tumors have been observed after gamma knife treatment (Abstract 20-4). In some centers, fractionated radiosurgery has been used with encouraging results (Abstract 20-6). In some cases, radiosurgical treatment of arteriovenous malformations has led to symptomatic vasogenic edema, which usually is transitory (Abstract 20-5).

Endovascular therapy has advanced with improvements in angiography and catheter technology. Particularly exciting are the encouraging results reported in the treatment of intracranial aneurysms with platinum alloy Gugliemi detachable coils. Preoperative embolization with polyvinyl alcohol appears to be quite safe before excision of intracranial arteriovenous malformations (Abstract 20-7).

In contrast with minimally invasive treatments, *skull base microsurgery* has become ever more invasive, pursuing tumors into the cavernous sinus and other zones that previously were thought to be inoperable. By the application of refined surgical anatomy, detailed imaging, and refined microsurgery, remarkable total excisions have been achieved in this way. Examples are found in the combined supra- and infratentorial total resection of petroclival tumors (Abstract 21-16) and in the removal of clinoidal meningiomas that may involve the cavernous sinus (Abstract 21-17). In the vascular field, elective cardiopulmonary bypass and cardiac arrest have given good results for very difficult aneurysms (Abstract 23-7), and a transoral approach has permitted obliteration of mid-basilar aneurysms (Abstract 23-10).

Statistical studies are helping to establish indications for modern therapies by comparing the natural history and clinical results. Despite a welter of studies, the role of aggressive resection for gliomas remains poorly defined (Abstract 21-1). By contrast, it has required only a small number of successful total excisions of choroid plexus carcinoma to demonstrate the superiority of this approach (Abstract 21-10). A large statistical study has demonstrated clearly that intra-arterial 1, 3-bis-(2-chloroethyl)-1-nitrosourea is of no value for intracranial glioma (Abstract 21-4). For a number of adjunctive tumor treatments, data is insufficient to establish many therapies, such as brachytherapy (Abstracts 21–2 and 21–3), hyper-fractionation for glioma (Abstract 21–6) and chemotherapy for oligo-dendroglioma (Abstract 21–9). A sizable follow-up study of acoustic neu-roma has suggested that conservative therapy may be a very satisfactory option in some cases (Abstract 21–24). In *ischemia*, ongoing statistical studies should help define indications for endarterectomy of asymptom-atic carotid stenosis (Abstracts 22–1, 22–2, and 22–3). For *intracranial hemorrhage*, a large multicenter study has demonstrated superiority in North America for early operation of intracranial aneurysms (Abstract 23–4). Statistical studies have suggested a higher risk for hemorrhage from arteriovenous malformations with intranidal aneurysms (Abstract 23–19) and limited venous drainage (Abstract 23–18). The natural his-tory of cavernous angioma suggests a very benign outlook for asymptom-atic lesions (Abstract 23–23), but progressive downhill course from cer-tain brain stem lesions warrants surgical resection, which may improve status (23–24, 23–25). *Venous anomalies* appear to have an extremely low rate of hemorrhage, possibly nil (Abstract 23–26).

Physiologic studies have also helped the development of neurosurgical therapies. For *spinal cord trauma*, GM-1 ganglioside produced a statisti-cally significant benefit in controlled studies (Abstract 25–15). *Temporal lobectomy* guided by MRI and physiologic studies appears to offer sig-nificant benefit in patients older than 45 years of age (Abstract 28–1) and in the setting of reoperation after failed surgery (Abstract 28–2). For head injury, careful physiologically controlled studies have shown that *hyperventilation* may be harmful in some patients (Abstract 24–6). Re-garding *implantation* into the brain, adrenal-medullary transplantation for parkinsonism provides little useful benefit, with substantial complica-tions (Abstract 28–10), whereas fetal tissue implants (Abstract 28–8) and nerve growth factor (Abstract 28–9) yielded encouraging results in early studies.

Robert M. Crowell, M.D.

19 Diagnostics

MRI

Three-Dimensional In Vivo Mapping of Brain Lesions in Humans

Damasio H, Frank R (Univ of Iowa, Iowa City)
Arch Neurol 49:137–143, 1992
19–1

Background.—During the past 10 years, the study of patients with brain lesions has again become a principal means of elucidating the neural basis of cognition. A multistep technique for 3-dimensional reconstruction and analysis of brain lesions in vivo has been developed.

Technique.—The method is based on (1) obtaining raw MRI data with a particular protocol, in which the type of pulse sequence and the thickness of the cut play an important role; (2) a program to generate 3-dimensional reconstruction from 2-dimensional data; and (3) several programs to allow manipulation and cross-referencing of 3-dimensional and 2-dimensional data sets. The method involves both automated and interactive steps. First, a thin-cut MR scan is obtained with T1-weighted pulse sequence using 1 of 2 techniques. The raw MR data are transferred to magnetic tape, and each MR cut is brought on-line. The contour of the brain is traced to eliminate all nonbrain structures, and target structures are extracted from the raw slices using special software. The hemispheres are reconstructed. Voxel images can be generated after rotation over any coordinate axes. The image of damaged cortical tissue can then be clearly seen. When a particular sulcus is identified, it can be marked with color-coded points in the 3-dimensional voxel image. These points are then projected into the raw slice data. The marks can be used as a reference to define areas of interest. The reconstructed brain volume can be resliced in any plane, revealing the anatomical structures of the exposed section.

Conclusion.—This technique, which is based on the manipulation of MR raw data obtained in a special protocol, allows the direct visual identification of neuroanatomical landmarks in each brain specimen. It also eliminates the need to rely on averaged templates of human brain sections, which can be a source of error in localizing lesions. In addition, it allows for bidirectional cross-referencing between data points in 2-dimensional slices and volume reconstruction, and for subcortical structure projection onto the 3-dimensional cortical surface.

▶ The techniques of surface rendering that are so nicely demonstrated in Figure 2 in the original article undoubtedly will be of help to neurosurgeons planning an attack on superficial lesions. This is especially true for lesions related to eloquent gyral structures, such as the speech and motor cortex.—R.M. Crowell, M.D.

Magnetic Resonance Imaging of Human Spinal Cord Infarction

Nagashima C, Nagashima R, Morota N, Kobayashi S (Saitama Med School, Moro; Saitama-ken, Japan; Kobayashi Neurosurgical Hosp, Ueda, Nagano-ken, Japan)
Surg Neurol 35:368–373, 1991   19–2

Background.—Spinal cord infarction is rare. The thoracic cord is involved most often, followed by the cervical and lumbar areas. The literature contains no studies of surgically proven hemorrhagic spinal cord infarction on MRI, nor does it contain studies with sequential MR scans from the beginning to the late stage of ischemic cord infarction. Two patients were examined.

Patients.—The patients were 2 men, aged 50 and 52 years. One had hemorrhagic thoracic cord infarct, and the other had ischemic cervical cord infarct with sequential MR images. An enlarged cord with strand-shaped or longitudinal hypointensity on both T1- and T2-weighted images was seen in the hemorrhagic infarct (Fig 19–1). Hypointensity on the T2-weighted image was thought to result from hemosiderin, which shortens T2 relaxation. In the ischemic infarct, a small, round area of hypointensity on T1-weighted images and of hyperintensity on T2-weighted images seen 9 hours after ictus changed on day 22 to a cephalocaudal strandlike hypointensity on T1-weighted image enhanced by Gd-DTPA. This hypointensity suggested pencil-like softening in the infarct of medium age. On day 49 after ictus, it demonstrated an extensive homogeneous hypointensity involving several segments of the cord on T1-weighted images and hyperintensity on T2-weighted images with negative Gd-DTPA enhancement. This suggests "late transverse infarct."

Conclusion.—Magnetic resonance images obtained in 2 patients with spinal cord infarction were studied. The sequential changes seen from the beginning to the late stage may be valuable in diagnosing ischemic cord infarction and assessing the age of the cord infarct in individual patients.

▶ This study indicates that it is possible to image human spinal cord infarction. Other reports confirming this concept have appeared.—R.M. Crowell, M.D.

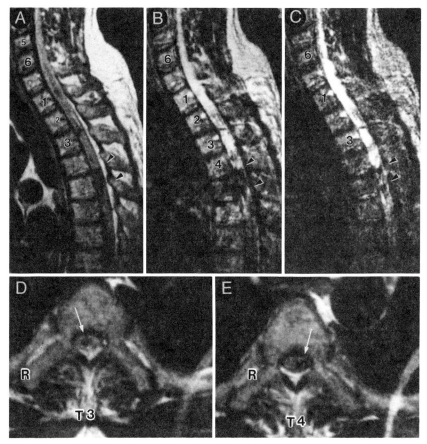

Fig 19–1.—A, midsagittal T1-weighted (TR/TE = 500/40 ms). **B**, proton density (TR/TE = 1,800/50). **C**, T2-weighted (TR/TE = 1,800/100) spin-echo MR images. Note the enlarged cord from C-6 to Th-6 levels, with multiple strand-shaped hypointensities in the cord from C-7 to Th-1, Th-2 to Th-3, and Th-4 to Th-5. In **A**, Th-4 to Th-5 hypintensity (*black arrowheads*) is the largest and is also hypointense on proton density and T2-weighted images (**B** and **C**, *black arrowheads*), caused by hemosiderin, which shortens the T2 relaxation time, producing a dark area on T2-weighted and proton density images. In **B** and **C**, the areas of enlarged cord from C-7 to Th-6 are hyperintensities. **D** and **E**, axial T1-weighted (TR/TE = 500/40) MR images at the Th-3 and Th-4 levels. Note the round (**D**) and irregularly round (**E**) hypointensity in the cross section of the cord (*white arrows*). (Courtesy of Nagashima C, Nagashima R, Morota N, et al: *Surg Neurol* 35:368–373, 1991).

Magnetic Resonance Imaging Contrast Agents: Theory and Application to the Central Nervous System
Bronen RA, Sze G (Yale Univ School of Medicine, New Haven, Conn)
J Neurosurg 73:820–839, 1990   19–3

Background.—The Food and Drug Administration recently approved gadopentetate dimeglumine (known formerly as Gd-DTPA) as a para-

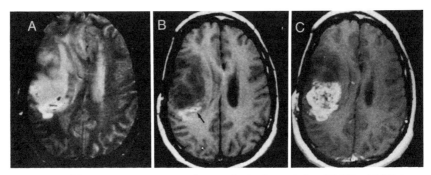

Fig 19–2.—Magnetic resonance images of an anaplastic glioma. **A,** long-TR/TE axial MR image showing increased signal abnormality and associated mass effect in the right frontal and parietal lobes. It is impossible to separate "gross" lesion from edema. **B,** short-TR/TE coronal image demonstrating the mass effect on the right frontal sulci and right lateral ventricle. It is again difficult to separate the lesion from edema. Hyperintensity (*arrow*) at the posterior margin is consistent with tumor. **C,** gadolinium-DTPA-enhanced short-TR/TE image revealing an enhancing lesion consistent with the tumor. This contrast-enhanced scan clearly separates gross tumor from edema. Hemorrage cannot be distinguished from enhancement. (Courtesy of Bronen RA, Sze G: *J Neurosurg* 73:820–839, 1990.)

magnetic contrast agent. This is an effective contrast agent because of its hydration number, its magnetic moment, its correlation time, its proximity to water protons, and its low toxicity in both animal and clinical trials. In MRI, contrast agents act on adjacent protons to shorten T_1 and T_2 relaxation times, resulting in signal intensity changes. Historically, MR studies were able to detect more abnormalities but were less able to characterize them. The use of contrast agents for MRI allows MRI to surpass CT for the evaluation of most CNS lesions. Whereas contrast-enhanced CT can detect abnormalities, the multiple planes on MRI can provide invaluable information. In the brain, contrast MRI with Gd-DTPA is useful in the evaluation of intracranial metastases, pituitary microadenomas, acoustic neurinomas, meningeal disease, primary brain tumors, and some skull-base lesions (Fig 19–2). In spinal imaging, MR diagnosis with Gd injection is used routinely for failed-back syndrome or when intradural and intramedullary lesions are suspected.

Conclusions.—The FDA's approval of Gd-DTPA has provided the only currently approved contrast agent for MRI. Gd is a safe, efficacious paramagnetic contrast agent with no significant side effects. Future applications for MR contrast agents include new uses for accepted agents like Gd-DTPA and development of new contrast agents. It seems that Gd-DTPA may be especially useful in dynamic scanning, a fast scanning technique that is easily coupled with the use of 3-dimensional Fourier transform imaging. It may also be used in fat-suppression MRI techniques in which contrast enhancement is not masked by fat. Other developments of contrast materials include nongadolinium compounds, intrathecal contrast media, cerebral blood flow and volume evaluation, and antibody-labeled contrast agents.

▶ In clinical neuroscience, MRI with contrast enhancement has been firmly established as the diagnostic method of choice for a wide variety of conditions. It is astonishing how the method can diagnose conditions that previously were so difficult to pinpoint, such as multiple epidural abscesses in the spine. It also is remarkable how the approach can help with the differential diagnosis of conditions, e.g., epidural scar vs. recurrent herniated disc in the postoperative spine. Consideration of the physical bases of contrast enhancement together with pathophysiology leads one to suspect that further developments of an impressive nature will continue. Of particular current interest are investigations in cerebral blood flow and volume, and antibody labelling.—R.M. Crowell, M.D.

MR Angiography

3DFT MR Angiography of the Carotid Bifurcation: Potential and Limitations as a Screening Examination
Masaryk AM, Ross JS, DiCello MC, Modic MT, Paranandi L, Masaryk TJ
(Univ Hosps of Cleveland; Cleveland Clinic Found, Ohio)
Radiology 179:797–804, 1991   19–4

Introduction.—There are doubts about the ability of some MR flow techniques to approximate vascular stenoses. Preliminary experience with 3-dimensional Fourier transform time-of-flight MR angiography suggests that artifacts can be minimized and accurate, reproducible results are obtainable. Three-dimensional Fourier transform time-of-flight carotid MR angiography was compared with intra-arterial digital subtraction angiography (DSA) in 38 patients suspected of having arteriosclerotic disease of the anterior cerebrovascular circulation.

Methods.—Magnetic resonance imaging was carried out with multiecho, T2-weighted axial and T1-weighted sagittal pulse sequences. Magnetic resonance angiographic studies of both carotid arteries were done using simultaneously acquired sagittal 3-dimensional Fourier transform volumes. These studies and DSA were carried out within a week of one another. The method of correlating bifurcational anatomy is illustrated in Figure 19–3.

Findings.—Technically adequate MR angiograms were acquired in 65 of the 75 carotid arteries evaluated by DSA. When 2 independent observers made readings on 2 occasions, consistent interpretations were made within and between the observers. The 2 methods were comparably able to depict changes in the percent area of stenosis. The median percent stenosis as determined by MR angiography and intra-arterial DSA did not differ significantly, for either the right or left carotid artery. A cutoff of 70% stenosis made MR angiography highly sensitive and specific in detecting hemodynamically significant lesions.

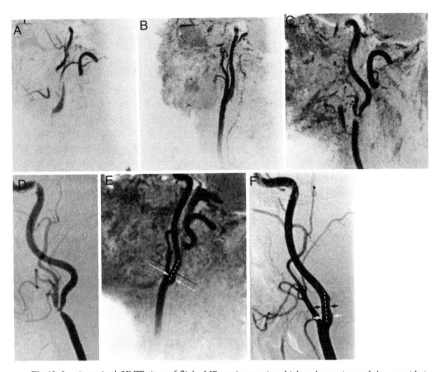

Fig 19–3.—A, sagittal 3DFT time-of-flight MR angiogram in which only portions of the carotid sinus, internal carotid artery, and external carotid branches are included in the imaging volume. Such cases were deleted from the comparative analysis. **B,** sagittal 3DFT time-of-flight MR angiogram of a nonstenotic carotid bifurcation. Such normal cases were included in the comparative analysis. In the absence of a definable stenosis, measurements were taken at the proximal internal and distal common carotid arteries. **C and D,** sagittal 3DFT time-of-flight angiogram **(C)** and intra-arterial DSA image **(D)** in a patient with severe stenosis at the carotid bifurcation. Note that, despite a small focal area of vessel discontinuity or signal void at the stenosis on the MR angiogram, distal flow is obvious and precludes a diagnosis of occlusion. Such "gap" lesions were arbitrarily assigned a 99.9% area of stenosis on MR angiograms. **E,** sagittal 3DFT time-of-flight MR angiogram and intra-arterial DSA image **(F)** demonstrate comparable filling defects on the posterior wall of the carotid sinus. Arterial diameter measurements were made approximately perpendicular to the vessel axis (*dashed line*) on hard-copy images with use of vernier calipers. The *black arrows* designate the point of maximum luminal compromise (D_{sten}); *white arrows* indicate diameter of the nearest proximal normal arterial segment (D_{norm}). (Courtesy of Masaryk AM, Ross JS, DiCello MC, et al: *Radiology* 179:797–804, 1991.)

Conclusion.—Magnetic resonance angiography may prove to be a sensitive screening procedure for carotid stenosis.

▶ This careful study indicates an excellent correlation between MR angiographic estimation and angiographic estimation of internal carotid artery stenosis caused by carotid occlusive disease. The receiver-operating characteristic analysis is a useful approach to the problem. However, it is also important to keep in mind that the anatomical plaque itself may be used as the source of data. We have done this at the Massachusetts General Hospital and have found that there is an excellent (but not perfect) correlation of MR angiographic residual lumen diameter and the true anatomical residual lumen. We can also state that, contrary to what is stated in this article, signal drop-out regularly occurs in arteries smaller than 2 mm in diameter (not in arteries that are 99.9% stenosed). Further information correlating radiographic, clinical, and surgical anatomical pathologic data will be required before the role of MR angiography can be firmly established in this area.—R.M. Crowell, M.D.

MRI in Spontaneous Dissection of Vertebral and Carotid Arteries: 15 Cases Studied at 0.5 Tesla
Gelbert F, Assouline E, Hodes JE, Reizine D, Woimant F, George B, Hagueneau M, Merland JJ (Lariboisière Hosp, Paris)
Neuroradiology 33:111–113, 1991   19–5

Background.—The definitive diagnosis of vertebral or carotid artery dissection is currently based on angiographic findings. Some physicians

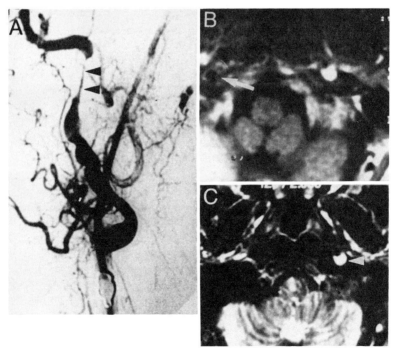

Fig 19–4.—Carotid artery dissection. **A,** left carotid angiogram showing a severe dissection of the petrous portion of the internal carotid artery (ICA) (*arrowheads*). **B,** axial T1-weighted images (600/30) showing a semilunar signal hyperintensity (*arrowhead*) narrowing the residual lumen of the ICA. The right CA has a normal signal void (*arrow*). **C,** axial T2 (2,000/120)-weighted image showing the persistence of the signal hyperintensity (*arrowhead*). (Courtesy of Gelbert F, Assouline E, Hodes JE, et al: *Neuroradiology* 33:111-113, 1991.)

have described the use of MRI, which can show flow and bleeding, in the diagnosis of cervical vessel dissection. The magnetic resonance diagnosis of vertebral and carotid artery dissection was examined in 1 series.

Patients and Findings.—Between 1987 and 1990, 15 patients were observed. Six had angiographically confirmed vertebral artery dissection, and 9 had carotid artery dissection. The findings showed a concordance between MRI and angiography in all but 1 case. The dissected part consistently demonstrated a semilunar hyperintensity narrowing the residual eccentric signal void of the lumen when the artery occlusion was not complete. Magnetic resonance imaging indicated a small signal void within the hyperintensity, indicating incomplete occlusion, in 1 angiographically occluded vessel. Magnetic resonance imaging clearly demonstrated the length of the dissected portion. Follow-up MRI and angiographic assessment confirmed the regression of the dissection and allowed evaluation of the cerebral parenchyma (Fig 19–4).

Conclusion.—Magnetic resonance imaging can now be considered a routine complementary assessment in cases of suspected vessel dissection. Information obtained from MRI studies appears to be complementary to that found on angiography. Direct visualization of the mural hematoma, better visualization of the length of the dissection, and visualization of a residual signal void indicating severe stenosis rather than complete thrombosis are possible. At present, MRI is complementary to angiography in the dissection of vertebral and carotid arteries; with the introduction of new sequences and coils, it may become the evaluation of choice.

▶ That magnetic resonance angiography can detect dissection of cranial cervical vessels is emphasized once again. This also permits follow-up in a noninvasive fashion and can guide treatment.—R.M. Crowell, M.D.

Intracranial MR Angiography: A Direct Comparison of Three Time-of-Flight Techniques
Lewin JS, Laub G (Cleveland Clinic Found, Ohio)
AJR 158:381–387, 1992   19–6

Objective.—Three methods of intracranial time-of-flight (TOF) MR angiography were compared under equivalent imaging conditions. The subjects were 32 healthy volunteers, 12 of whom served for evaluation and adjustment of the imaging parameters, and 20 for direct comparison of the 3 techniques.

Methods.—For all studies, a superconducting 1.5-tesla whole-body system with a 10-mT/m gradient capability was used. The single-volume method used a 3-dimensional Fourier transformation gradient-echo sequence, as did the multiple thin-volume method. The sequential 2-di-

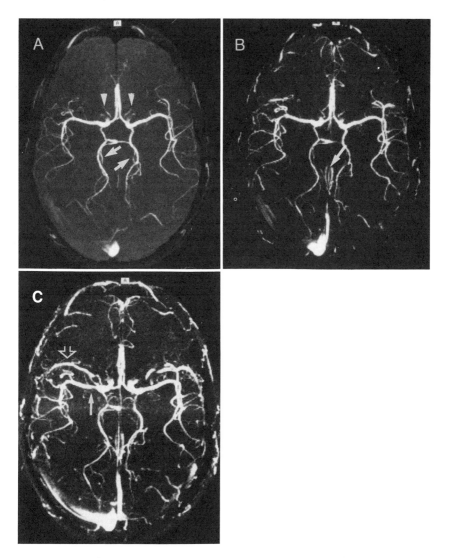

Fig 19–5.—Axial maximum-intensity-projection reconstructed angiograms. **A,** single-volume method. Good signal is noted in proximal portions of anterior, middle, and posterior cerebral arteries. Many cortical branches in middle and posterior cerebral distributions are noted, along with bilateral posterior communicating arteries, proximal ophthalmic arteries (*arrowheads*), and superior cerebellar arteries (*arrows*). **B,** multiple thin-volume method. Again, proximal portions of anterior, middle, and posterior cerebral arteries are well visualized, along with posterior communicating arteries and portions of ophthalmic and superior cerebellar arteries. More small cortical branches are noted as compared with single-volume technique. Signal within internal cerebral veins and straight sinus is also noted (*arrows*). **C,** sequential 2-dimensional slice method. Slight artifactual narrowing is noted in region of the right supraclinoid carotid bifurcation (*solid arrow*), but the remainder of the proximal large arteries is well visualized. Numerous cortical vessels, posterior communicating arteries, and portions of the ophthalmic and superior cerebellar arteries are seen. In addition to internal cerebral veins and straight sinus, sphenoparietal (*open arrow*) and right transverse sinus are visualized much better than with other methods. However, more slowly flowing in-plane spins in the left transverse sinus are not visualized because of persistent spin saturation. Note that the anterior limb of carotid siphon is not entirely included in the region of interest, precluding adequate evaluation for flow void in this region in this research subject. (Courtesy of Lewin JS, Laub G: *Am J Roentgenology* 158:381–387, 1992.)

mensional (2-D) slice technique incorporated a 2-D Fourier transformation gradient-echo sequence.

Findings.—Large-vessel bifurcations were best defined using the volume inflow methods (Fig 19–5). The multiple thin-volume method was best for demonstrating small vessel detail. Examining individual partitions or slices from data sets before postprocessing yielded relatively good definition of small communicating arteries. In most cases, small middle cerebral artery branches were best shown by the multiple thin-volume method. Venous sinuses and subependymal veins were visualized well using the sequential 2-D slice method. No motion artifacts occurred with the single-volume technique.

Discussion.—Progressive saturation of inflowing spins is a problem in TOF MR angiography, but several methods are available to minimize this effect. Both thinner imaging volumes and 2-D slices are helpful. The clinical results can be optimized by tailoring the technique to the abnormality suspected of being present on the basis of requirements for spatial resolution and slow-flow sensitivity.

▶ The authors present data with 3-dimensional TOF techniques for MR angiography of the intracranial vessels. Rather attractive images are presented, along with possible artifacts and their explanations. It should be pointed out that this is a rapidly developing field. At a presentation in June 1992, Robert Edelman and his colleagues at the Beth Israel Hospital in Boston presented images of stunning clarity and reliability on a routine basis, using new programming sequences, with reliable depiction of structures such as the anterior inferior cerebral artery, on a routine basis. This is clearly a wave of the future. In units such as that at the Beth Israel Hospital, this is already a very useful method for screening patients for intracranial aneurysm. It may become more valuable in a wider range of patients with possible unruptured intracranial aneurysm, but it seems unlikely to supplant conventional angiography in cases of subarachnoid hemorrhage. Stay tuned for further developments.—R.M. Crowell, M.D.

Three-Dimensional Computerized Tomography Angiography in the Diagnosis of Cerebrovascular Disease
Harbaugh RE, Schlusselberg DS, Jeffery R, Hayden S, Cromwell LD, Pluta D
(Dartmouth-Hitchcock Med Ctr; Aesculys Research Group, Lebanon, NH)
J Neurosurg 76:408–414, 1992   19–7

Background.—Three-dimensional CT angiography uses contrast-enhanced CT brain scan data to generate 3-dimensional images of the intracranial vasculature. Three-dimensional CT angiography was used in 20 patients with known or suspected cerebrovascular disease.

Methods and Findings.—Diagnoses were made using computer-generated 3-dimensional reconstruction of the intracranial vascular system. The color prints and videotape images obtained aided in the diagnosis of intracranial aneurysms, arteriovenous malformations, and venous angiomas. They were also helpful in excluding structural abnormalities in patients with suspected intracranial vascular pathologic conditions and in screening patients who had a strong family history of intracranial aneurysm. The diagnostic correlation between 3-dimensional CT angiography and intra-arterial angiography was 100% in the 11 patients undergoing both procedures. There were no complications resulting from the procedure or from incorrect diagnosis.

Conclusion.—Both MRI and 3-dimensional CT angiography are currently useful for imaging the intracranial vasculature with minimal risk to the patient. Although more clinical experience is needed to determine whether either of these methods is a clinically acceptable substitute for intra-arterial angiography, early experience suggests that 3-dimensional CT angiography is a potentially valuable tool in diagnosing cerebrovascular disease.

▶ This study uses sophisticated imaging enhancement techniques for the diagnosis of cerebrovascular anomalies using CT scanning. The pictures are impressive; however, one must emphasize that even very small lesions may hemorrhage, particularly in the setting of familial aneurysms and multiple aneurysms. Such lesions might fall below the threshold for CT detection, even using the sophisticated approach. The gold standard for diagnosis of these lesions is still conventional angiography. When the index of clinical suspicion is high and the CT study is negative, conventional angiography should be considered.

In addition, one should mention the widespread and growing availability of MR angiography (MRA) for the detection of intracranial arterial lesions without angiography. This continues to improve and, in certain leading centers, lesions in the range of 2–3 mm can be detected. It will be interesting to see how these noninvasive techniques, advanced CT and MRA, can be used for noninvasive identification of aneurysms and arteriovenous malformations.—R.M. Crowell, M.D.

Stereoscopic Display of MR Angiograms
Wentz KU, Mattle HP, Edelman RR, Kleefield J, O'Reilly GV, Liu C, Zhao B (Beth Israel Hosp, Boston, Mass)
Neuroradiology 33:123–125, 1991   19–8

Background.—Recent advances in MRI permit high-resolution imaging of blood flow. Projection angiograms can be produced to overcome the tomographic nature of conventional MR scans. These angiograms are similar to plain x-ray film or digital subtraction angiograms in their demonstration of blood vessels, but the 3-dimensional information inherent in them is partially lost in single projections. A method of 3-dimensional display consisting of stereo pairs of MR angiograms was examined.

Methods.—Magnetic resonance angiograms were obtained in normal subjects and patients with vascular disorders. A 1.5-tesla whole body magnet was used. Two sequence designs were used. In the first, a volume of tissue was imaged using a 3-dimensional flow-compensated fast low angle shot pulse sequence. This method was best used in regions where motion is not a prominent feature, (e.g., the cerebrovascular system). In the second design, a series of 2-dimensional flow-compensated fast low angle shot images were obtained. This was used in the abdomen and chest during breath-holding, where motion may limit image quality. Also, it can be used for MR venography of the head and extremities. The angiograms were stereoscopically displayed by photographing projection images obtained with a difference in angle of 6–10 degrees.

Results.—Stereoscopic image pairs allowed the clinician to perceive the relative distance of vessels to one another. Two examples were given to illustrate how MR angiograms permitted perception of vascular anatomy in 3 dimensions.

Conclusion.—Stereoscopic display of MR angiograms using image pairs is a simple way to recover some of the 3-dimensional information inherent in these projection images. Like conventional stereo contrast angiograms, these angiograms can enhance the perception of normal and pathologic vascular anatomy if viewed with a stereoscope or by an examiner familiar with the "cross-eyed" method.

▶ This novel approach to MR angiography truly permits recovery of stereoscopy. The examples offered clearly illustrate that lesions such as aneurysms can be seen to project out of the field of 2-dimensional presentation, thus allowing retrieval of important diagnostic information, such as the relation of an aneurysm to local areas. Using either the "cross-eyed technique" or a stereoscope, the viewer can recapture important diagnostic information. This would seem to be an important advance in MR angiography, particularly in understanding aneurysms and arteriovenous malformations.—R.M. Crowell, M.D.

Other Techniques

Radiation Necrosis vs High-Grade Recurrent Glioma: Differentiation by Using Dual-Isotope SPECT With ^{201}Tl and ^{99m}Tc-HMPAO

Schwartz RB, Carvalho PA, Alexander E III, Loeffler JS, Folkerth R, Holman BL (Brigham and Women's Hosp, Boston)

AJR 158:399–404, 1992

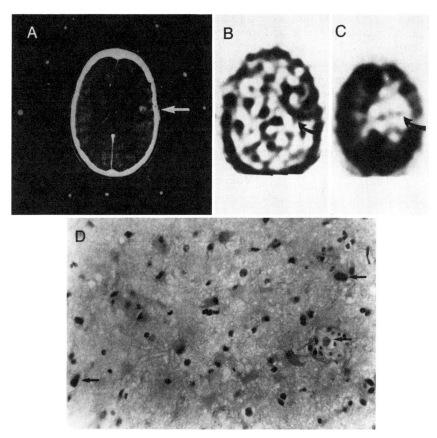

Fig 19–6.—Patient who was well and without recurrence 8 months after resection and brachytherapy for left temporal lobe glioblastoma. **A,** transaxial enhanced CT scan obtained with patient in a stereotaxic head frame shows low-attenuation lesion with focus of peripheral enhancement in the left temporal lobe (*arrow*) with slight edema and mass effect. **B,** a ^{201}Tl scan at level of CT scan shows a ring of low thallium uptake (*arrow*) corresponding to abnormality on CT. **C,** [99M]Tc-HMPAO scan shows decreased perfusion to this area (*arrow*). **D,** photomicrograph of biopsy specimen from region of greatest tracer uptake shows radiation necrosis, with intact cerebral white matter containing astrogliosis and edema. Scattered astrocytes with enlarged atypical nuclei (*arrows*) represent cells with limited growth potential. (H and E, original magnification × 1,000.) (Courtesy of Schwartz RB, Carvalho PA, Alexander E III, et al: *AJR* 158:399-404, 1992.)

Objective.—Patients who have deterioration after radiotherapy for high-grade glioma may have either recurrent tumor or radiation necrosis. Because the distinction is very important, dual-isotope high-resolution single photon emission tomography (SPECT) imaging, using radiothallium and technetium-labeled hexamethylpropyleneamine oxime (HMPAO), was performed in 15 patients with deterioration after irradiation of high-grade symptomatic glioma.

Methods.—The SPECT imaging was performed using the ASPECT imager after injection of 3 mCi of ^{201}Tl-chloride. Subsequently, 15–20 mCi of ^{99m}Tc-HMPAO were injected and imaging was repeated. Computed tomography was performed on the morning of the scheduled biopsy.

Findings.—Computed tomography consistently demonstrated a large intraparenchymal mass lesion of mainly low attenuation internally, with peripheral enhancement and surrounding edema. All 4 patients with foci of ^{201}T1 uptake died of locally recurrent tumor. All 3 patients with low ^{201}T1 uptake had reactive changes only on biopsy (Fig 19–6). Among patients having an intermediate level of ^{201}T1 activity in the tumor bed, 3 of 4 in whom perfusion was preserved or increased had solid tumor. None of 4 patients with reduced perfusion had locally recurrent tumor.

Conclusion.—Dual-isotope SPECT scanning may prove very useful in detecting the sites of likely tumor recurrence in patients who remain symptomatic after irradiation of high-grade glioma. The findings can help guide brain biopsy so that a definitive diagnosis will be possible.

▶ This report suggests that dual-isotope SPECT scanning can differentiate radiation necrosis from high-grade recurrent glioma. Although the data indicate correct diagnosis in 14 of 15 pathologically proven cases, they will require confirmation by other investigators. This method is attractive because it is easier to apply than PET scanning, which is a more complex and costly procedure.—R.M. Crowell, M.D.

Intracerebral Penetration of Infrared Light: Technical Note
McCormick PW, Stewart M, Lewis G, Dujovny M, Ausman JI (Henry Ford Hosp, Detroit, Mich)
J Neurosurg 76:315–318, 1992   19–10

Background.—There is increasing interest in using in vivo optical spectroscopy to noninvasively estimate cerebral oxyhemoglobin concentration and cerebral hemoglobin oxygen saturation. It remains uncertain whether infrared light in the range of 650–1100 nm can penetrate the adult human scalp and skull, undergo attenuation specific to intracerebral tissues, and return to the scalp to be detected.

Methods.—A bolus of 1 mg of indocyanine green dye in 1 mL of normal saline was placed in the exposed internal carotid artery in 5 adults undergoing carotid endarterectomy. The external carotid artery was occluded as transmission spectroscopy was done over the ipsilateral frontal bone with a nonpulsed 803-nm light. Infrared light signals were collected 1 cm and 2.7 cm from the point source.

Findings.—Vital signs did not change significantly after dye injection. Major changes in optical density were recorded in the channel with a 2.7-cm source-receiver separation distance after tracer infusion. The bolus was detected washing into and out of the cerebral vessels, with an activity curve consistent with a nondiffusible tracer. Change in optical density was very reproducible in all 5 patients. The signal-to-noise ratio for detecting dye in the cerebral vasculature exceeded 100:1.

Conclusion.—Depth resolution of cerebral infrared transmission spectra was demonstrated in humans. It seems feasible to use this technique to map mean cerebral transit times. With multiple receivers, it should be possible to resolve cerebral and extracranial transit times.

▶ In this study, the authors show that infrared transmission spectroscopy done over the hemisphere of a patient can detect bolus transit through the ipsilateral cerebral circulation with a signal-to-noise ratio of > 100:1. This technology will soon be adapted to measure local cerebral hemoglobin saturation for a sort of pulse oximetry of the brain. The usefulness of this technology for clinical practice in an intensive care unit setting is obvious.—R.M. Crowell, M.D.

The Clinical Application of Neurogenic Motor Evoked Potentials to Monitor Spinal Cord Function During Surgery
Owen JH, Bridwell KH, Grubb R, Jenny A, Allen B, Padberg AM, Shimon SM (Washington Univ, St Louis)
Spine 16:S385–S390, 1991   19–11

Objective.—Although somatosensory evoked potential (SEP) monitoring has proven to be an effective safety measure during surgery for spinal deformity, there is concern about its failure to detect purely motor lesions or deficits. Therefore, neurogenic motor evoked potentials (NMEPs) were monitored intraoperatively in 177 children and 123 adults undergoing spinal surgery in 1987–1989, in most cases for posterior spinal deformity requiring instrumentation.

Methods.—In posterior spinal cases, NMEPs are elicited by stimulating the cord with 2 24-gauge steel electrodes. Recording is made by subdermal needle electrodes in the area of the sciatic nerve at the popliteal fossa. Somatosensory evoked potentials are elicited by stimulating the posterior tibial nerve at the ankle, and they are recorded at the popliteal fossa, over C4-5, and cortically.

Findings.—The somatosensory evoked potential recordings were more variable than NMEPs, presumably because of anesthesia and other factors. The neurogenic motor evoked potentials were a more reliable indicator of postoperative motor status than were the SEPs. No motor paralysis occurred in patients with normal NMEPs, and no sensory loss occurred in the presence of normal SEPs. Both potentials occasionally were reduced in patients who lost motor function. If both types of potential remained stable, no postoperative deficit occurred.

Recommendation.—Both SEPs and NMEPs should be used to monitor spinal cord function during surgery that places the spinal cord at risk.

▶ The Washington University Group reports favorable results with neurogenic motor evoked potentials (NMEPs) for spinal cord surgery. In a substantial volume of cases, 300 patients with a variety of problems NMEPs were studied. The correlation of NMEP changes with outcome was superior to that for SEPs. For example, in vascular surgical cases, the 2 (of 28) patients who awoke with motor deficits both had NMEP abnormalities (but no SEP abnormalities) during surgery. The NMEPs appear to offer an advantage over SEPs for monitoring spinal cord function during surgery.—R.M. Crowell, M.D.

Transcranial Doppler Monitoring During Carotid Endarterectomy
Naylor AR, Wildsmith JAW, McClure J, Jenkins AM, Ruckley CV (Royal Infirmary, Edinburgh)
Br J Surg 78:1264–1268, 1991   19–12

Introduction.—Preexisting ischemic damage and impaired hemodynamic reserve may make the brain more susceptible to minor embolism or a modest reduction in cerebral perfusion pressure during carotid endarterectomy. Doppler monitoring of flow velocity in the middle cerebral artery was therefore used during the procedure.

Study Design.—Transcranial Doppler monitoring of middle cerebral arterial flow was undertaken in 30 consecutive patients undergoing carotid endarterectomy in an 18-month period. A hand-held probe was used in a majority of patients. The end-tidal CO_2 tension was maintained at 32–40 mm Hg during surgery.

Observations.—Flow velocity decreased significantly when carotid clamps were applied. An internal carotid artery stump pressure less than 50 mm Hg, taken as an indication for shunting, corresponded to a systolic middle cerebral artery flow velocity less than 42 cm/s and to a mean velocity less than 30 cm/s. Embolization was more frequent than expected, especially after placement of a shunt and final restoration of blood flow. Doppler monitoring identified a probable cause of minor neurologic deficit in both patients who were affected. The Doppler study showed good flow in the internal carotid artery, precluding the need for reexploration in both patients.

Implications.—Transcranial Doppler monitoring is of use during carotid endarterectomy, because it can provide warning of developing problems before cerebral ischemia is established. Monitoring may be especially revealing during mobilization of the carotid bifurcation, during placement of a shunt, and after flow is restored.

▶ This interesting report describes transcranial Doppler monitoring during 30 consecutive carotid endarterectomies. Although individual data are not provided for the various patients, the authors note that systolic middle cerebral artery (MCA) velocity decreased from 56 (56–62) to 35 (28–42), both being statistically significant decreases. Systolic MCA velocities were also correlated with internal carotid artery stump pressures, and the reportedly critical stump pressure of 50 mm Hg was correlated with 42 cm/s of critical velocity. On the basis of stump pressures, 15 patients were treated with an intraoperative shunt. (This is a high proportion in comparison with the literature; in our own experience, only 10% of patients need a shunt.) Thus far, one cannot use PCV as a clear indication for shunting. Further correlation of outcome with PCV values after clamping would be required to achieve this standard.

Further information of value to be obtained from this study includes the remarkable alterations in MCA flow velocity during mobilization of the carotid bifurcation, probably as a result of manipulation of the carotid artery and alterations in carotid flow. In addition, after release of cross-clamping, multiple moments of abnormal signal were recorded, possibly indicating a burst of embolization. In addition, in patients with neurologic deficit following carotid endarterectomy, PCV was able to provide information suggesting patency of the carotid and thus avert potentially dangerous emergency reexploration. These data are interesting overall, but the data are not yet sufficient to establish transcranial Doppler monitoring as a substitute for electroencephalogram monitoring during carotid endarterectomy.—R.M. Crowell, M.D.

20 Techniques

Stereotaxis

Stereotactic Management of Colloid Cysts: Factors Predicting Success

Kondziolka D, Lunsford LD (Univ of Pittsburgh, Pittsburgh, Pa)
J Neurosurg 75:45–51, 1991
                                                                    20–1

Background.—Used alone or with microsurgical resection, stereotactic aspiration is a useful operative alternative for colloid cyst treatment. The management of 22 consecutive patients with colloid cysts, all of whom were treated initially with stereotactic methods, was evaluated.

Patients.—The patients underwent CT-guided stereotactic surgery between 1981 and 1990. The colloid cysts were located in the third ventricle. Presenting symptoms included headache in 15, mental status change in 6, and sudden coma in 5. Gaze palsies, syncope, and hemisensory loss were less common.

Outcomes.—Stereotactic aspiration alone was successful in 50% of the patients. Among the 11 patients in whom aspiration failed, stereotactic endoscopic resection was attempted in 3 and was successful in 1. Seven patients needed craniotomy and microsurgical removal of the cyst through a transcortical approach. The preoperative CT appearance of a hypodense or isodense cyst in 8 patients correlated well with successful aspiration in 6. A hyperdense preoperative CT appearance was associated with subtotal aspiration in 13 of 14 patients, 5 of whom required craniotomy. In 8 patients, preoperative MRI provided excellent anatomical definition of the cyst and its relationship to other third ventricle structures. However, correlating successful aspiration with MR appearance was not possible with short or long relaxation time sequences.

Conclusion.—Preoperative CT studies accurately determine size, predict viscosity, and help to define a group of patients with colloid cysts for whom stereotactic aspiration is likely to be successful. In this series, unsuccessful stereotactic aspiration was related to the high viscosity of the intracystic colloid material and deviation of the cyst away from the aspiration needle because of small cyst volume. Stereotactic surgery should be offered to selected patients as the initial procedure of choice, with craniotomy reserved for those whose imaging studies predict failure and whose cysts cannot be aspirated.

▶ Surgical excision of symptomatic colloid cysts can often be accomplished with a good outcome and avoidance of shunt, but there is a significant risk factor that cannot be eliminated because of the deep location of the lesion. On the other hand, stereotactic aspiration of colloid cysts can sometimes be highly effective; however, it is hard to know which cases will respond.

This communication indicates that patients with CT cysts of hypodensity or isodensity greater than 1 cm in size often will respond to cyst aspiration. On the other hand, patients with smaller lesions or hyperdensity are much less likely to respond, and other treatments (surgical excision or shunting) appear more appropriate in this group.—R.M. Crowell, M.D.

Stereotactic Suboccipital Transcerebellar Biopsy Under Local Anesthesia Using the Cosman-Roberts-Wells Frame: Technical Note

Spiegelmann R, Friedman WA (Univ of Florida, Gainesville)
J Neurosurg 75:486–488, 1991   20–2

Background.—Suboccipital transcerebellar stereoactic biopsy methods reported previously, done with the patient in the prone position, have required general endotracheal anesthesia. A technique for doing such biopsies with the patient in the lateral decubitus position and using local anesthesia has been developed.

Technique.—The surgeon uses standard parts of the Brown-Roberts-Wells system combined with the Cosman-Roberts-Wells arc, applying the base ring to the patient's skull using local anesthesia. The ring is positioned as low as possible in the nuchal area, with the anterior part directed toward the patient's ear on the side of the lesion. The posts are placed so that the surgeon has clear access to the suboccipital area on the side of the lesion. Contrast-enhanced axial CT scans are obtained, the lesion is visualized, and a target and suitable entry point are selected on the same CT slice. An entry point that is clearly below the transverse sinus is selected, permitting a safe trajectory to the target. In the operating room, the patient is placed in the lateral decubitus position. The lesion side is uppermost. The base ring is fixed to the Mayfield adaptor, and target and entry point Cartesian coordinates are obtained. The surgeon mounts the Cosman-Roberts-Wells arc in the sagittal position, allowing a plane-of-target entry point. The pointer is set at the target coordinates in the Cosman-Roberts-Wells arc-compatible phantom. The arc is then applied to the phantom, and a biopsy probe is advanced to corroborate setting accuracy. The phantom pointer is repositioned to the entry-point coordinates, and the arc is rotated into a horizontal position on the entry-point side. The probe-holder is displaced along the arc as needed so the biopsy needle shaft touches the phantom pointer at a 90° angle. The surgeon reads the angular values for the arc and probe and secures the positions, assuring that the probe will traverse the desired entry point and reach the desired target.

The arc is applied to the base ring, and the skin is prepared for surgery. Nuchal muscles are dissected bluntly, and the biopsy needle is advanced to the target.

Conclusion.—This technique for posterior fossa biopsy through the transcerebellar route is precise and rapid. Avoiding general anesthesia may significantly reduce the time needed for the procedure and the potential complications. The surgeon may base his or her choice of transfrontal or transcerebellar approach exclusively on the location and characteristics of the lesion.

▶ The authors present a straightforward technique for transcerebellar biopsy using both local anesthesia and the standard Cosman-Roberts-Wells frame. For many years, neurosurgeons were hesitant to perform biopsy on structures in the posterior fossa using the stereotactic technique; however, standard modern technology has indicated that this area can also be safely approached through a stereotactic biopsy.—R.M. Crowell, M.D.

Brain Tumor Resection Aided With Markers Placed Using Stereotaxis Guided by Magnetic Resonance Imaging and Computed Tomography
Hassenbusch SJ, Anderson JS, Pillay PK (Cleveland Clinic Found, Ohio)
Neurosurgery 28:801–806, 1991   20–3

Background.—Defining and locating the edges of deep-seated tumors or those with indistinct color and consistency can be difficult in the operative resection of brain tumors. A simple, precise method for placing visual markers to aid in tumor resections is examined.

Technique.—The basic Brown-Roberts-Wells or Cosman-Roberts-Wells stereotactic frame was used. With routine CT or MRI after application of the frame, multiple points along the tumor edges were used as target points. Standard techniques were used in the operating room for skin incision, bone-flap removal, and opening the dura. After opening the dura and using stereotactic coordinates and equipment, "micropatties," or small catheters with pledgets or catheter tips, were placed at each target point at the tumor edges (Fig 20–1). After the arc was removed, the tumor was resected in a conventional nonstereotactic fashion, following string tails or catheters to the tumors. Gross tumor edges were established from the positions of the patties or catheter tips.

Conclusion.—These simple, precise methods enable tumor resection under stereotactic guidance with equipment that is readily available to most neurosurgeons. The accuracy of marker placement in relation to

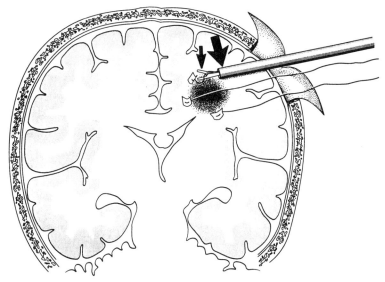

Fig 20–1.—Diagrammatic representation of the stereotactic placement of a "micropatty" with an attached "tail" extending out through the brain and the site of the durotomy and craniotomy. Two patties have already been placed at the edges of the CT or MRI contrast-enhanced brain tumor (*stippled area*). The tips of the biopsy forceps (*small arrow*) are extending out from the biopsy needle tube (*large arrow*) to place a third patty. The needle tube is attached to and directed by the stereotactic arc (not shown). The bone flap has been removed, and the dura has been opened. The protrusion of the tips of the biopsy forceps past the end of the needle tube has been exaggerated for illustrative purposes. (Courtesy of Hassenbusch SJ, Anderson JS, Pillay PK: *Neurosurgery* 28:801–806, 1991.)

tumor edges is maintained despite shifts in the tumor and/or brain as cystic areas are drained or large amounts of tumor are resected.

▶ The authors provide information on a technique of stereotactic brain tumor resection using a limited number of data points for operative guidance. This represents, in essence, a scaled-down version of Kelly's approach to stereotactic resection of intracranial tumors (1).

There are significant questions regarding this approach. One could argue that the method is unnecessary for most tumors, because the surgeon can adequately define using microsurgical control the margins of the tumor for dissection. On the other hand, it may be suggested that for truly volumetric resection à la Kelly, only the Kelly system will suffice. According to Dr. Kelly, implementation of his system is not as daunting or extensive as many surgeons have expected. One must consider yet another possibility: stereotactic biopsy followed by appropriate treatment, often radiation, has been shown to be extraordinarily low risk and may be just as effective as these more invasive approaches.

Applying these principles to the cases presented, one could argue that the patient in Figure 3 in the original article could be operated on without stereotactic technique; instead, the tumor might be localized at surgery by ultrasonic methodology. One might also argue that, because the case in Figure 4 in the original article is obviously a butterfly glioma, it is not curable (as was proved by the postoperative scan showing persistent tumor). Therefore, it is reasonable to carry out an open careful microsurgical left frontal tumor resection with safety but with no effort at total removal. For the present, the careful judgment of the operating neurosurgeon is crucial. In our institution, most patients with accessible tumors in good condition undergo an effort at microsurgical resection of the lesion. On the other hand, for deep seated lesions, most patients are subjected to stereotactic biopsy with later treatment determined on the basis of pathologic findings.—R.M. Crowell, M.D.

Reference

1. Kelly PJ, Alker GJ Jr: *Surg Neurol* 15:331, 1981.

Stereotactic Radiosurgery With the Cobalt-60 Gamma Unit in the Treatment of Growth Hormone-Producing Pituitary Tumors

Thorén M, Rähn T, Guo W-Y, Werner S (Karolinska Hosp, Stockholm, Sweden)
Neurosurgery 29:663–668, 1991   20–4

Objective.—No entirely satisfactory way has been found to normalize growth hormone (GH) secretion in patients with acromegaly. Stereotac-

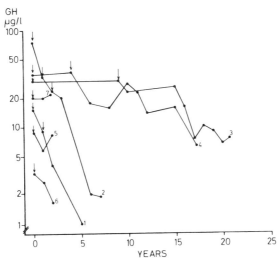

Fig 20–2.—The plasma GH levels before and after stereotactic pituitary irradiation as the primary treatment in patients 1 through 7 with acromegaly. *Arrows* indicate points in time for radiosurgery. (Courtesy of Thorén M, Rähn T, Guo W-Y, et al: *Neurosurgery* 29:663–668, 1991.)

tic radiosurgery with the cobalt-60 gamma unit was evaluated in 21 patients with GH-producing pituitary adenomas and acromegaly.

Patients.—All but 1 of the patients had locally invasive macroadenomas, and a majority exhibited parasellar growth. Radiosurgery was the initial treatment for 7 patients, whereas 14 had previously undergone pituitary surgery. Eight of the latter patients also had received external pituitary irradiation. All patients had clinical signs of active acromegaly at the time of radiosurgery.

Management.—The patients who had not been given radiotherapy previously received 40–70 Gy as many as 3 times, whereas those who *were* previously treated received 30–50 Gy once or twice. Follow-up extended for as long as 21 years after radiosurgery.

Results.—The plasma GH response was quite variable in patients who underwent stereotactic pituitary irradiation as the primary treatment (Fig 20-2). In only 8 cases did both the plasma GH and clinical activity decrease. Of the 21 patients, 11 had no substantial effect from treatment. Pituitary insufficiency developed in 2 patients who had not undergone conventional external irradiation previously. No adverse visual effects were noted.

Conclusion.—The lack of impressive results in this series may in part reflect the treatment of invasive macroadenomas and the use of reduced radiation doses in previously treated patients. Better results might be achieved by using MRI with contrast enhancement to visualize the target volume.

▶ This paper from a very experienced unit reports the results of stereotactic radiosurgical treatment of GH-producing pituitary tumors. The authors selected 21 very difficult cases in which there was local invasion by macroadenomas and often parasellar growth. It is clear that such patients are difficult to treat by any methodology; however, this represents a good place to start in the definition of effectiveness and safety of radiosurgical treatment. It is a testament to the care and expertise of the authors that so few complications were encountered. On the other hand, only approximately half the patients showed successful responses, despite substantial doses of radiation. It seems appropriate to undertake a prospective dose-seeking study in patients with advanced or life-threatening acromegaly so as to determine an effective radiosurgical dose. Moreover, combined therapy, with preoperative surgery to reduce mass and compression effects, may also have some role.—R.M. Crowell, M.D.

Radiation-Induced Edema After Radiosurgery for Pontine Arteriovenous Malformation: A Case Report and Detection by Magnetic Resonance Imaging

Yamamoto M, Jimbo M, Lindquist C (Tokyo Women's Med College Dai-ni

Hosp, Tokyo; Karolinska Hosp, Stockholm)
Surg Neurol 37:15–21, 1992   20–5

Background.—Stereotactic radiosurgery is considered the treatment of choice for small, deep-seated arteriovenous malformations (AVMs); however, experience with this treatment in brain stem AVMs is limited. A pontine AVM seen with radiation-induced edema surrounding the nidus after successful obliteration of the AVM evaluated.

Case Report.—A pregnant woman, 29, experienced a change in taste sensation, a right-sided facial muscle weakness, and periodic vomiting. At a local hospital, CT showed a small hemorrhage within the pons. The patient's symptoms worsened during the next week, and she was referred. Her pregnancy was terminated 2 weeks after admission. A new CT scan showed a hyperdense right dorsal pontine lesion enhanced by contrast medium. Angiography showed a small pontine AVM fed by the anterior inferior cerebellar artery draining into the petrous sinus. Medical treatment produced complete remission, and after 12 months free of symptoms, the patient underwent stereotactic radiosurgery. Twelve months after radiosurgery, she had no signs of neurologic deficit. However, 19 months after irradiation, she had sudden onset of facial nerve palsy with trigeminal nerve disturbance. Magnetic resonance imaging showed significant radiation-induced edema around the nidus. Angiography showed total obliteration of the AVM 24 months after irradiation. Magnetic resonance studies done 28 months after treatment showed that the radiation-induced edema had subsided, despite the persistance of symptoms.

Conclusion.—In this case, the dose given was not considered to be dangerously high. Part of the pons may have been vulnerable to the ischemia accompanying AVM obliteration because of previous damage by the hemorrhage.

▶ Unfortunately, radiosurgery done with the gamma knife can be associated with radiation-induced neurologic deficit from sensitive structures. This is true even with a dose as low as 24 Gy. Radionecrosis must be considered a part of the risk in dealing with these lesions. In addition, one must calculate the potential for bleeding during the latency period (12–24 months) as also being part of the overall risk.—R.M. Crowell, M.D.

Fractionated Stereotactic Radiation Therapy for Intracranial Tumors
Souhami L, Olivier A, Podgorsak EB, Villemure J-G, Pla M, Sadikot AF (McGill Univ, Montreal)
Cancer 68:2101–2108, 1991   20–6

Background.—Stereotactic radiosurgery involves the delivery of a single, large radiation dose to a small, well-defined, stereotactically localized intracranial tumor. Unlike with conventional radiation therapy, radiosurgery makes no attempt to spare normal cells within the target volume by fractionating tumor dose. A program of fractionated stereotactic radiation therapy for selected lesions involving sensitive brain structures was begun at 1 center to improve the therapeutic index and to study the feasibility of the fractionated method.

Methods.—Fifteen patients underwent the multifraction regimen, which typically consisted of 6 fractions of 700 cGy each, given on alternate days for 2 weeks. All patients were treated with the dynamic stereotactic radiosurgical method. The patients' heads were immobilized using a head ring, or "halo frame," set up during the radiation treatments. The median follow-up was 27 months.

Outcomes.—Most patients' symptoms were improved clinically at follow-up evaluation. Improvement was usually noticed within a few weeks after treatment was completed. However, the radiologic response occurred much more slowly. Only 2 patients have had complete radiologic disappearance of their tumors. Most have had only a reduction in tumor size. The patients tolerated the treatment well. There were no acute complications. One patient who had a vasogenic edema 11 months after therapy recovered fully after steroid treatment.

Conclusion.—Fractionated stereotactic radiation therapy is feasible for selected patients with intracranial tumors. Although these preliminary findings are encouraging, the technique should still be considered experimental. A larger patient series and longer follow-up are needed to determine whether the results of this method are actually better than those of conventional radiation therapy.

▶ This novel approach to radiosurgery has been used for tumors involving sensitive brain structures. The volumes are relatively low, with the tumor diameter in the range of 3 mm or less. However, the total treatment fractions add up to 420,000 cGy. A number of different tumor types have been treated, including meningioma, low-grade astrocytoma, and high-grade astrocytoma. There also is no permanent morbidity and apparent tumor control in most cases. Although the results of this approach should be regarded as preliminary, they are encouraging.—R.M. Crowell, M.D.

Endovascular

Treatment of Cerebral Arteriovenous Malformations With PVA: Results and Analysis of Complications

Schumacher M, Horton JA (Univ of Freiburg, Germany; Univ of Pittsburgh, Pa)
Neuroradiology 33:101–105, 1991   20–7

Background.—There is still considerable risk when performing microsurgical procedures in larger or deeply placed arteriovenous malformations (AVMs). Preoperative embolization is used as an alternative in the treatment of AVMs. To define the risk-benefit ratio for embolization be-

Technical Problems and Neurological Complications

Case	AVM-localization	Embolization	Neurological complication	Outcome of complication
66 Y, M, L. hemiparesis	R. par.-occip.	PVA. silk	Slight dysmetria l. arm	Recovered
42 Y, F, Ataxia	L. temporal	PVA. silk Prox. occlusion of feeders	Ataxia. dizziness	Recovered
22 Y, M, Ataxia	Cerebellar vermis	PVA. silk Hemorrhage	Ataxia	Recovered
26 Y, M, Dizziness	R. fronto-par.	PVA	Hypesthesia l. leg	Recovered
28 Y, M, Seizure	L. frontal	PVA	Alopecia 8 days after embol.	Recovered

(continued)

Table (*continued*)

12 Y, M, Hemiparesis Hemihypesthesia	L. parietal	PVA. vessel perforation. hemorrhage l. thalamus a. mid-brain	Increased hemiparesis. dysphasia	Mild spastic hemiparesis. dysphasia. partially recovered
52 Y, M, Hemiparesis Aphasia	L. tempor.-par.	PVA. silk coils	Astereognosia agraphia	Partially recovered
63 Y, F,	R. par.-occip.	PVA. silk. coils	L. hemianopsia weakness l. arm	Partially recovered
55 Y, M,	R. temp.-par	PVA. vessel perforation. sah. hemorrhage	No complication	—
24 Y, M, Seizure, aphasia	L. temporal	PVA. l. temporal hemorrhage, sah	No complication	—
37 Y, F,	R. thalamic	PVA. silk. catheter Disconnection	No complication	—

(Courtesy of Schumacher M, Horton JA: *Neuroradiology* 33:101–105, 1991.)

fore surgery or sterotactic radiotherapy, data from 35 patients with cerebral AVMs treated by endovascular embolization were examined.

Patients.—The patients' ages ranged from 10 to 66 years. The signs and symptoms before embolization included parenchymal hemorrhage, seizure, motor deficit, subarachnoid hemorrhage, speech disorder, and visual deficit (table). The most common location of the AVM was in the temporal lobe, extending to the parietal and occipital regions. The AVM measured more than 4 cm in 22 patients, between 2 and 3.9 cm in 11, and less than 2 cm in 2.

Treatment.—Sixty-three embolizations by the transfemoral route were performed. Treatment was performed with polyvinyl alcohol in most patients, with additional applications of silk, coils, gelfoam, or detachable balloon in some patients.

Results.—The size of the AVM was reduced by one third in 20 patients and between one third and two thirds in 12. Subtotal embolization (more than 90%) was only possible in 3 patients. Eight patients had mild-to-moderate neurologic deficits, which persisted in 3 (8.6%). In most patients, the complications were caused by technical problems (e.g., vessel perforation after guidewire manipulation). There were no correlations between complications and history of bleeding, neurologic deficit, AVM localization, AVM size, angioarchitecture, amount of size reduction, and duration of the procedure. There were no deaths.

Conclusion.—Compared with previously reported studies, the complication rate associated with embolization of deep and large AVMs is lower. The use of bucrylate for embolization in the previous studies may be more hazardous than the use of polyvinyl alcohol. The rate of complications depends on the technical factors of the embolization itself.

▶ The authors report 35 cases of AVM embolized with polyvinyl alcohol. They found 8 complications with 3 lasting deficits (8.6%). Two of the 3 deficits were probably related to ischemia, whereas 1 involved hemorrhage for a perforation. None of the complications were life threatening. In our unit, we have had similarly low morbidity with this approach using butyl cyanoacrylate. In 48 patients we found 1 moderate persisting deficit and 2 minor obsessing deficits. This approach appears to have a low risk factor, and it is often helpful in terms of adjunctive treatment of these cases.—R.M. Crowell, M.D.

Other

An Extensive Transbasal Approach to Frontal Skull-Base Tumors: Technical Note
Kawakami K, Yamanouchi Y, Kubota C, Kawamura Y, Matsumura H (Kansai Med Univ, Moriguchi, Japan)
J Neurosurg 74:1011–1013, 1991   20–8

Introduction.—A lesion deep in the anterior skull base requires adequate retraction of the frontal lobes to provide a sufficiently large operative field. A new approach, based on en bloc bilateral osteotomy of the orbital roofs and frontal sinus, has been developed for these lesions. This "extensive transbasal approach" is a modification of that described by Derome and Guiot.

Technique.—A wide craniotomy is done to develop a pedicled dural flap from the frontal convexity should dural repair be necessary. A microsagittal bone saw is used to osteotomize the frontal skull base to the extent necessary. The dura is repaired (if necessary) after removing the tumor, and the osteotomized frontal bar is then fixed so that no dislocation takes place. The pericranial flaps taken from the forehead are affixed to the frontal skull base to close off communication between the nasal cavity and the inside of the skull.

Complications.—The olfactory, frontal, supraorbital, and oculomotor nerves are vulnerable to damage during the procedure. The olfactory nerve may be preserved by limiting the osteotomy to the anterior part of the crista galli and by leaving part of the dura mater affixed in the central anterior skull base. Damage to the frontal and supraorbital nerves may be avoided by carefully freeing the periorbital membrane and performing the osteotomy under direct vision.

▶ This report details a modification of the Derome approach to subfrontal tumors. Of special note is the closure, using dural grafting as well as pericranial pedicle fascial coverage of the posterior frontal sinus.—R.M. Crowell, M.D.

Rapid Polymerizing Fibrin Glue From Autologous or Single-Donor Blood: Preparation and Indications

Stechison MT (Ohio State Univ, Columbus)
J Neurosurg 76:626–628, 1992   20–9

Objective.—The risk of transmitting blood-borne disease has limited the use of fibrin glue in neurosurgery. In addition, self-mixed preparations generally are runny mucoid products unsuitable for use in the presence of CSF. A fibrin glue that polymerizes within several seconds of ejection from the syringe has been developed. The material is made from single-donor rather than pooled cryoprecipitate, and it can be prepared from the patient's own blood.

In Vitro Studies.—The preparation with the briefest polymerization time and the firmest consistency used 2,000 units/mL thrombin solution and a 3:1 cryoprecipitate:thrombin solution. The glue remained intact and retained the shape of the mold containing it for 5 days when stored uncovered at room temperature.

Summary of 38 Cases With Use of Fibrin Glue

Surgical Procedure	No. of Cases
transsphenoidal resection of pituitary tumor	18
(includes intraop repair of CSF leak)	(5)
transpetrosal resection of skull-base tumor	2
orbitozygomatic/frontal craniotomy for tumor	4
cavernous sinus aneurysm/tumor	3
microvascular decompression†	6
lumbar discectomy, CSF leak	2
bilat C-2 decompression-occipital neuralgia	1
anterior cervical discectomy, CSF leak	1
Chiari malformation/pseudomeningocele repair	1

† Involvement of the 5th, 7th, and 9th cranial nerves.
(Courtesy of Stechison MT: *J Neurosurg* 76:626–628, 1992.)

In Vivo Studies.—The fibrin glue was used when a dural defect could not be repaired in a watertight manner; it also was used as a sealant over Gelfoam packing of the paranasal sinuses (table). No postoperative CSF leakage has occurred in any of 38 patients treated. Five patients in whom glue was used to repair iatrogenic CSF leaks, incurred during transsphenoidal pituitary resection, had no CSF rhinorrhea during follow-up. An early recipe of glue failed in 1 instance. Use of the fibrin glue caused no complications.

Conclusion.—This fibrin glue preparation may reduce the need for later surgery to repair CSF leaks that occur intraoperatively. Single-donor cryoprecipitate carries a relatively low risk of transmitting disease.

▶ This report describes a practical method of preparing fibrin glue from cryoprecipitate and thrombin, which are commonly used and are easily accessible components in clinical practice. With the use of cryoprecipitate from a single donor, an extremely low risk of infection with virulent infectious agents is possible. The preparation of the material (as described) is simple, and the results are (as described) almost always effective in preventing CSF leakage. On the Neurosurgical Service at the Massachusetts General Hospital, we have used a very similar approach in approximately 30 cases with similar results. Although further data are required, the information available to date supports this approach as a useful adjunct in the prevention of CSF leakage.—R.M. Crowell, M.D.

Experimental Evaluation of a Collagen-Coated Vicryl Mesh as a Dural Substitute

San-Galli F, Darrouzet V, Rivel J, Baquey C, Ducassou D, Guérin J (Hôpital Pellegrin; Université de Bordeaux II, Bordeaux, France)

Neurosurgery 30:396–401, 1992   20–10

Background.—Absence of the dura mater can result from congenital malformation, tumor or trauma, or surgical removal. Effective dural substitutes must provide immediate restitution of a membranous covering for the brain without provoking adverse host reactions or adhesions to underlying nerve tissues. Ideally, this material would disappear completely, being replaced by tissues similar to dura mater. The in vivo biologic compatibility and function of a dura mater prosthetic replacement consisting of collagen-coated vicryl mesh were evaluated after implantation in dogs.

Methods and Results.—Parietal dural defects were created in 12 beagle dogs and were closed with a vicryl mesh prosthesis. The prosthesis was made watertight by a film of bovine collagen. Clinical and biologic tolerance was judged to be satisfactory. Early local infection developed in 1 dog. Gross and microscopic assessments were performed 7 days to 9 months after implantation. The prosthetic mesh was degraded, and the connective tissue growth into the implant mimicked dura mater as soon as 15 days after implantation. No attendant inflammatory reaction or cortical adhesions or other adverse reactions occurred.

Conclusion.—A collagen-coated vicryl mesh, implanted as a dural substitute in beagle dogs, had satisfactory biologic function and compatibility. Degradation of the prosthetic mesh and connective tissue growth into the implant mimicking dura mater were noted as early as 15 days after the prosthesis was implanted.

▶ This communication draws attention to the association between cerebral arterial fenestrations and intracranial saccular aneurysms. The fenestration of an anterior communicating artery (duplication or triplication) is relatively common with nearby aneurysm. The authors point out that this situation can also occur with the basilar artery, middle cerebral artery, vertebral artery, and even carotid artery. The anatomy can be worked out with oblique angiographic views, and MRI is sometimes helpful to the surgeon in planning the surgical approach. It is particularly true when special approaches are required, as in transclival approach to a midline basilar aneurysm.—R.M. Crowell, M.D.

Postoperative Deficits and Functional Recovery Following Removal of Tumors Involving the Dominant Hemisphere Supplementary Motor Area

Rostomily RC, Berger MS, Ojemann GA, Lettich E (Univ of Washington, Seattle)
J Neurosurg 75:62–68, 1991   20–11

Background.—The supplementary motor area (SMA) is a segment of premotor cortex on the mesial aspect of the frontal lobe that may have a role in planning or initiating motor activity, including speech.

Methods.—The function of the SMA was investigated by reviewing the findings in 6 patients with tumors of the dominant hemisphere who underwent removal of the dominant SMA in the course of tumor resection. All the patients initially had seizure activity. Three of the 6 had a mild right hemiparesis. The SMA was localized by direct stimulation mapping of the primary motor cortex.

Observations.—Five patients with glial tumors became mute within 24 hours of resection but had no disorder of sensation or comprehension. Fluent speech returned within 12 days of surgery, but the patients continued to hesitate and have trouble initiating speech. Some patients had transient difficulty finding words and exhibited verbal perseveration for a time. Motor deficits were more variable. All the patients had slight dyspraxia and impaired fine motor control, which resolved within a year after surgery.

Conclusion.—It appears possible to ablate the SMA (after identifying the primary motor cortex) without significant permanent loss of speech function or motor activity.

▶ Dr. George Ojemann and his colleagues have extended their work in the characterization of the functional anatomy of the brain, as documented by cortical stimulation studies in patients who underwent surgery using local anesthesia. In this study, they show that tumors involving the dominant hemisphere of the SMA may be extensively removed with good results. In the 6 patients described, very substantial temporary deficits involved impairment of speech initiation and contralateral limb movements; however, the deficits receded, with good results in all. Surgeons operating in this area should be aware of the anatomy, the techniques of mapping, and the transient postoperative deficits.—R.M. Crowell, M.D.

Successful Use of a Vascularized Intercostal Muscle Flap to Seal a Persistent Intrapleural Cerebrospinal Fluid Leak in a Child
Azizkhan RG, Roberson JB Jr, Powers SK (Univ of North Carolina, Chapel Hill)
J Pediatr Surg 26:744–746, 1991   20–12

Introduction.—Prolonged CSF leak after spinal trauma or surgery is an unusual occurrence. The successful closure of a dural fistula was achieved using a vascularized intercostal muscle flap.

Case Report.—Girl, 4 years, with severe upper respiratory infection, underwent left posterior lateral thoracotomy to excise an 8-cm posterior mediastinal mass that was displacing the left upper lobe and was extending into the spinal cord through the T2 and T3 neural foramina. During this operation, a large dural opening was encountered where the tumor had grown 2–3 mm intradurally along the T2 nerve root. The leaves of dura on either side of the root sleeve had to be removed with the tumor, and they were approximated with metal vascular clips. The tumor proved to be a ganglioneuroma. Two weeks after surgery, the child had tachypnea and a large left hydrothorax, which drained 900 mL initially and 300 mL of clear but slightly xanthochromic fluid per day during the next 2 weeks. Reaccumulation of this pleural fluid did not respond to repeated lumbar punctures. Leakage of CSF with extravasation of contrast medium into the pleural cavity at T2–T3 was demonstrated on CT myelography. The tube was removed 14 days later because of dysfunction and minimal drainage, but a significant loculated left hydrothorax recurred within 5 days, necessitating reoperation. The chest incision was reopened, and a CSF leak that looked like an extension of the original torn root sleeve was seen coming from a 4- to 5-mm dural defect. An 8-cm intercostal muscle flap based on the dorsal intercostal artery and vein was created and sutured without tension to the area of the leak. The leak ceased immediately—a postoperative lumbar subarachnoid drain was removed on the third postoperative day and chest tubes were removed on the fifth and sixth days. There were no further problems 1 year later.

Discussion.—Persistent thoracic dural-pleural fistula with recalcitrant CSF hydrothorax is an uncommon problem. Diagnosis and management may be difficult, and direct surgical approaches are needed when nonoperative methods fail. Use of a vascularized intercostal muscle flap to repair such a defect has not previously been reported.

▶ Transthoracic surgery has become more common for spinal problems. This communication shows how CSF leakage into the chest may be precisely diagnosed with CT scanning and contrast material. In many cases, the defect may be closed directly, either with suture technique or by the use of fibrin glue and patch technique. This report describes a clever pedicle-based muscle flap for a large leak, and this would be particularly appropriate in circumstances in which the leak cannot be adequately exposed.—R.M. Crowell, M.D.

21 Tumors

Gliomas

The Relationship Between Survival and the Extent of the Resection in Patients With Supratentorial Malignant Gliomas
Quigley MR, Maroon JC (Allegheny Gen Hosp, Pittsburgh, Pa)
Neurosurgery 29:385–389, 1992   21–1

Background.—The radical surgical removal of supratentorial gliomas, when possible, is favored. It is believed that this treatment improves patient survival; however, the efficacy of this approach is still debated. The literature was reviewed to determine the relationship between survival and resection extent in patients with supratentorial malignant gliomas.

Methods.—All published series in the English language literature pertaining to the surgical treatment of supratentorial malignant gliomas in the past 30 years involving at least 75 patients were reviewed. Twenty reports including 5,691 patients were found. Of the cases, 85% involved glioblastoma multiforme, although this varied markedly among the series. Gross total resection was accomplished an average of 21% of the time. All series used the surgeon's impression rather than objective scan criteria.

Findings.—Only 4 studies found that the extent of resection was related to patient survival. In 2 of those studies, extent of resection followed age, histologic findings, and performance status in importance. The other 2 studies did not rank prognostic variables. However, closer examination suggested that there is a subgroup of young patients with favorable histologic findings and good performance status for whom surgery is beneficial.

Conclusion.—None of the reported series represents a valid comparison of surgery vs. biopsy in patient survival. All were flawed statistically, because the selection bias favored surgical candidates. Overall, extent of resection extent alone does not seem to predict outcome. In a small subgroup of patients, however, a radical resection probably does enhance survival and quality of life compared with biopsy. Future research on survival after treatment needs to stratify results on the basis of the known prognostic variables of age, performance status, and histologic findings if that subgroup of patients benefiting from surgery is ever to be characterized correctly.

▶ This review highlights the uncertain effectiveness of cytoreductive surgery in the treatment of gliomas. The central question is: Should one take out what tumor is possible accepting the morbidity of the procedure, or should one do a minimally invasive biopsy with adjunctive therapy? The available data do not permit a clear answer to this question. Only a properly designed prospective randomized study can answer the question.

In normal pressure hydrocephalus, the results included complications in 50% of the cases with a 1% mortality; shunt malfunction was the most common complication (31%), followed by infection (19%). Moreover, the preoperative evaluation cannot reliably indicate which patients will improve from treatment. Thus, the complication rate cannot be reduced significantly by patient selection.—R.M. Crowell, M.D.

Long-Term Outcome of 89 Low-Grade Brain-Stem Gliomas After Interstitial Radiation Therapy

Mundinger F, Braus DF, Krauss JK, Birg W (Neurosurgical Hosp, Freiburg, Germany)
J Neurosurg 75:740–746, 1991   21–2

Background.—Brain stem gliomas are common, comprising 14% to 28% of all infratentorial neoplasms. They are a heterogeneous group of tumors, different in their clinical incidence, appearance on CT, microscopic features, and biologic behavior. However, most of these tumors are ultimately lethal, regardless of their initial histologic class. Therefore, the management of low-grade brain stem gliomas was debated. The long-term benefit of stereotactic treatment was assessed in 89 patients with histologically confirmed, nonresectable low-grade astrocytomas in the brain stem treated between 1974 and 1985.

Methods.—Iodine 125 was implanted in 29 patients, and iridium 192 was implanted in 26. According to CT, 78% of the tumors were located chiefly in the mesencephalic region, 70% were circumscribed, and 78% were contrast-enhanced. Thirty-four patients had biopsy without prior aggressive tumor-specific treatment. Among these cases, 70% of the tumors were mainly in the pons, 74% were diffuse, and 59% were hypodense or isodense after contrast enhancement.

Outcomes.—There was no significant difference in life expectancy between patients with grade I and grade II brain stem gliomas. The mortality among all patients with brain stem tumors, with or without radiation therapy, was 2.4%. Six percent of the total number had complications; 2.4% of the 6% involved hemorrhage with hemipareses and cranial nerve palsy. Long-term follow-up showed that life expectancy after interstitial radiation therapy with ^{125}I implanted directly by catheter either permanently or temporarily tended to be more favorable than life expectancy after treatment with ^{192}Ir.

Conclusion.—Interstitial radiation therapy with ^{125}I appears to be effective against slowly proliferating, differentiated, well-delineated, non-resectable brain stem gliomas. With this method, it is possible to achieve radiosurgical tumor control. When carefully applied, it represents the least traumatic treatment. Reducing the tumor mass improves clinical symptoms. Further research on the biologic behavior of brain stem gliomas and prospective randomized long-term follow-up studies are now needed to assess the different kinds of treatment available for these patients.

▶ This interesting study compares results in patients with low-grade astrocytomas managed with biopsy only, interstitial treatment with ^{125}I and interstitial treatment with ^{192}Ir. However, the criteria for selection of the treatment method were not assigned randomly; specifically, biopsy only was carried out when patients refused interstitial radiation or when the lesion was irregular in its margin. Iridium-192 was implanted only after it became available in 1979. Thus, Figure 3 in the original article is somewhat misleading, because it suggests that interstitial radiation is superior to biopsy. In addition, the small numbers make it impossible to achieve statistical significance in differences between any of the groups. Moreover, it may be noted that the same kind of high-intensity, local irradiation can be achieved without opening the skull through stereotactic radiosurgery.—R.M. Crowell, M.D.

Selection Bias, Survival, and Brachytherapy for Glioma
Florell RC, Macdonald DR, Irish WD, Bernstein M, Leibel SA, Gutin PH, Cairncross JG (Univ of Western Ontario, London, Ont; Univ of Toronto, Ont; Mem Sloan-Kettering Cancer Ctr, New York; Univ of California, San Francisco)
J Neurosurg 76:179–183, 1992   21–3

Purpose.—For patients with malignant glioma, interstitial irradiation with high-activity Iodine-125 (^{125}I) sources is a promising treatment. Adjuvant brachytherapy has come into use as a result of longer-than-expected survivals after treatment for recurrent tumors. The effects of patient selection on survival was studied in 101 adults with supratentorial malignant glioma treated at 1 regional cancer treatment facility during a 2-year period.

Methods.—The initial treatment consisted of maximum feasible surgical resection and external beam radiation, with individualized treatment for progressive or recurrent tumors. The decision as to whether patients were eligible for adjuvant brachytherapy was made by 2 surgeons and a radiation oncologist on the basis of imaging studies and performance status. Survival and prognostic factors in the eligible and ineligible groups were compared.

Results.—A total of 32% of the patients were judged eligible for brachytherapy. This group survived for 17 months vs. 9 months for the ineligible group, its members were younger—50 vs. 57 years. They also had larger resections and better Karnofsky scores. A total of 40% of the patients with glioblastoma were eligible. They survived 14 months vs. 6 months for those who were ineligible. Because of their small numbers, no conclusions could be drawn for patients with anaplastic glioma.

Conclusion.—The improved outcome with adjuvant brachytherapy for glioma appears to result at least partly from patient selection. This therapy is not suitable for most patients with malignant glial tumors. Proof that longer survival is a result of treatment will require randomized trials of comparably selected patients.

▶ This important study illustrates that the apparent benefit for patients with brachytherapy is at least in part the result of patient selection. Although brachytherapy has been around for more than a decade, it remains an innovative approach that has yet to achieve full scientific validation. In addition, there is a theoretical basis for the recommendation that radiosurgery can accomplish the same effects without opening the skull. Further studies will be required to permit general use of this technique.—R.M. Crowell, M.D.

A Randomized Comparison of Intra-Arterial Versus Intravenous BCNU, With or Without Intravenous 5-Fluorouracil, for Newly Diagnosed Patients With Malignant Glioma

Shapiro WR, Green SB, Burger PC, Selker RG, VanGilder JC, Robertson JT, Mealey J Jr, Ransohoff J, Mahaley MS Jr (St Joseph's Hosp and Med Ctr, Phoenix, Ariz)
J Neurosurg 76:772–781, 1992   21–4

Background.—Previous experience suggests that surgery plus radiotherapy and intravenous administration of 1,3-bis (2-chloroethyl)-1-nitrosourea (BCNU) significantly promotes the survival of patients with malignant glioma, compared with treatment without chemotherapy. Increased levels of BCNU probably can be achieved in tumor tissue using regional chemotherapy.

Objective.—A phase III trial was planned to compare intra-arterial administration of BCNU and intravenous treatment, with and without intravenous 5-fluorouracil, in 448 patients seen at 7 centers with histologically confirmed supratentorial malignant glioma. All the patients were 15 years of age and older. All received radiotherapy in addition to chemotherapy.

Treatment.—The dose of BCNU was 200 mg/m² every 8 weeks, and that of 5-fluorouracil was 1 g/m² 3 times daily, 2 weeks after administration of BCNU. A total of 315 patients who were able to receive intra-arterial BCNU were randomized.

Percent Surviving

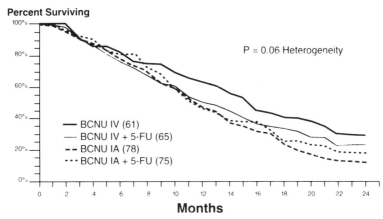

P = 0.06 Heterogeneity

━━ BCNU IV (61)
── BCNU IV + 5-FU (65)
╌╌ BCNU IA (78)
••• BCNU IA + 5-FU (75)

Months

Fig 21–1.—Graph showing patient survival time from randomization correlated with the chemotherapy group for the 279 patients eligible to receive intra-arterial (IA) BCNU in the Valid Study Group. The *numbers in parentheses* denote the number of patients in each group. IV = intravenous; *5-FU* = 5-fluorouracil. (Courtesy of Shapiro WR, Green SB, Burger PC, et al: *J Neurosurg* 76:772–781, 1992.)

Outcome.—The patients given intra-arterial BCNU had reduced survival (Fig 21-1). The median survival times were 11 months for that group and 14 months for those patients treated intravenously. Irreversible encephalopathy developed in 10% of the patients treated intra-arterially, and 15% of the patients had visual loss ipsilaterally. The use of 5-fluorouracil did not influence survival. The difference in survival between intra-arterial and intravenous treatment was seen in patients with anaplastic astrocytoma but not in those with glioblastoma multiforme. There was neuropathologic evidence of white matter necrosis after intra-arterial BCNU treatment.

Conclusion.—Intra-arterial administration of BCNU is not a safe treatment for malignant glioma, and it is no more effective than intravenous administration.

▶ This important study lays to rest the possible use of intra-arterial BCNU for malignant glioma. Although there are theoretical and laboratory bases for expecting efficacy from locally infused BCNU in the treatment of malignant gliomas, a large controlled study has shown no such effectiveness. In fact, in a number of subgroups, the patients who received intra-arterial BCNU actually fared worse than those receiving intravenous BCNU. In addition, the incidence of toxic effects resulting from the treatment was noteworthy: approximately 10% of the patients had irreversible encephalopathy develop, and nearly 15% had visual loss. Thus, this large, well-designed study shows that the use of intra-arterial BCNU for gliomas should be discarded. There is some chance that other agents might be effective by this route; however, a large sophisticated study would be necessary to prove this point.—R.M. Crowell, M.D.

Experimental Therapy of Human Glioma by Means of a Genetically Engineered Virus Mutant

Martuza RL, Malick A, Markert JM, Ruffner KL, Coen DM (Harvard Med School, Boston)
Science 252:854–856, 1991 21–5

Introduction.—Gliomas comprise a large percentage of brain tumors in the United States. Glioblastomas are almost always fatal, and no present therapeutic modality has changed the outcome for patients with this type of cancer. The use of a genetically engineered virus found to destroy glioma cells but spare normal brain cells was examined.

Methods.—Twenty nude mice were inoculated with cell inoculum that caused 100% mortality within 1.5 months in a pilot study. The mice were then divided randomly into 3 groups: group 1 received 10^3 plaque-forming units (pfu) of *dls*ptk, a thymidine kinase-negative mutant of herpes simplex virus 1; group 2 received 10^5 pfu of *dls*ptk; a control group received DME+ (Dulbecco's modified Eagle's medium with 10% fetal bovine serum and antibiotics) alone.

Outcomes.—Growth inhibition of tumor was noted in mice with subrenal U87 human gliomas given *dls*ptk; in mice with intracranial U87 gliomas given *dls*ptk, survival was longer (Fig 21–2). In cell culture, human glioblastoma cells were destroyed.

Conclusion.—Genetically engineered viruses may play an important role in the treatment of some resistant tumors, such as malignant human

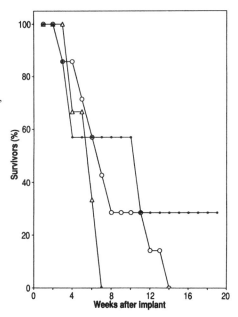

Fig 21–2.—Ten days after intracerebral injection of 1.6×10^5 U87 cells into each of 20 nude mice, the tumors were treated with either 10^3 pfu of *dls*ptk (*open circles*), 10^5 pfu of *dls*ptk (*filled circles*), or DME + alone (*triangles*). (Courtesy of Martuza RL, Malick A, Markert JM, et al: *Science* 252:854–856, 1991.)

gliomas. These viruses merit evaluation as new antineoplastic agents and should be investigated further.

▶ This sophisticated basic study shows how molecular strategies against glioma can be evaluated in the laboratory. A genetically engineered virus mutant of herpes simplex was introduced into mouse gliomas with a remarkable cytotoxic effect on tumor cells, which rapidly reproduce but have little effect on the brain with its slower metabolism. Whether this particular method is helpful clinically, the approach nonetheless demonstrates the usefulness of the basic oncologic laboratory for testing new concepts of brain tumor therapy.—R.M. Crowell, M.D.

Hyperfractionated Radiation Therapy in Brain Stem Tumors: Results of Treatment at the 7020 cGy Dose Level of Pediatric Oncology Group Study number #8495
Freeman CR, Krischer J, Sanford RA, Cohen ME, Burger PC, Kun L, Halperin EC, Crocker I, Wharam M (McGill Univ, Montreal; Univ of Florida, Gainesville; St Jude Children's Research Hosp, Memphis, Tenn; Roswell Park Mem Inst, Buffalo, NY; Duke Univ, Durham, NC; et al)
Cancer 68:474–481, 1991   21–6

Introduction.—In radiation therapy for brain stem tumors, hyperfractionation exploits the differences in repair capacity between early-reacting normal tissues and tumors and late-reacting normal tissues. In 1984, the Pediatric Oncology Group began a study of hyperfractionated radiotherapy (HRT) in a total dose of 6,600 cGy, given in 60 fractions over 6 weeks; the results were comparable to those of conventional treatment, with acceptable acute toxicity and no late complications. In 1986, the trial was reopened using a dose level of 7,020 cGy; the results of this treatment were evaluated.

Methods.—From 1986 to 1988, 57 patients with high-risk brain stem tumors were entered into the study. There were 27 males and 30 females (median age, 6.5 years). The total dose of 7,020 cGy was delivered to local fields in 117 cGy fractions given twice a day, for a total of 60 fractions for 6 weeks. The minimum interaction interval was 6 hours. Information on clinical status during HRT was available for 55 patients. The CT and/or MRI results were available for 52 patients.

Results.—During HRT, clinical status improved in 44 patients, was stable in 6, and deteriorated in 5. Neuroimaging studies revealed 1 complete and 3 partial responses, with 40 patients remaining stable. Thus, the total response rate was 77%. The median time to progression was 6 months, and the median survival 10 months. One-year survival was 40%, and 2-year survival was 23%.

Complications.—Six patients had an enhanced skin reaction and 9 had otitis media and/or externa. Bleeding into the tumor after HRT occurred in 1 case, and intralesional necrosis occurred in 3. In 5 patients who took steroids for extended periods, complications included opportunistic infections, impaired glucose tolerance, hypertension, osteoporosis, and mood changes. No late injuries were ascribed to the HRT regimen.

Conclusions.—A trial of HRT at a dose of 7,020 cGy shows a trend toward improved survival with lower dose levels, even though the patient characteristics are less favorable at the higher level. The outcome appears to be related to type of neurologic deficit. A trial using a total dose of 7,560 cGy for 6 weeks is under way.

▶ This abstract represents a further study of HRT for brain stem tumors in children. A dose of 117 cGy was given twice daily, to a total dose of 7,020 cGy. Of 55 patients, 80% improved, 6 were stable, and 5 deteriorated. The complications were minor, and 5 patients required steroids for protracted periods. Compared with patients treated at a lower dosage, there appeared to be a trend toward improved survival. There is good rationale for this type of approach (to permit a higher safe dosage), and these encouraging results warrant further follow-up study.—R.M. Crowell, M.D.

The Prognostic Significance of Postoperative Residual Tumor in Ependymoma

Healey EA, Barnes PD, Kupsky WJ, Scott RM, Sallan SE, Black PM, Tarbell NJ (The Children's Hosp, Boston, Mass)
Neurosurgery 28:666–672, 1991   21–7

Background.—Ependymoma, an uncommon CNS tumor, originates from the ependymal cells that line the cerebral ventricles and central canal of the spinal cord. The prognostic significance of residual tumors after surgery was assessed.

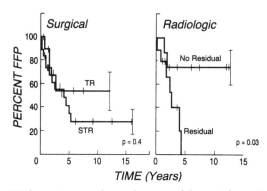

Fig 21–3.—The FFP for patients according to the extent of the surgical resection as determined by the operating neurosurgeon compared with postoperative neuroimaging (no residual disease vs. residual disease) (*TR*, total resection; *STR*, subtotal resection; *Bx*, biopsy). *Vertical bars* indicate standard error. (Courtesy of Healey EA, Barnes PD, Kupsky WJ, et al: *Neurosurgery* 28:666–672, 1991.)

Patients.—Fifteen male and 14 female patients were treated for intracranial ependymomas between 1970 and 1989. Ten were infants, 12 were children, and 7 were adults as old as 66 years of age. The median follow-up was 82 months. Twenty-five patients were given initial postoperative radiotherapy with a median tumor dose of 5,360 cGy.

Outcomes.—The 5- and 10-year actuarial survival rates were 61% and 46%, respectively. Anaplastic histologic findings were seen in only 2 cases. Local failure was the primary pattern of relapse, with a median time to recurrence of 22 months. The most important prognostic factor was the presence of radiographic residual disease seen on postoperative MRI or CT. Analysis of the 19 patients undergoing postoperative imaging showed a 75% 5-year freedom from progressive disease for 9 patients with no residual disease. None of the 10 patients with gross residual disease was free from progressive disease. The surgical evaluation of residual disease was nonsignificant. Age at presentation was a significant prognostic variable. The overall actuarial survival rate at 12 years for patients who were age 24 months or younger at diagnosis was 0%, whereas that for older patients was 62% (Fig 21–3).

Conclusion.—Complete surgical resection followed by local-field, high-dose radiotherapy appears to offer the best chance for the long-term survival of patients with nonanaplastic ependymomas. Patients with radiologically apparent postoperative disease have a markedly reduced survival. Therefore, maximal surgical resection and novel therapeutic approaches are merited for this high-risk group. Future protocols should use postoperative imaging rather than operative reports to stratify patients.

▶ The results indicate quite clearly that radiologic evidence of tumor is a very bad prognostic sign for these patients. Some authors believe that radiation should be offered only to those patients with residual disease, because recurrence has not yet been noted in that group.—R.M. Crowell, M.D.

Posterior Fossa Ependymomas: Report of 30 Cases and Review of the Literature
Lyons MK, Kelly PJ (Mayo Clinic and Found; Mayo Graduate School of Medicine, Rochester, Minn)
Neurosurgery 28:659–665, 1991   21–8

Introduction.—In 1976–1988, 30 patients with a median age of 44 years were operated on for histologically confirmed primary ependymoma of the posterior fossa. Ataxia, nausea/vomiting, and headache were the most frequent symptoms. The median duration of symptoms was 6 months in adults. Nearly two thirds of the patients initially had ataxia and nystagmus; dysmetria and reflex abnormalities were less frequent.

Methods.—In 8 patients, all gross tumor was removed, 21 had subtotal resection, and 1 had only a biopsy. All but 3 tumors occupied the fourth ventricle, and most of them extended beyond the confines of this structure. Reoperation was performed in 5 patients for residual or recurrent tumor. In 8 patients there were high-grade ependymomas. All but 3 patients received radiotherapy postoperatively. A full course of chemotherapy was completed by 5 children and 2 adults.

Results.—There was 1 operative death. The 16 surviving patients were followed up for a median time of 86 months. All but 1 of the surviving patients were doing well when last seen; 10 patients were alive after subtotal tumor removal. All patients who died had residual or recurrent tumor at the primary site. Neither the preoperative clinical features nor the duration of symptoms predicted the outcome.

Conclusion.—Posterior fossa ependymomas should be removed as completely as is technically feasible. If the postoperative myelogram or MRI is negative for spinal seeding, prophylactic spinal irradiation is not necessary.

▶ This experience of the Mayo Clinic and review of the literature indicate that the young patient with ependymoma has a poor prognosis. The 5-year survival has improved with gross total resection. Recurrence is at the primary intracranial site, and asymptomatic spinal seating is uncommon. Surgical resection is warranted, even in eradicating tumor from the lateral recess, and even from the peduncle (but not, of course, from the floor of the fourth ventricle)—R.M. Crowell, M.D.

The Treatment of Oligodendrogliomas and Mixed Oligodendroglioma-Astrocytomas With PCV Chemotherapy

Glass J, Hochberg FH, Gruber ML, Louis DN, Smith D, Rattner B (Massachusetts Gen Hosp, Boston)
J Neurosurg 76:741–745, 1992   21–9

Introduction.—More than half the patients operated on for oligodendroglioma fail to live 5 years. Recent reports have suggested that anaplastic oligodendrogliomas are quite sensitive to chemotherapy. Systemic chemotherapy was evaluated in 7 patients with oligodendroglioma or anaplastic oligodendroglioma and in 14 others with mixed oligodendroglioma-astrocytoma.

Management.—Fourteen patients received chemotherapy before radiotherapy, and 7 received it afterward. The PCV (procarbazine, CCNU, vincristine) therapy was given in 2–5 cycles at 6-week intervals.

Results.—Eleven of the 14 patients who were given chemotherapy before radiotherapy had at least a 50% reduction in tumor mass when evaluated 20 weeks to more than 100 weeks after treatment. Two patients with anaplastic lesions and 9 with mixed tumors responded, and 1 in each group had a complete response. Three of the 7 patients given chemotherapy after radiotherapy had partial responses. Four patients had stabilization of tumor growth after PCV treatment. There were no serious treatment complications.

Conclusion.—Administration of PCV chemotherapy before irradiation may benefit patients with anaplastic oligodendroglioma or malignant mixed glioma.

▶ In this study, which albeit is small, data are presented that indicate a useful response in 14 of 21 patients with oligodendroglioma or anaplastic oligodendroglioma. Further studies are indicated to confirm these findings, but on the basis of this information, one can now recommend that chemotherapy with procarbazine, CCNU and vincristine be given before radiation in this subset of patients with glioma.—R.M. Crowell, M.D.

Choroid Plexus Carcinoma of Childhood
Packer RJ, Perilongo G, Johnson D, Sutton LN, Vezina G, Zimmerman RA, Ryan J, Reaman G, Schut L (Children's Natl Med Ctr, Washington, DC; Children's Hosp of Philadelphia)
Cancer 69:580–585, 1992   21–10

Introduction.—Choroid plexus carcinoma (CPC) is a rare primary choroid tumor found in children. Its biologic behavior is poorly defined, and there is no consensus as to treatment—including the need for postoperative adjuvant therapy. The presentation, growth patterns, and therapeutic response were analyzed in 11 children with CPC, and the results were compared to those of other reported series.

Patients.—The children were 6 boys and 5 girls (median age, 26 months). Three were older than 7 years of age when CPC was diagnosed. Eight patients had ventricular tumors with some attachment to the subependymal area, 2 had primary thalamic tumors, and 1 had a primary posterior fossa tumor. Gross total resection was done in 5 patients, with 1 having radiation therapy; 6 patients had subtotal resection, 3 having radiation therapy and 1 having chemotherapy.

Outcomes.—A median of 48 months after diagnosis, 5 children were in continuous progression-free remission. Four of them had gross total resection; relapse occurred in all but 1 child treated with subtotal resection. Only 1 patient treated with radiation therapy or chemotherapy responded—this patient received etoposide. Including patients from other reported series, 11 of 14 children with gross total resection had prolonged progression-free survival vs. 2 of 20 children with less than total resection. These results occurred regardless of the type of adjuvant therapy.

Conclusion.—The benefits of adjuvant chemotherapy for children with CPC remain to be proven. This finding should be borne in mind when trials of alternative treatments for these patients are analyzed, particularly for patients with totally resected tumors. With current treatment methods, patients with subtotal resection do not have good results.

▶ This is a very important paper. It shows that gross total resection of CPC is dramatically superior to partial resection for this lesion. These uncommon lesions are likely to be fatal with subtotal resection. Treatment adjuncts to make total resection possible are highly desirable. These may include embolization, chemotherapy, or radiotherapy. Protocols to demonstrate superiority for any of these adjuvant treatments are still being evaluated.—R.M. Crowell, M.D.

Intracranial Tumours and Blood Groups
Sowbhagya P, Sastry Kolluri VR, Subba Krishna DK, Das S, Das BS, Narayana Reddy GN (Natl Inst Mental Health and Neurosciences, Bangalore, India)
Eur J Cancer 27:221–222, 1991   21–11

Introduction.—The association between blood groups and diseases has been verified. The distribution of different blood groups in patients with intracranial tumors was studied and compared with the general population.

Study Design.—A total of 1,287 patients were treated for intracranial tumors during a 5-year period. Tumor types included glioma (668), meningioma (310), schwannoma (215), and medulloblastoma (94). Blood group distribution in this group of patients was compared with that of the general population.

Results.—Significantly more tumor patients had type A blood, whereas more individuals in the general population had type O. In the glioma group, there were significantly more patients with type A than type O. For medulloblastoma, more patients were in types B and AB than in the general population, and the proportion was significantly higher in group B. There was a significantly less number of type O patients in the schwannoma group, but most patients with meningioma were in blood groups O or A. All of these determinations were based upon the general population.

Conclusion.—Significant blood types appear more often in individual tumor groups. The effect of these findings requires further investigation.

▶ This interesting study has demonstrated a preponderance of type A blood in patients with intracranial tumors, especially those in the glioma group. Although the precise meaning of this observation is not yet clear, it certainly bolsters the notion that genetic mechanisms are operative in the development of intracranial tumors.—R.M. Crowell, M.D.

Genes for Epidermal Growth Factor Receptor, Transforming Growth Factor α, and Epidermal Growth Factor and Their Expression in Human Gliomas *in Vivo*
Ekstrand AJ, James CD, Cavenee WK, Seliger B, Pettersson RF, Collins VP
(Ludwig Inst for Cancer Research, Stockholm; Henry Ford Hosp, Detroit; Ludwig Inst for Cancer Research, Montreal)
Cancer Res 51:2164–2172, 1991   21–12

Background.—Malignant human gliomas appear to harbor anomalies of the epidermal growth factor receptor (EGFR) gene in vivo. The EGFR molecule is a tyrosine kinase functioning transmembrane protein, and it may participate in an autocrine growth stimulation process. The results of tumor tissue analysis from 62 human glioma patients, including dosage, structure, and expression of the EGFR gene in these tumors, were evaluated.

Methods.—Fifty-six primary tumors and 10 recurrent human gliomas were assessed for nucleic acid content and DNA and RNA content, using complementary DNA and messenger RNA radioactive probe techniques, southern blot hybridization methods, and protein analysis.

Findings.—Of the 62 gliomas, 27 primary and 3 recurrent human gliomas were studied. Of these 29 tumors, only 1 had detectable EGFR gene amplification. No tumors demonstrated rearrangements of the EGFR gene. Using brain tissue as the control, 3 of the tumors expressed reduced EGFR messenger RNA levels, 13 had equal EGFR messenger RNA expression, 8 demonstrated slightly greater expression, and 6 had significantly greater expression of the EGFR messenger RNA. The EGFR gene was amplified from 10 to 100 times in 16 of the 32 glioblastomas. Two of the EGFR oligonucleotide probes demonstrated the existence of restriction fragment length polymorphisms (PC17 with *Hind* III and PC55 with *Sac* I). Monoallelic amplification was found in samples in which the amplification of the EGFR gene occurred in a heterozygous patient. Of the 13 samples with amplified EGFR genes, all had increased levels of EGFR messenger RNA. A total of 62.5% of the glioblastomas with amplified EGFR genes also demonstrated co-amplification of the rearranged EGFR genes along with expression of the aberrant messenger RNA.

Conclusion.—These results indicate that the activation of the EGFR-mediated growth stimulation may be possible in human glioma tumors. This mechanism could include the expression of a structurally changed receptor that eluded normal physiolgic controls, while various stimulating pathways, such as those involving co-expression of the receptor and its ligands, come into play.

▶ This sophisticated investigation illustrates how comprehensive evaluation of the genetics of tumors may shed light on tumor growth and development. It is not enough to simply show an abnormal gene. It is necessary to evaluate the functional expression of this abnormality. In this particular study, the investigators have shown that glioma tumors demonstrate EGFR gene amplification in half the cases, some with restriction fragment length polymorphisms or increased EGFR messenger RNA. There are many examples of co-amplification of rearranged EGFR genes. All of these details taken together indicate that genetic abnormalities in the tumor are capable of significant modification of the epidermal growth factor receptor, which can provide positive feedback (autocrine) for tumor growth.—R.M. Crowell, M.D.

Nucleolar Organizer Regions in Vascular and Neoplastic Cells of Human Gliomas

Hara A, Sakai N, Yamada H, Hirayama H, Tanaka T, Mori H (Gifu Univ, Gifu, Japan)
Neurosurgery 29:211–215, 1991   21–13

Background.—Vascular cell proliferation is a characteristic histologic feature of glial tumors. The proliferative potential of vascular cells and glioma cells was studied using staining of nucleolar organizer regions (NORs) by means of the argyrophilia of their associated proteins (Ag-NORs).

Methods and Findings.—The number of NORs in vascular cells and neoplastic cells in human gliomas was counted using a combined stain-

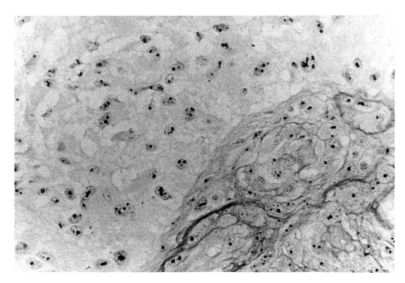

Fig 21–4.—Glioblastoma multiforme. The section stained with silver colloid for nucleolar organizer region–associated argyrophilic proteins (AgNORs) and periodic acid-Schiff contains vascular cells forming glomerular-shaped vessels. Numerous AgNORs are present in the tumor cells and vascular cells. The AgNOR score of the vascular cells is lower than that of the tumor cells. (Courtesy of Hara A, Sakai N, Yamada H, et al: *Neurosurgery* 29:211-215, 1991.)

ing method, consisting of 1-step silver colloid for AgNOR and periodic acid-Schiff staining for basement membrane of vascular components. The number of AgNORs in the vascular and neoplastic cells was determined in various tumors. In benign astrocytoma, this number was 1.52 and 1.8, respectively; in anaplastic astrocytoma, 1.98 and 2.87; in glioblastoma multiforme, 2.05 and 3.13 (Fig 21-4). The vascular cells of benign astrocytomas, anaplastic astrocytomas, and glioblastomas had significantly higher AgNOR scores than those in low-grade gliomas.

Conclusion.—The proliferative activity of both vascular and neoplastic cells in gliomas increase as histologic malignancy advances. Quantifying AgNORs was useful in assessing proliferative activity in vascular cells and malignancy in neoplastic tissue.

▶ This work shows a nice correlation of the neoplastic state with presence of nucleolar organizing regions. Vascular and tumor cells appear to have increased rates of proliferation in tumors of all grades. Neoplastic astrocytes presumably produce a factor that is mitogenic to endothelial cells. Interestingly, vascular cells from low-grade astrocytomas show an increased number of nucleolar organizing regions. This suggests that secretion of an endothelial cell mitogen might be an early event in the development of such tumors.—R.M. Crowell, M.D.

Radiation Necrosis vs High-Grade Recurrent Glioma: Differentiation by Using Dual-Isotope SPECT With ^{201}Tl and ^{99m}Tc-HMPAO
Schwartz RB, Carvalho PA, Alexander E III, Loeffler JS, Folkerth R, Holman BL (Brigham and Women's Hosp, Boston)
AJNR 12:1187–1192, 1991   21–14

Introduction.—Patients who have received radiation therapy for high-grade gliomas often suffer clinical deterioration because of radiation necrosis or recurrent tumor progression. In symptomatic patients, however, the conventional imaging modalities are not always sufficient to distinguish between these 2 entities. A series of such patients was evaluated with high resolution dual-isotope single-photon emission computed tomography (SPECT) using thallium-201 (^{201}T1) and ^{99m}Tc-hexamethyl-propyleneamine oxime (HMPAO).

Methods.—The subjects were 15 patients with high-grade gliomas who had progressively worsening symptoms after radiation therapy. Each underwent both SPECT with ^{201}T1 and ^{99m}Tc-HMPAO 1 day before biopsy and resection were done. The 2 radionuclide studies were correlated with CT images to provide 3-dimensional coordinates for biopsy.

Results.—In all cases but 1, the SPECT findings correlated with the biopsy findings. Local tumor recurrence was present in all patients with high ^{201}T1 uptake, and radiation changes only, with no evidence of solid tumor, were present in all patients with low ^{201}T1 uptake. When ^{210}T1 uptake in the tumor bed was intermediate, the uptake of ^{99m}Tc-HMPAO was able to differentiate patients with and without active tumor. Biopsy specimens revealed solid tumor in 3 of 4 patients with preserved or increased perfusion vs. none in 4 patients with decreased perfusion.

Conclusion.—In patients who receive radiation therapy for malignant glioma, dual SPECT imaging using ^{201}T1 and ^{99m}Tc-HMPAO may help to distinguish probable tumor growth from nonspecific radiation changes. It can also help direct the surgeon as to which area to biopsy. Dual-isotope SPECT should be further investigated as a management tool for patients with high-grade glioma.

▶ This preliminary report on 15 patients with documented gliomas indicates that dual-isotope SPECT in 14 of 15 patients correctly differentiated between radiation necrosis and recurrent glioma. This differential diagnosis is a common clinical problem. Thus far, only positron emission tomography scanning was able to reliably differentiate the diagnosis. If other studies can bear out this finding, SPECT, which is more commonly available, may become the study of choice for this clinical problem.—R.M. Crowell, M.D.

Metastases

Metastatic Brain Tumors: Review of a Surgical Series of 81 Patients
Delarive J, de Triboler N (Centre Hospitalier Universitaire Vaudois, Lausanne, Switzerland)
Neurochirurgie 38:89–97, 1992   21–15

Introduction.—Approximately 30% of all patients with cancer subsequently have clinical signs of an intracranial recurrence. Excision of a solitary intracranial metastasis in patients with controlled primary cancer can prolong and improve the quality of survival. The role of postoperative radiotherapy to decrease the risk of a recurrence is less clear in view of the potential for important morbidity. The records of 81 patients who underwent craniotomy for cerebral metastases were reviewed.

Patients.—There were 58 men and 23 women aged 34–76 years, (mean age, 56.3 years). Clinical signs were recorded for 61 patients, of whom 79% had mostly neuropsychologic symptoms, 43% had symptoms of intracranial hypertension, and 31% had epilepsy. Two patients were asymptomatic; recurrence was discovered during follow-up with CT. Seventy-two patients (89%) had solitary intracranial metastases, of which 33.3% were located in the frontal lobe. Nine patients (11%) had multiple lesions. Pulmonary carcinoma was the most common primary diagnosis (46%). The primary tumor was unknown in 18% of patients.

Results.—Tumor excision was judged complete in 70% of cases, subtotal in 19%, and partial in 11%. The immediate postoperative course was rated excellent in 58% of cases, favorable in 20%, and poor in 22%. The perioperative mortality was 7.4%. A group of 55 patients who survived for 30 days after craniotomy underwent whole brain radiation therapy in doses ranging from 15 to 40 Gy given in fractional doses of 200–650 cGy; 10 patients with poor prognosis did not undergo irradiation. Chemotherapy was not given.

Survival.—The mean overall survival was 10.2 months. Ten patients (12%) survived for more than 18 months, and 1 patient was still alive almost 4 years after craniotomy. The mean survival in the 10 patients who did not have postoperative radiation was 4.9 months. There was no relation between histologic type of the primary tumor and survival. Patients with solitary or multiple lesions had similar survival.

Conclusion.—In younger patients whose primary systemic disease is under control and who have no associated pathologic conditions, craniotomy plus postoperative focal radiotherapy will prolong and improve the quality of survival. Daily radiation doses should not exceed 180–200 cGy, and the total dose should not exceed 40–45 Gy.

▶ This retrospective study of 81 patients in 1 clinic revealed several interesting points: bronchial adenocarcinoma in 19%, squamous carcinoma of the lung in 11%, and melanoma in 12% were the most common metastases to brain. (Interestingly, breast carcinoma was not judged to be common.) A total of 22% of the patients had worsening of neurologic deficits after excision, and this substantial risk must be kept in mind when operating on these patients. The mean survival was only 10.2 months. Only 10 patients survived more than 18 months, and a single patient was alive at 4 years. Interestingly, in this study, the survival was not linked to the histology. These features must be kept in mind before we recommend surgery for these lesions.—R.M. Crowell, M.D.

Meningiomas

The Combined Supra- and Infratentorial Approach for Lesions of the Petrous and Clival Regions: Experience With 46 Cases
Spetzler RF, Daspit CP, Pappas CTE (Barrow Neurological Inst, Phoenix, Ariz)
J Neurosurg 76:588–599, 1992   21–16

Introduction.—Very difficult lesions in the region of the clivus and in the petrous area may be managed with a combined supratentorial and infratentorial approach, providing exposure from the sphenoid ridge and cavernous sinus to the foramen magnum and anterior cervical spinal cord.

Variations.—A translabyrinthine approach, which involves petrous bone resection, entails a loss of hearing. Where applicable, a retrolabyrinthine approach may be used with less petrous bone resection, thereby preserving hearing. A transcochlear variation entails maximum petrous drilling and transposition of the facial nerve. With all these procedures, the clivus/petrous region is well exposed, with minimal or no brain retraction. The superior petrosal sinus is always sacrificed, and the tentorium is totally cut. The sigmoid sinus may sometimes be preserved, depending on how much exposure is needed.

Experience.—Forty-six patients had the combined procedure for large lesions extending above and below the tentorial incisura. The mean patient age was 45 years. Meningiomas and schwannomas were the most frequent lesions. All but 4 patients did well postoperatively and returned to their previous work. Four meningiomas were removed incompletely. Facial nerve paresis developed in 30% of patients, and CSF leakage developed in 13%. There were no intraoperative deaths.

Conclusion.—The combined supra- and intratentorial approach allows relatively safe surgery for lesions involving the clivus and petrous region. Among the possible procedures are tumor resection, removal of an arteriovenous malformation, and aneurysm clipping.

▶ This paper shows the value of collaboration of a neurosurgeon versed in skull base and vascular surgery and a neuro-otologist versed in transmastoid-transcochlear procedures. This is a tour-de-force, with gross total removals in almost all the tumor cases. On the other hand, almost 40% of the patients had some kind of difficulties (often 7th cranial nerve or other cranial nerve dysfunctions). Although this aggressive form of treatment may be warranted in some cases, one should carefully weigh the alternatives of total removal, radiosurgery, or even no surgery at all. Less aggressive measures may well be appropriate in older patients or those with limited symptoms.—R.M. Crowell, M.D.

Clinoidal Meningiomas
Al-Mefty O (Univ of Mississippi, Jackson, Miss)
J Neurosurg 73:840–849, 1990   21–17

Background.—Meningiomas of the anterior clinoid frequently are grouped with suprasellar meningiomas or with meningiomas of the sphenoid ridge. Significant surgical mortality resulting from injury to the major cerebral vessels, high morbidity rates, failure of total removal, and a high rate of recurrence characterize the anterior clinoidal meningioma. The best chance for cure is radical total removal, but because of the risk of injury to the encased cerebral vessels, subtotal removal with subsequent repeat surgery and radiation therapy is more common. However, recent advances in cranial-base exposure and cavernous sinus surgery facilitate radical total removal.

Methods.—The orbitocranial approach was used in 24 cases of surgery for anterior clinoidal meningiomas. A microsurgical technique has improved operative mortality and morbidity by allowing the surgeon to dissect adherent or encased structures caused by the cleavage of the arachnoid membrane. Three subgroups were distinguished on the basis of the presence of interfacing arachnoid membranes between the tumor and

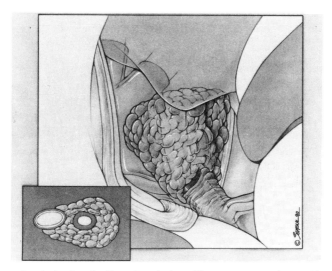

Fig 21–5.—Artist's drawing of a Group I meningioma. The tumor encases the carotid artery and its branches, with direct attachment to the adventitia. The optic nerve maintains an arachnoid plane from the chiasmatic cistern. (Courtesy of Al-Mefty O: *J Neurosurg* 73:840-849, 1990.)

cerebral vessels. The presence or absence of arachnoid membranes depends on the origin of the tumor and its relation to the naked segment of carotid artery lying outside the carotid cistern.

Results.—When the arachnoid membrane was absent (group 1), dissection was impossible, and none of the tumors were removed totally (Fig 21-5). Total tumor removal was possible in group 2, despite total encasement of the arteries and nerves. In group 3 patients, the tumors were totally removed without complications.

Conclusion.—Anterior clinoidal meningiomas are characterized by high surgical mortality and morbidity from injury to encased cerebral vessels. The high surgical risk often necessitates subtotal removal with subsequent recurrence. Radiation therapy is a useful adjuvant in treating nonremovable or recurring tumors. Microsurgical techniques have facilitated radical total removal. The surgeon is able to dissect adherent or encased structures resulting from the cleavage of the arachnoid membrane. When the membrane was absent, none of the tumors were removed totally.

▶ Al-Mefty presents his classification and results with anterior clinoid meningiomas. Using an orbitocranial approach and strict microsurgical technique, the author was able to achieve total removal in 20 of 24 cases, with 2 deaths and 1 hemiplegia. Al-Mefty emphasizes the importance of resection because of the likelihood of late recurrence and neurologic deterioration. Unfortunately, reliable data regarding the role of radiation therapy and stereotactic radiosurgery for these lesions have not yet been obtained. It will be important to have such information to decide how aggressive surgical resection ought to be in selected cases. For lesions with more extensive involvement of the optic nerve and carotid artery, such as in group 1, one must be content with a subtotal resection, and radiation might be considered. Clearly, the smaller, less adherent lesions can be resected with good results. The major discussion will be regarding the intermediate group 2 lesions. Patient condition, age, and symptomatology should be important considerations, as should the experience of the surgeon.—R.M. Crowell, M.D.

A t(4;22) in a Meningioma Points to the Localization of a Putative Tumor-Suppressor Gene

Lekanne Deprez RH, Groen NA, van Biezen NA, Hagemeijer A, van Drunen E, Koper JW, Avezaat CJJ, Bootsma D, Zwarthoff EC (Erasmus Univ, Rotterdam, The Netherlands)
Am J Hum Genet 48:783–790, 1991   21–18

Introduction.—The loss of all or part of a specific chromosome, which suggests the involvement of a tumor-suppressor gene, has been implicated in cancers such as meningioma, a common benign mesenchymal intracranial or intraspinal tumor. This paper reports on the cytogenetic analysis of meningioma cells from a particular patient who had the stem-line karyotype 45, XY, −1, 4p+, 22q−, 22q+, which ultimately meant a rearrangement of both chromosomes 22.

Case Report.—Man, 64, had a second meningioma (MN32) that was removed from the right temporal side of his brain. He had a history of head inju-

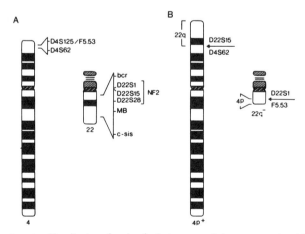

Fig 21–6.—**A,** regional localization of probes for loci on normal chromosomes 4 and 22. The area in which the NF2 gene has been mapped is indicated. **B,** schematic representation of reciprocal t(4;22), creating 4p+ and 22q− marker chromosomes in meningioma MN32. The breakpoints (*arrows*) are shown according to DNA probes for chromosomes 4 and 22. (Courtesy of Lekanne Deprez RH, Groen NA, van Biezen NA, et al: *Am J Hum Genet* 48:783–790, 1991.)

ries and had had an olfactorial meningioma removed 21 years earlier. The second meningioma was syncytial, transitional, and fibroblastic.

Methods.—Tissue culture, hybrid cell lines, and cytogenetics were all used to characterize the tumor tissue. Analysis of DNA included extraction, Southern blotting, and hybridization to delineate the gene and the involved loci.

Results.—Cytogenetic analysis of the meningiomas that were surgically removed demonstrated an alteration of both copies of chromosome 22, including abnormal karyotype and basic stem line of 45, XY, −1, 4p+, 22q−, 22q+. The marker chromosome 22q+ had been translocated with chromosome 1, leading to a dicentric chromosome 22pter→ q11::1p11→qter. The hybridization signals indicated that 2 copies of D22S1 were present, but only 1 copy each of D22S15 and D22S201 were present. The karyotype of the tumor showed that both the 22q− and 22q+ marker chromosomes lost sequences distal to band q11. Figure 21-6 demonstrates the outline of the position of the DNA probes on chromosomes 4 and 22 and their position on the translocation products.

Implications.—These findings suggest that a tumor-suppressor gene was deleted at the 22q+ marker site; this led to the disruption of this gene's second allele by the t(4;22). Such a translocation mapped between D22S1 and D22S15, measured 1 cm on the linkage map of this chromosome, and appeared to be located within the area near the gene that predisposes to neurofibromatosis.

▶ Here is another sophisticated genetic investigation. In this case, a defective putative tumor-suppressor gene has been located in a meningioma. This is support for the concept that suppressor genes exist, and that their deletion can lead to expression of the tumor. The concept may well have application in diagnosis and treatment.—R.M. Crowell, M.D.

Prediction of Biologic Aggressiveness in Human Meningiomas: A Cell Kinetic Study Using Bromodeoxyuridine in Cells of Primary Explant Culture
Kharbanda K, Karak AK, Sarkar C, Dinda AK, Mathur M, Roy S (All India Inst of Med Sciences, Ansari Nagar, New Delhi, India)
J Natl Cancer Inst 84:194–195, 1992   21–19

Background.—On their own, histopathologic criteria are insufficient for accurate assessment of biologic aggressiveness in meningiomas. Preliminary reports of in vivo bromodeoxyuridine labeling index (BrdU LI) and DNA flow cytometric proliferative index show good correlation with biologic aggressiveness, regardless of histologic heterogeneity. Aggressiveness was assessed by estimating BrdU LI in cells of primary explant culture after 1 week of culture.

Methods.—Twenty-six meningiomas were analyzed, including 5 recurrent tumors and 3 that had invaded the brain parenchyma. The remaining 18 tumors were considered benign. The tumors were subjected to routine histologic studies, and small samples were explanted for culture. At the end of 1 week, coverslips with the cultured cells were exposed to 10 μm of BrdU and were stained with monoclonal anti-BrdU antibody. At least 1,000–2,000 cells were counted to calculate BrdU LI.

Results.—First-week BrdU LI was not correlated with age, sex, site of the tumor, duration of symptoms, and histologic subtypes. However, the values of the recurrent and malignant tumors were significantly different than those of the benign tumors. The LI was greater than 5% in all recurrent or malignant tumors and less than 5% in 12 of 18 benign tumors.

Conclusion.—In meningioma, BrdU LI of the primary explant culture is a useful alternative to in vivo BrdU LI and DNA flow cytometry for correlation with biologic aggressiveness. This procedure should encounter no problems with acceptability and widespread use. Tumors with a first-week BrdU LI greater than 5% should be carefully followed up for early detection of recurrence.

▶ This small study adds weight to the data that BrDU LI values less than 5% strongly suggest a benign character in meningioma.—R.M. Crowell, M.D.

Pituitary

Positron Emission Tomography of Pituitary Macroadenomas: Hormone Production and Effects of Therapies

Francavilla TL, Miletich RS, DeMichele D, Patronas NJ, Oldfield EH, Weintraub BD, Di Chiro G (Natl Inst of Neurological Disorders and Stroke, Bethesda, Md; George Washington Univ, Washington, DC; Clinical Ctr; Natl Inst of Diabetes and Digestive and Kidney Diseases, Bethesda, Md)
Neurosurgery 28:826–833, 1991   21–20

Background.—Positron-emission tomography (PET) with [18F] fluorodeoxyglucose (FDG) is useful for predicting and defining the growth potential of some intracranial tumors. The measure of glucose use may also be a useful indicator of the biologic behavior of pituitary macroadenomas. The energy metabolism of pituitary macroadenomas under various circumstances using PET-FDG was studied.

Methods.—Twenty-four patients with pituitary macroadenomas underwent 32 PET-FDG studies. The ratio of FDG uptake of tumor to a whole brain slice, called the adenoma metabolic index, was determined. In each PET study, the adenoma was visually identified as an area of moderate to high FDG uptake in the region of the sella turcica. Tumor uptake of FDG and hormone and treatment responses were compared.

Findings.—The macroadenoma was easily identified in each PET study as an area of increased FDG uptake near the region of the sella. Nonfunctional adenomas had the highest FDG uptakes. The prolactin, growth hormone, and thyroid-stimulating hormone-producing groups showed similar levels of glucose metabolism. The average adenoma metabolic index for all tumors was 1.3, with a range of .3 for a thyroid-stimulating hormone adenoma to 3.5 for a nonfunctional tumor. The tumors did not have metabolic rates characterizing the type of hormone produced. Recurrent macroadenomas had metabolism comparable to tumors that did not undergo surgery. Irradiated adenomas displayed lower glucose uptake than nonirradiated tumors. Drug treatment with bromocriptine or octreotide also reduced tumor glucose use. The amount of hormone produced was not correlated with the adenoma metabolic index. However, patients scanned more than once had changes in hormone levels that changed or did not change in parallel with tumor metabolism.

Conclusion.—Positron-emission tomography may be able to predict and define pituitary adenoma growth. This may be especially valuable when plasma hormone assays and conventional imaging modalities are not adequate for monitoring patient response to treatment.

▶ This communication describes an experience in 24 patients studied with PET scans of pituitary macroadenomas. A number of interesting observations on tumor metabolism have been made in relation to a variety of hormone productions and therapies. At present, the data do not warrant the use of this technology in a clinical sense, because imaging studies and hormone titers will be much more cost-effective and practical. Nonetheless, further investigations in this direction are justified as a research endeavor.—R.M. Crowell, M.D.

Radiologic Characteristics and Results of Surgical Management of Rathke's Cysts in 43 Patients
Ross DA, Norman D, Wilson CB (Univ of Michigan, Ann Arbor; Univ of California, San Francisco)
Neurosurgery 30:173–179, 1992   21–21

Objective.—Rathke's cysts are sellar and suprasellar structures found in as many as one third of autopsies; they rarely are symptomatic. The management of Rathke's cysts was reviewed in 43 patients operated on during a 13-year period.

Patients and Management.—Forty patients underwent transsphenoidal surgery with drainage of the cyst contents and biopsy of the cyst wall. Biopsy confirmed a Rathke's cyst in 26 of these patients. Patients with a Rathke's cyst recognized at surgery were followed up for a mean of 62 months.

Appearances.—Nineteen of the 30 cysts visualized on CT study and MRI were 3–10 mm in diameter. Two thirds of the cysts were at an intrasellar site, and one third were suprasellar lesions. A majority of the larger lesions had both intrasellar and suprasellar components. Most contrast CT studies demonstrated a low-density cyst. Two thirds of the MRI studies showed a high-signal intensity cyst on short TR/TE images. Magnetic resonance studies done with contrast enhancement demonstrated both the intrasellar and suprasellar components. Imaging using long-TR/TE parameters yielded variable signal intensity values.

Recommendations.—Simple drainage by the transsphenoidal route and biopsy of the cyst wall are suggested for symptomatic Rathke's cysts. A single follow-up MRI study is appropriate unless symptoms or signs develop.

▶ This report of 43 patients with Rathke's porch cysts indicated a number of important features. The most prominent symptom is headache; other symptoms include amenorrhea, visual field defects, and hypopituitarism. Both CT and MRI have features that defy confident radiologic diagnosis. Forty patients had transsphenoidal surgery, and 3 had craniotomy. The complications were minor and generally cleared with appropriate therapy in a short period of time. Simple cyst drainage appeared to be effective in the relief of symptoms. Biopsy of the wall (when safe) is recommended for confirmation of diagnosis. Because of the very benign nature of the lesions, until there is a progression of symptoms, a conservative course of management is appropriate.—R.M. Crowell, M.D.

Results of Transsphenoidal Extirpation of Craniopharyngiomas and Rathke's Cysts

Landolt AM, Zachmann M (Univ of Zürich, Switzerland)
Neurosurgery 28:410–415, 1991   21–22

Background.—The best way to treat craniopharyngiomas is with primary total surgical resection. The surgical approach is determined by the location and extension of the tumor. The endocrine results of transsphenoidal extirpation of a craniopharyngioma or Rathke's cyst were studied.

Methods.—Three female and 11 male patients, aged 6–43 years, underwent endocrinologic assessment before and after transsphenoidal extirpation. The patients were followed up for as long as 16 years (average follow-up, 8.5 years).

Outcomes.—One patient died of uncontrollable arterial bleeding during surgery. Another patient had tumor recurrence 12 years after the procedure. A third patient died 2 years after transsphenoidal extirpation; this was the only patient operated on because of a recurrent craniopharyngioma after previous radiotherapy. None of the patients recovered pituitary functions that were lost before surgery. A patient with an isolated growth-hormone deficiency and another with panhypopituitarism with sustained antidiuretic hormone secretion had no changes from their preoperative endocrine status. The other 11 patients lost pituitary function and needed drug replacement of 1–4 pituitary hormones.

Conclusion.—The transsphenoidal approach should be used to treat all patients with a primarily intrasellar craniopharyngioma or Rathke's cyst. This approach is associated with a low tumor recurrence rate, a low risk of surgical mortality, and insignificant incidence of complications. However, with the possible exception of diabetes insipidus cases, the results obtained with this approach (in terms of endocrine function) are no better than those achieved with a craniotomy.

▶ This interesting paper emphasizes that certain craniopharyngiomas (those that are primarily within an enlarged sella) can be approached by the transsphenoidal route with a low rate of recurrence. However it should be emphasized that one should expect a high incidence of postoperative endocrine deficiency, and that even catastrophic bleeding can be encountered by this route. Thus, craniotomy is likely to remain the standard surgical approach for craniopharyngiomas. On the other hand, the transsphenoidal approach may be appropriate in selected patients such as the elderly or those patients with large cystic components.—R.M. Crowell, M.D.

Acoustic

Intracanalicular Acoustic Neurinomas
Samii M, Matthies C, Tatagiba M (Nordstadt Hosp, Hannover, Germany)
Neurosurgery 28:189–199, 1991   21–23

Background.—It is unknown whether the origin, growth, and pathophysiologic changes of purely intracanalicular neurinomas are meaningfully different from those of neurinomas with both intracanalicular and extracanalicular growth. A retrospective study of a group of patients with exclusively intracanalicular acoustic neurinoma was reviewed.

Patients.—Sixteen patients comprising 2.7% of 600 patients with acoustic neurinomas treated at the Neurosurgical Clinic at Nordstadt Hospital during the past 8 years were studied. The 16 patients had exclusively intracanalicular acoustic neurinoma diagnosed by air CT cisternography or MRI. The study group had a comparatively earlier onset of vestibular symptoms and signs, which precipitated diagnosis. Magnetic resonance imaging was performed secondarily to CT in a patient with bilateral widening of the internal auditory canal showing only thickening of the neurovascular bundle on the left; therefore, air CT was performed for evaluation of both auditory canals.

Outcomes.—In all patients, complete tumor removal was achieved through the suboccipital approach. There was 100% preservation of facial nerve and facial function. The cochlear nerve was preserved anatomically in all patients and functionally in 57%. None of the patients have had recurrences.

Conclusion.—Intracanalicular acoustic neurinoma is a separate clinical entity. Early, predominant manifestation of vestibular signs and symptoms are characteristic. Prompt MRI is indicated by the clinical presentation of vestibular signs, acoustic disturbances, and neurophysiologic effects. High-resolution bone window CT scanning of the posterior fossa is important for preoperatively visualizing the internal auditory canal, the semicircular canals, and the jugular bulb. The suboccipital approach is the access of choice when the surgeon is experienced. Ideally, surgery should be accompanied by monitoring of acoustic evoked potentials as a parameter of acoustic and brain stem functions.

▶ This remarkable study presents 16 patients with intracanalicular acoustic neuromas that were totally excised by the suboccipital route. The authors report 100% preservation of facial function, 57% preservation of cochlear nerve function, and no recurrence. The suboccipital route is the approach of choice for such patients, and preservation of the vascular supply is critical.—R.M. Crowell, M.D.

Conservative Treatment of Patients With Acoustic Tumors
Bederson JB, von Ammon K, Wichmann WW, Yasargil MG (Univ Hosp, Zurich, Switzerland; Montefiore Med Ctr/Albert Einstein College of Medicine, Bronx, NY)
Neurosurgery 28:646–651, 1991   21–24

Background.—Several authors have estimated the growth rate of acoustic tumors. Most have reported slow growth, and spontaneous regression has been seen. However, a certain percentage of these tumors grow unexpectedly fast. More effective treatment of acoustic neurinomas will require a better understanding of the growth rates of these tumors.

Methods.—Of 178 patients with acoustic tumors, 70 were initially treated conservatively and were followed up for a mean of 26 months. Computed tomography (CT) or MRI scans were obtained sequentially throughout follow-up, and tumor size was determined by the mean maximum anteroposterior and mediolateral diameters.

Findings.—The average tumor growth was 1.6 mm in the first year and 1.9 mm in the second. Four tumors appeared to regress; 40% had no detectable growth, and 53% did grow. In individual patients, tumor growth rate determined in the first year of follow-up predicted the tumor growth rate in the following year. Rapid tumor growth or clinical deterioration in 9 patients initially receiving conservative therapy necessitated surgery at a mean of 14 months after presentation. These patients had a larger tumor size initially and a faster 1-year growth rate than the 61 patients who did not need surgery. However, 2 patients had neurologic deterioration necessitating surgery, even though their tumors did not grow.

Conclusion.—Surgeons must consider the high incidence of acoustic tumors that have no detectable growth or apparent spontaneous regression when evaluating the indications for surgery and the efficacy of radiotherapy. Because acoustic tumors generally grow slowly, a trial of conservative treatment is possible in selected patients. Serial radiologic studies are needed in these patients.

▶ This fascinating study shows that as much as 40% of acoustics have no detectable growth, and that most of the remainder have slow growth, whereas 13% have rapid growth. In older patients with minimal symptomatology, a course of watchful waiting with serial seems quite reasonable.—R.M. Crowell, M.D.

Bilateral Acoustic Neurofibromatosis (Neurofibromatosis 2): A Disorder Distinct From von Recklinghausen's Neurofibromatosis (Neurofibromatosis 1)
Flexon PB, Nadol JB Jr, Schuknecht HF, Montgomery WW, Martuza RL (Massachusetts Eye and Ear Infirmary; Massachusetts Gen Hosp, Boston)
Ann Otol Rhinol Laryngol 100:830–834, 1991   21–25

Introduction.—Central neurofibromatosis, NF-2, is distinct from classic von Recklinghausen's disease (NF-1). Bilateral eighth nerve schwannomas are common in NF-2, whereas acoustic schwannoma is rare in NF-1.

Case Report.—Man, 20, was seen with hearing loss and tinnitus in the left ear 11 years after neurofibromatosis had been diagnosed from resection of a brachial plexus neurofibroma. Cervical laminectomy was done at age 13 years for schwannomas of the spinal cord. No café au lait spot was found. Computed tomography revealed a 2.5-cm mass in the left cerebellopontine angle and a large, heavily calcified mass on the right side (Fig 21–7). A left-sided eighth nerve schwannoma was removed subtotally. Another cord lesion was removed the following year; later, an intramedullary astrocytoma was irradiated. Hearing in the right ear deteriorated, and a schwannoma was removed completely at age 24 years. A meningioma also seen in the right cerebellopontine angle was subtotally removed. Continued problems from brain stem compression necessitated a second craniectomy for gross removal of residual schwannoma. Hearing was not preserved. The patient had respiratory distress caused by tracheal and spinal cord compression by cervical masses, and he died of respiratory failure.

Discussion.—Most patients with NF-2 have other CNS tumors in addition to eighth nerve schwannomas. The diagnosis should be considered when an apparently unilateral eighth nerve schwannoma appears before 30 years of age; in a child having a meningeal or Schwann-cell tu-

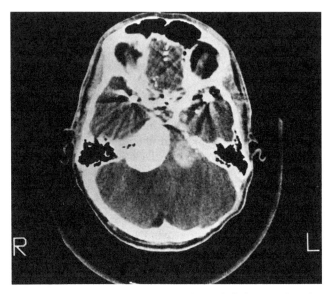

Fig 21–7.—Axial CT through petrous apices showing large calcified mass at the right cerebellopontine angle (CPA) and a 2.5-cm mass at the left CPA. (Courtesy of Flexon PB, Nadol JB Jr, Schuknecht HF, et al: *Ann Otol Rhinol Laryngol* 100:830–834, 1991.)

mor; and in an individual lacking a family history of NF-1 who had neurofibromas but few or no café au lait macules and no Lisch nodules.

▶ Distinct clinical and genetic features of NF-2 show it to be distinct from classical Von Recklinghausen's Disease (NF-1). Neurofibromatosis 2 should be suspected in a patient with apparent unilateral 8th nerve Schwannoma before 30 years of age; in a child with a meningeal or schwann cell tumor; in a patient without a family history of NF-1 but with 1 or more neurofibromas and few or no café au lait spots and no Lisch nodules; or in a close relative of a patient with known NF-2. The best screening test is Gd-enhanced MRI. Once the diagnosis is made, the patient is best cared for by a team experienced in the management of these complex patients.—R.M. Crowell, M.D.

22 Ischemia

Carotid Endarterectomy

Carotid Endarterectomy and Prevention of Cerebral Ischemia in Symptomatic Carotid Stenosis

Mayberg MR, for the Veterans Affairs Cooperative Studies Program 309 Trialist Group (Univ of Washington, Seattle)

JAMA 266:3289–3294, 1991   22–1

Background.—Patients with symptoms of cerebral or retinal ischemia in the distribution of a hemodynamically significant internal carotid artery stenosis are believed to represent a distinct subgroup that is at increased risk for stroke. Whether carotid endarterectomy provides protection against subsequent cerebral ischemia in men with ischemic symptoms in the distribution of significant ipsilateral internal carotid artery stenosis was investigated.

Methods and Findings.—Sixteen university-affiliated Veterans Affairs medical centers participated in the prospective, randomized trial. Ninety-one men received carotid endarterectomy plus best medical care, and 98 received best medical care alone. The follow-up was an average of 11.9 months. Stroke or crescendo transient ischemic attacks occurred in significantly fewer patients in the endarterectomy group than in the nonsurgical group of patients, those percentages being 7.7% and 19.4%, respectively. This represents an absolute risk reduction of 11.7%. The benefit of surgery was more pronounced in those with internal carotid artery stenosis of more than 70%.

Conclusion.—Carotid endarterectomy can reduce the risk of subsequent ipsilateral cerebral ischemia in selected patients with symptoms of cerebral or retinal ischemia in the distribution of a high-grade internal carotid artery stenosis. In this subgroup, the risk of cerebral ischemia is much higher than was once believed.

▶ This study from the Veterans Administration adds further support for carotid endarterectomy as effective prevention against cerebral ischemia in symptomatic carotid stenosis. A statistically significant benefit of surgery was demonstrated in patients with stenosis greater than 70%. A reasonable surgical complication rate of approximately 5% was achieved in this study. This is particularly important in view of the high-risk nature of the typical VA patient. Of some concern is the fact that death occurred in 3 of the surgical cases and in none of the non surgical cases.—R.M. Crowell, M.D.

Selection Process for Surgeons in the Asymptomatic Carotid Athero-sclerosis Study

Moore WS, Vescera CL, Robertson JT, Baker WH, Howard VJ, Toole JF (Univ of California, Los Angeles; Univ of Tennessee, Memphis; Loyola Univ Med Ctr, Maywood, Ill; Wake Forest Univ, Winston-Salem, NC)
Stroke 22:1353–1357, 1991   22–2

Background.—The Asymptomatic Carotid Atherosclerosis Study is a prospective, multicenter trial designed to show whether prophylactic carotid endarterectomy plus aspirin improves the outlook compared with aspirin alone in patients with hemodynamically significant but asymptomatic carotid stenosis.

Selection of Surgeons.—For inclusion in the study, a surgeon had to have performed 12 or more carotid endarterectomies annually. The combined neurologic morbidity and mortality in the last 50 consecutive operations had to be no greater than 5% for all indications or 3% for operations on asymptomatic patients.

Observations.—Thirty-eight centers were active participants in the study. Of 164 surgeons applying for approval, 117 were approved, 17 were rejected, and 30 were not reviewed. Approved surgeons had a combined mortality and neurologic morbidity of 2.3% for 5,641 endarterectomies. The mortality for unapproved surgeons was nearly 3 times that for those who were approved, and perioperative strokes were twice as frequent for unapproved surgeons.

Conclusion.—The surgeon selecting process appears to have achieved its goal. The performance of approved surgeons was well within the range of what is considered acceptable by the Stroke Council of the American Heart Association.

▶ This communication represents a note of progress for the study of asymptomatic carotid atherosclerosis. It is a credentialing process for surgeons entering the study. A total of 117 approved surgeons undertook 5,641 endarterectomies; the combined mortality and neurologic morbidity rate was 2.3%, with a variety of indications for surgery. This very low rate of complications should be kept in mind as a guide for those undertaking this kind of surgery. It also attests to the quality of the study, which will bolster the eventual results.—R.M. Crowell, M.D.

Carotid Endarterectomy for Asymptomatic Carotid Stenosis: An Update

Thompson JE (Baylor Univ Med Ctr, Dallas)
J Vasc Surg 13:669–676, 1991   22–3

Background.—The advisability of performing arteriography and carotid endarterectomy on patients with asymptomatic carotid stenosis is

Long-Term Follow-Up Data on Patients Operated On or Not Operated On for
Asymptomatic Carotid Bruits (Author's Series)

	Asymptomatic	*TIAs*	*Nonfatal stroke*	*Fatal stroke*	*Length of follow-up*
Operated on (132 patients)	120	6	3	3	6 to 184 mo
	90.9%	4.5%	2.3%	2.3%	(mean, 55 mo)
Not operated on: (138 patients)	77	37	21	3	to 199 mo
	55.8%	26.8%	15.2%	2.2%	(mean, 55 mo)
Significance	$p < 0.01$	$p < 0.01$	$p < 0.01$		

(Courtesy of Thompson JE: *J Vasc Surg* 13:669–676, 1991.)

controversial. The factors that currently seem to predict an increased incidence of stroke in patients with asymptomatic carotid stenoses were reviewed in an attempt to better define the indications for carotid endarterectomy. Two series of patients, an operated group and a nonoperated group, were followed prospectively over the years (table).

Discussion.—After noninvasive screening and arteriography, several specific indications for carotid endarterectomy can be identified. These indications are the presence of severe unilateral stenosis of greater than 70%; bilateral stenoses greater than 50%; unilateral stenosis and contralateral occlusion; stenosis progressing to more than 50%; positive noninvasive tests, such as duplex scan, spectral analysis, ocular pneumoplethysmography (OPG), and possibly CT and MRI; and a markedly ulcerated plaque. Carotid endarterectomy should be done before other major surgery when the noninvasive tests and arteriography are strongly positive.

Conclusion.—When patients are selected properly, angiography is done by skillful clinicians, and appropriate surgery is performed by experienced operators, the operative mortality and morbidity rates associated with carotid endarterectomy are low and the immediate results are excellent. When these conditions are met, asymptomatic patients seem to have better outcomes than their nonoperated counterparts in terms of subsequent cerebral ischemic episodes.

▶ In this report, a number of published data are reviewed relative to the question of the use of carotid endarterectomy for the treatment of asymptomatic carotid stenosis. In essence, these studies suggest a stroke rate of nearly 5% per year for hemodynamically significant asymptomatic carotid stenosis. The operative statistics for many surgical teams are shown to indicate a 2% morbidity/mortality rate for endarterectomy in this same group. Data are presented, with historical controls, that suggest a reduction in the annual stroke incidence in patients undergoing endarterectomy.

Thompson suggests the following indications for endarterectomy in asymptomatic patients: unilateral stenosis greater than 70%; bilateral stenoses greater than 50%; unilateral stenosis and contralateral occlusion; and progressive stenosis to greater than 50%. This is useful information, however, the results of the ongoing randomized controlled trials will be of greater importance in establishing the role, if any, of carotid endarterectomy in asymptomatic patients.—R.M. Crowell, M.D.

Risk Factors for Intra-operative Neurological Deficit During Carotid Endarterectomy

Ross Naylor A, Merrick MV, Vaughan Ruckley C (Royal Infirmary, Edinburgh; Western Gen Hosp, Edinburgh)
Eur J Vasc Surg 5:33–39, 1991   22–4

Introduction.—The risk factors for patients undergoing carotid endarterectomy were assessed. By identifying these factors, a more discriminating approach to patient selection for operation can be practiced, and intraoperative protection can also be better administered.

Methods.—Sixty patients were assessed preoperatively by medical history, angiography, CT scan, and quantification of the mean cerebral transit time (MCTT). Carotid endarterectomy was done by the same surgeon using a standard technique.

Results.—Six of the 60 patients had either a new neurologic deficit or worsening of a preoperative condition after carotid endarterectomy. Those patients older than 65 years of age and those with residual neurologic deficit before surgery had a significantly greater risk of intraoperative neurologic deficit (IOND) developing. Separately, impaired cerebral vascular reserve and CT scan evidence of infarction were not significant predictors of risk, but they presented a significant risk for IOND in combination. Intraoperatively, complex plaque morphology was significantly associated with an increased risk for IOND.

Conclusion.—Patient selection for carotid endarterectomy can be enhanced in view of the risk factors determined in this study. Additionally, closer intraoperative monitoring in higher risk patients can be planned for preoperatively.

▶ This interesting study emphasizes the concept of cerebral vascular reserve as it regards the likelihood of intraoperative deficit occurring during carotid endarterectomy. An isotopic method was used to study the mean cerebral transit time. Impaired cerebrovascular reserve and a cerebral infarct on CT showed a high correlation with postoperative deficit. In addition, other risk factors for new deficit were age older than 65 years, prior deficit, and complex plaque. The high incidence of patients with new deficits among 60 consecutive cases (10%) is of some concern in this communication. To offer significant benefit by endarterectomy, most authorities suggest that the combined morbidity/mortality should be less than 5%.—R.M. Crowell, M.D.

Carotid Surgery: Is Regional Anesthesia Always Appropriate?

Becquemin J-P, Paris E, Valverde A, Pluskwa F, Mellière D (Hospital Henri

Mondor, Créteil, France)
J Cardiovasc Surg 32:592–598, 1991   22–5

Background.—Although local anesthesia for carotid surgery has been reported to decrease the rate of postoperative complications and hospital stay, it can also make the procedure more difficult. There have been only limited comparative studies from institutions using both local and general anesthesia. A series of 385 carotid endarterectomies performed using general or local anesthesia were reviewed.

Methods.—The procedures were performed in 352 patients, mean age 63 years, during a 5-year period. A total of 242 procedures were done using general anesthesia—thiopental and fentanyl for induction and isoflurane and nitrous oxide 50% in oxygen for maintenance. A total of 145 were done using regional anesthesia—cervical epidural anesthesia in 114 cases and deep cervical block in 31. The type of anesthesia was chosen individually after discussion by the patient, surgeon, and anesthesiologist. Cerebral function was monitored with local, but not general, anesthesia. The 2 groups were compared for rates of perioperative morbidity and mortality and for the factors influencing choice of anesthesia.

Findings.—The preoperative risk factors were similar for the 2 groups. They also had similar rates of transient ischemic attacks, stroke, death, combined mortality, and severe neurologic and cardiac morbidity. Of the general anesthesia group, 17% had shunts inserted, compared with 7% of the regional anesthesia group; 5% of the patients given general anesthesia had myocardial infarctions vs. 0% of the regional anesthesia group. However, thrombosis attributable to technical error occurred in 2.7% of the regional anesthesia group vs. .4% of the general anesthesia group.

Conclusion.—For patients undergoing carotid surgery who either have coronary artery disease or are at risk of intolerance to cross-clamping, regional anesthesia appears to be the best choice. For those who are poorly cooperative or for whom technical problems are expected, general anesthesia is better. Regional anesthesia is generally preferred, because it is less expensive and because it provides a reliable means of monitoring cerebral function.

▶ This interesting study compares the results for carotid endarterectomy done using regional anesthesia and general anesthesia at 1 institution during a 5-year period. Although the study is neither randomized nor prospective, some interesting results emerge. The rate of myocardial infarction was statistically significantly higher in the general anesthesia group, although there was a tendency for overall higher combined mortality and morbidity with general anesthesia. This study was performed without special attention to silent myocardial infarction. At Massachusetts General Hospital, we have found that careful postoperative monitoring of serial electrocardiograms and enzyme studies can disclose a number of silent myocardial infarctions after carotid surgery. In addition, with modern techniques for patient selection and preoperative care, surgeons are forcing the operative complication rate downward to remarkably low levels, in some institutions to 1% or 2%. Myocardial ischemia and infarction appear to be a part of this latter and seemingly irreducible complication rate. Perhaps the French suggestion of using regional anesthesia for patients with high-risk cardiac disease is especially appropriate in this effort.

Many surgeons have hesitated to use regional anesthesia for carotid endarterectomy because of its inconvenience and perceived difficulty. With a solid regional block and careful preparation, most patients are quite cooperative, and surgery can proceed without interference. One difficult situation is ischemia occurring during cross-clamping in a patient who is uncooperative and moving but in whom a shunt may become necessary.—R.M. Crowell, M.D.

Correlation of Contralateral Stenosis and Intraoperative Electroencephalogram Change With Risk of Stroke During Carotid Endarterectomy
Redekop G, Ferguson G (Univ of Western Ontario, London, Ontario)
Neurosurgery 30:191–194, 1992   22–6

Background.—Carotid endarterectomy is done to reduce the risk of future stroke. There have been many refinements to the technique to reduce the risk of operative complications. However, physicians disagree about the best way to monitor cerebral function during carotid cross-clamping, the indications for indwelling shunt use, and the specific risks associated with carotid artery surgery in patients with contralateral carotid occlusion. The correlation of contralateral stenosis and intraoperative electroencephalogram (EEG) change with the risk of stroke during carotid endarterectomy was determined.

Methods and Outcomes.—A total of 293 carotid endarterectomies were done with EEG monitoring but without shunts. Two hundred sixteen patients had contralateral carotid stenosis of less than 70%, and 45 had contralateral stenosis of 70% to 99%. Thirty-two patients had contralateral occlusion, and 6 patients (2%) had perioperative strokes. Two patients died, for an incidence of .7%. Major EEG changes occurred in 14.3% of the patients with significant contralateral stenosis or occlusion and in 5.1% of those without it. The patients with major EEG changes had a significantly higher risk of immediate postoperative deficit than those without such changes. The risk in patients with less than 70% contralateral stenosis did not differ significantly from that in patients with greater contralateral stenosis or occlusion.

Conclusion.—Carotid endarterectomy can be done safely without a temporary shunt. Contralateral stenosis or occlusion alone does not indicate a higher risk. Major EEG changes occurred infrequently in this series. Such changes identified a subgroup of patients at significantly increased risk of intraoperative stroke.

► This interesting study indicated that the risks of intraoperative stroke were not different in patients with contralateral stenosis or occlusion. Of even more interest may be the finding that the risk of immediate postoperative deficit was significantly higher in the subgroup with major EEG changes (18.2%) than in those patients without changes (1.8%) (peak, less than .005). At our institution, we use the information only to determine whether to place an in-line shunt when such EEG changes are identified. Although scientific proof is lacking that such a shunt improves postoperative outcome, we believe that if the shunting is done carefully to avoid dissection and embolization, then the likelihood of reducing the operative stroke rate is high.—R.M. Crowell, M.D.

Computerized Electroencephalographic Monitoring and Selective Shunting: Influence on Intraoperative Administration of Phenylephrine and Myocardial Infarction After General Anesthesia for Carotid Endarterectomy
Modica PA, Tempelhoff R, Rich KM, Grubb RL Jr, (Washington Univ, St Louis, Mo)
Neurosurgery 30:842–846, 1992   22–7

Introduction.—In an attempt to promote collateral blood flow and prevent cerebral ischemia, many centers infuse phenylephrine during carotid endarterectomy to induce hypertension while the carotid artery is clamped. This practice may increase the risk of intraoperative myocardial ischemia when general anesthesia is used.

Methods.—Data were reviewed on 159 patients who had 171 carotid endarterectomies using general anesthesia. Shunt placement was predicated on the identification of cerebral ischemia using a computerized EEG monitor. Phenylephrine was infused when ischemia was associated with persistent hypotension, and when ischemia failed to respond promptly to shunt placement or removal of the carotid clamp.

Results.—Cerebral infarction occurred in 2 (1.2%) patients; 3 patients died for reasons unrelated to myocardial infarction, but 2 nonfatal infarcts occurred. Overall, 35 patients had ischemic EEG events, and 12 of the 35 received phenylephrine infusions intraoperatively. None of the latter patients had a permanent deficit, but 1 of those not given phenylephrine had a late EEG event with significant hypertension and incurred a permanent deficit.

Conclusion.—Phenylephrine-induced hypertension may be used on a limited basis when cerebral ischemia develops during carotid endarterectomy and fails to resolve promptly.

► In this study of 171 endarterectomies done using general anesthesia with selective shunting and selective induced hypertension, the authors noted no fatal myocardial infarctions and only 2 (1.2%) nonfatal myocardial infarctions. They argue that this program of management serves to reduce the incidence of myocardial infarction during carotid endarterectomy. They also suggest that the frequency of myocardial infarction compares favorably with that observed for local anesthesia. Proof of this hypothesis would require a prospective, randomized, controlled study. At present, there is no scientific substantiation of any specific anesthetic regimen for carotid endarterectomy.—R.M. Crowell, M.D.

Vein Patch Rupture After Carotid Endarterectomy: A Survey of the Western Vascular Society Members

Tawes RL Jr, Treiman RL (San Mateo, Calif)
Ann Vasc Surg 5:71–73, 1991   22–8

Background.—Vein patch angioplasty is used for closure of the carotid artery after endarterectomy. Rupture or blowout of the patch is uncommon and, consequently, most surgeons have had little experience with this complication. Members of the Western Vascular Society were polled to determine the prevalence, demographics, morbidity, and mortality of vein patch ruptures.

Methods.—Forty-eight surgeons had experience in 23,873 carotid operations, of which 1,760 included the use of a vein patch in 1,760 operations. Rupture occurred from a split in the saphenous vein patch in 13 patients. Two ruptures occurred on the first postoperative day, 6 occurred on the second day, 3 took place on the third day, 1 occurred on the eighth day, and 1 took place on the 21st day.

Findings.—Four patients died of airway obstruction (1), hemorrhagic cerebral infarction (1), or myocardial infarction (2). Three patients survived a stroke, 1 had a retinal embolus, and 5 patients underwent uneventful reoperation.

Conclusion.—The incidence of vein patch rupture is low, but there is significant mortality and morbidity when it occurs. To facilitate immediate reoperation, patients with a vein patch should be observed in the hospital for 3 days postendarterectomy.

▶ This survey indicates that patch rupture is infrequent (less than 1%) but extremely dangerous (mortality, 30%). We believe this is a strong reason to limit the use of patch graft to those patients who have a strong need. We define these patients to be those with an extremely small carotid artery (3–4 mm in diameter) and those with recurrence.—R.M. Crowell, M.D.

Hyperperfusion Syndrome After Carotid Endarterectomy: CT Changes

Harrison PB, Wong MJ, Belzberg A, Holden J (St Paul's Hosp, Vancouver, BC)
Neuroradiology 33:106–110, 1991   22–9

Background.—Neurologic problems may occur during and after carotid endarterectomy (CEA) in as many as 10% of patients. The CT scans of 2 patients who had headache and seizures suggesting hyperperfusion syndrome after CEA were studied.

Case Report.—Woman, 79, had a 1-year history of lightheadedness, falling to the left, and a probable transient ischemic attack affecting her left arm. She was found to have severe bilateral internal carotid stenoses with a left subclavian occlusion. A right CEA was done without complication. After surgery, the patient complained of a mild headache. However, analgesics relieved the headache, and she was discharged on day 2. Three days later, she was found unconscious in her home. She had several seizures involving her left arm, which later generalized. Repeat angiography showed carotid patency. Unenhanced CT indicated low-density changes in the right frontal and parietal cortical and subcortical areas (Fig 22–1). She was discharged and began taking steroids 13 days after admission. The next day, however, she was readmitted with left-sided focal seizures. She had a dense, left hemiparesis. Repeat CT scan demonstrated low-density changes more extensively involving the right cerebral white matter associated with greater mass effect (Fig 22–2). Three days later, the woman had an intense headache. She then became comatose. A scan showed punctate regions of hemorrhage and a 3-cm right frontal pole hematoma. The substantial hemisphere mass effect and subcortical hypodensity had gotten worse, with the overlying cortex apparently less involved (Fig 22–3). The patient died 20 days after surgery. At autopsy, her brain had fibrinoid necrosis of the small arteries and arterioles

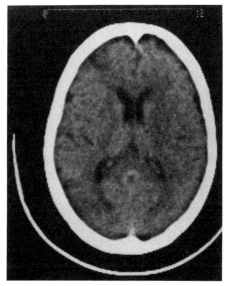

Fig 22–1.—Unenhanced CT scan demonstrates right frontal and parietal minor cortical and subcortical low density changes on day 5. (Courtesy of Harrison PB, Wong MJ, Belzberg A, et al: *Neuroradiology* 33:106–110, 1991.)

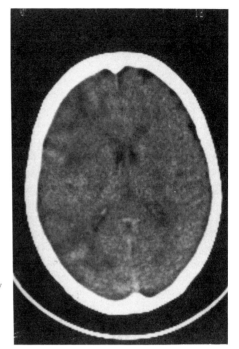

Fig 22–2.—A repeat CT scan on day 14 shows low density changes more extensively involving the right cerebral white matter, associated with greater mass effect. (Courtesy of Harrison PB, Wong MJ, Belzberg A, et al: *Neuroradiology* 33:106–110, 1991.)

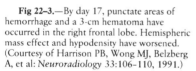

Fig 22–3.—By day 17, punctate areas of hemorrhage and a 3-cm hematoma have occurred in the right frontal lobe. Hemispheric mass effect and hypodensity have worsened. (Courtesy of Harrison PB, Wong MJ, Belzberg A, et al: *Neuroradiology* 33:106–110, 1991.)

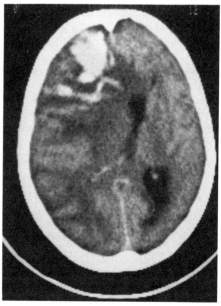

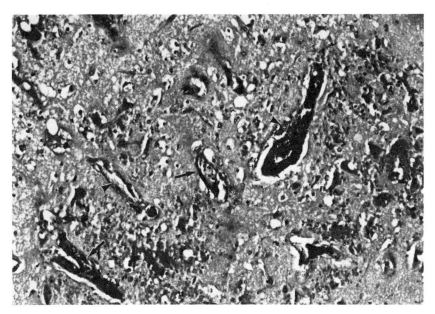

Fig 22–4.—In addition to the frontal hematoma, post-mortem examination shows fibrinoid necrosis of the small arteries and arterioles within the viable cortex adjacent to the hemorrhage (*arrows*). Intraluminal fibrin deposition, pronounced endothelial swelling, and red cell extravasation are present (*arrowheads*). The changes are similar to those of malignant hypertension. (Courtesy of Harrison PB, Wong MJ, Belzberg A, et al: *Neuroradiology* 33:106–110, 1991.)

within the viable cortex adjacent to the bleeding, as well as right frontal hematoma. Also, intraluminal fibrin deposition, marked endothelial swelling, and red blood cell extravasation were seen. These changes were comparable to those seen in malignant hypertension (Fig 22–4).

Conclusion.—The CT scans of the 2 patients showed ipsilateral mass effect and white matter hypodensity. Although infarction is said to be the most common neurologic event occurring after CEA, autopsy or cerebral blood flow studies in these patients suggested that the changes resulted from hyperperfusion rather than infarction.

▶ This study is in accord with much literature suggesting that nearly 1% of patients will have a significant hyperprofusion syndrome that may progress to hemorrhage. Identification of the problem before it results in catastrophic deterioration may be possible through the use of ultrasound, transcranial Doppler, or single-photon emission computed tomography (SPECT). Headache or seizures are often the tip-off. Prophylactic treatment should include careful control of blood pressure in an effort to avoid hemorrhage. Figure 2 in the original article suggests that the patient not mentioned in this abstract actually may have had amyloid angiopathy as a predisposing factor to hemorrhage.—R.M. Crowell, M.D.

Reduction in Thrombus Formation by Placement of Endovascular Stents at Endarterectomy Sites in Baboon Carotid Arteries

Krupski WC, Bass A, Kelly AB, Hanson SR, Harker LA (Emory Univ, Atlanta; Univ of California, San Francisco; Chaim Sheba Med Ctr, Tel-Hashomer, Israel)

Circulation 84:1749–1757, 1991   22–10

Objective.—Because both endarterectomy and angioplasty for atherosclerotic vascular disease produce thrombogenic sites, the effects of endovascular stenting were examined in baboons undergoing carotid endarterectomy.

Methods.—Platelet deposition was monitored by using autologous ^{111}In-labeled platelet in operated baboons given heparin but not antiplatelet agents. Some of the animals had self-expanding stainless steel wire endoprostheses inserted during endarterectomy. The wire mesh stents were free to pivot at lattice crossing points, and they became elastically extended when deployed.

Results.—Accumulation of platelets within 90 minutes of endarterectomy was much less marked at stented endarterectomy sites than at unstented sites. Deposition remained less in stented vessels as long as 48 hours after the procedure. Scanning electron microscopic studies of stented and control vessels at 30 days showed similarly confluent endothelium.

Conclusion.—Use of a vascular stent in conjunction with carotid endarterectomy may lessen acute thrombus formation at sites of luminal damage.

▶ This interesting experimental study demonstrates reduction in thrombus formation when endovascular stents are placed in endarterectomy sites. In relation to possible clinical application, it should be noted that such stents can be impregnated with anticoagulants to diminish further the local accumulation of thrombus. In addition, it has now been possible to place stents in a variety of vascular sites in the human body using endovascular techniques. However, whether this be done without dislodging plaque toward the brain has yet to be answered.—R.M. Crowell, M.D.

Other

Perioperative Complications of Encephalo-Duro-Arterio-Synangiosis: Prevention and Treatment

Matsushima Y, Aoyagi M, Suzuki R, Tabata H, Ohno K (Tokyo Med and Dental Univ)

Surg Neurol 36:343–353, 1991   22–11

Introduction.—Experience with encephalo-duro-arterio-synangiosis (EDAS) was reviewed in 81 patients with Moyamoya disease and in 8 patients having other ischemic disorders in the past decade. Most patients were Oriental and were living in Japan. The operative procedures totalled 169; the procedure was performed unilaterally in all the non-Moyamoya patients.

Complications.—In 6 patients, infarctive strokes occurred perioperatively (in 2 before surgery was performed). Severe hyperventilation and crying helped trigger infarction. In 2 patients, there was wound infection by gram-negative rods. An infected bone flap had to be removed, as did an acute epidural hematoma. In 5 patients, involuntary movements were temporarily aggravated after surgery. Mild fever and temporary hair loss were frequent sequelae. The donor arteries were injured in 7 instances.

Conclusion.—Although EDAS prevents some of the problems attending encephalo-myo-synangiosis and superior temporal artery-middle cerebral artery anastomosis, perioperative problems can occur.

▶ Professor Matsushima has introduced and continues to improve the operation of EDAS. In this study, 6 complications occurred in 169 procedures. The frequency of complications is lower than that recorded for other types of revascularization, such as superficial temporal artery to middle cerebral artery anastomosis, and long vein interposition grafting.—R.M. Crowell, M.D.

Post-Ischemic and Kainic Acid-Induced c-fos Protein Expression in the Rat Hippocampus

Jørgensen MB, Johansen FF, Diemer NH (Univ of Copenhagen, Denmark)
Acta Neurol Scand 84:352–356, 1991   22–12

Introduction.—The protein product of c-fos is a gene-regulatory third messenger involved in long-term cell responses to various stimuli, including signal transduction. Glutamate, a mediator of delayed ischemic necrosis, is a strong inducer of c-fos expression in the brain, and low levels of c-fos protein-like immunoreactivity have been found in neuronal nuclei. Seizures increase the expression of c-fos in specific brain regions.

Methods.—Rats were subjected to transient forebrain ischemia in a version of the 4-vessel occlusion model. The presence of c-fos protein (FP) 1 hour to 2 weeks after the imposition of a 10-minute ischemic episode was compared with that seen 3 hours after intraventricular injection of kainic acid, a glutamate analogue.

Findings.—Some CA1 pyramidal cells expressed FP the first day after ischemia, and this effect was more marked the following day. Many CA1 pyramidal cells were necrotic on day 3; FP expression was less intense and less widespread than the day before. Subsequently, gliosis increased without expression of c-fos in the CA1.

Conclusion.—Expression of c-fos was increased in hippocampal neurons after a 10-minute ischemic insult in rats. Delayed ischemic necrosis may be preceded by an increased level of cytosol calcium, possibly secondary to increased receptor stimulation.

▶ This experimental study shows that ischemia can induce c-fos protein expression. Other investigators have demonstrated similar findings. Although the significance is not clear, it is important that genetic mechanisms are now being studied with regard to various brain insults. This may lead to better understanding of pathophysiology and treatment.—R.M. Crowell, M.D.

23 Hemorrhage

Aneurysms

Screening for Unruptured Familial Intracranial Aneurysms: Subarachnoid Hemorrhage 2 Years After Angiography Negative for Aneurysms

Schievink WI, Limburg M, Dreissen JJR, Peeters FLM, ter Berg HWM (Univ of Amsterdam; Twenteborg Hosp, Almelo, The Netherlands)
Neurosurgery 29:434–438, 1991   23–1

Introduction.—It has been suggested that screening asymptomatic members of families with intracranial aneurysms can detect unruptured aneurysms before major hemorrhage occurs. A member of a large Dutch family with a documented history of intracranial aneurysms had a negative contrast digital subtraction angiographic study but, nevertheless, had subarachnoid bleeding 2 years later. Conventional angiography demonstrated 3 aneurysms measuring 3×3 mm (Fig 23-1).

Implications.—Even conventional arteriography does not demonstrate all intracranial aneurysms, and it does carry a real—although small—risk. Aneurysms can grow significantly over several days or weeks, and they

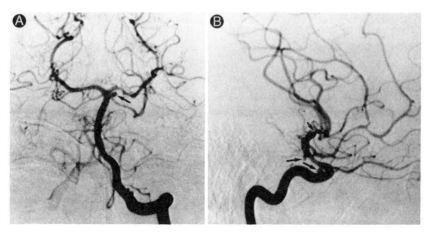

Fig 23–1.—**A,** a subtraction arteriogram of the left vertebral artery shows a small basilar aneurysm (*arrow*) located between the left cerebellar artery and the posterior cerebellar artery. **B,** subtraction arteriogram of the right internal carotid artery shows an aneurysm of the carotid siphon protruding into the cavernous sinus (*arrow*). A second aneurysm is visible at the origin of the posterior cummunicating artery (*arrow*). There is moderate narrowing of the vascular lumen of the middle cerebral artery (*short arrow*). (Courtesy of Schievink WI, Limburg M, Dreissen JJR, et al: *Neurosurgery* 29:434-438, 1991.)

324 / Neurosurgery

may develop at sites that previously appeared normal. It is appropriate to decide whether surgery would be indicated before screening for intact aneurysms. Both high-resolution CT with contrast enhancement and MR angiography are relatively sensitive ways of visualizing aneurysms, and they may prove valuable for screening large numbers of subjects, repeatedly if necessary.

Follow-Up Study of Unruptured Aneurysms Arising From the C3 and C4 Segments of the Internal Carotid Artery
Inagawa T (Shimane Prefectural Central Hosp, Izumo, Japan)
Surg Neurol 36:99–105, 1991   23–2

Background.—The indication for direct surgery for aneurysms at the C3 segment, especially when they are small and unruptured, is still debated. Patients with unruptured aneurysms at the C3 and C4 segments of the internal carotid artery were followed up to determine the natural history of these entities.

Patients and Outcomes.—Twenty-two patients with 24 aneurysms originating at C3 or C4 were seen from 1979 to 1989. They comprised 3% of all intracranial aneurysms and 11% of all internal carotid artery aneurysms diagnosed in that 10-year period. The patients were 18 women and 4 men, aged 34–82 years. A total of 55% had multiple aneurysms. Fifteen patients with 16 aneurysms were followed up without treatment, and 7 patients with 8 aneurysms underwent surgery or died soon after diagnosis. The average maximal dimension of the 16 aneurysms followed up was 5 mm, ranging from 2 to 17 mm. The follow-up ranged from 11 months to 10.5 years, with a mean of 4.7 years. None of the aneurysms ruptured during this time, and all but 1 had remained asymptomatic. This exception had been discovered as a result of the cavernous sinus syndrome.

Conclusion.—Some surgeons are operating on intracavernous carotid artery aneurysms, even if they are unruptured and small. This follow-up study shows that the risk of rupture of small unruptured aneurysms arising from the C3 or C4 segment of the internal carotid artery is apparently very low. Further research is needed to delineate the natural history of such aneurysms.

▶ This important study reports on 24 aneurysms of the C3 or C4 (cavernous) segment of the internal carotid artery (ICA). Seven of these patients were excluded because of surgery or death, leaving 15 patients with unruptured intracavernous aneurysms for long-term follow-up. During an average of 4.7 years, none of the 16 aneurysms in these patients ruptured. It should be noted that only 1 of these lesions was larger than 10 mm. Nonetheless, this information indicates a very low risk of rupture of small C3-4 ICA aneurysms. This report offers little encouragement to those who propose a direct attack for the treatment of such small lesions.

For large lesions, it is known that there is a more substantial possibility of subarachnoid hemorrhage; therefore, even in the unruptured asymptomatic patient, surgery might be considered. Under these conditions, direct attack, trapping with bypass, and proximal ICA balloon occlusion (with or without bypass) might be considered. Treatment is also warranted in patients who have had symptoms from such aneurysms, including headache, cranial nerve palsies, or carotid cavernous fistulas.—R.M. Crowell, M.D.

Early CT Features of Ruptured Cerebral Aneurysms of the Posterior Cranial Fossa

Kayama T, Sugawara T, Sakurai Y, Ogawa A, Onuma T, Yoshimoto T (Sendai Natl Hosp; Sendai Municipal Hosp; Inst of Brain Diseases; Tohoku Univ, Sendai, Japan)
Arch Neurochir (Wien) 108:34–39, 1991   23–3

Objective.—In a retrospective study, the CT findings on 34 patients with ruptured cerebral aneurysm of the posterior cranial fossa were reviewed to identify the early CT features of this condition. The CT scans were obtained within 3 days of hemorrhagic crisis.

Data Analysis.—Subarachnoid hemorrhage (SAH) extended to the supra- and infratentorial cisterns in 28 (82%) patients, but it was confined only in the infratentorial cistern in 6 (18%). Although SAH was observed in both supra- and infratentorial cisterns, thicker hematomas were also present in the cisterns at the periphery of the brain stem. Thicker hematomas were also noted in the infratentorial cisterns, even in the presence of thick, high-density hematomas in the supratentorial cisterns. In aneurysms located at the level of the posterior inferior cerebellar artery and vertebral artery, hematomas in the ambient cistern were thicker and of higher density of the aneurysm side. Thick, high-density hematomas also were observed in the interpeduncular cistern in patients with basilar artery bifurcation and basilar artery-superior cerebelli artery aneurysms. Only 1 (3%) patients had intracerebral hematoma, whereas 14 (41%) patients had intraventricular hemorrhage. All but 1 of the interventricular hemorrhages demonstrated a reflux pattern. Hydrocephalus occurred in 26 (76.5%) patients.

Conclusion.—The identification of acute-phase CT features may prove valuable in the diagnosis of ruptured cerebral aneurysms of the posterior cranial fossa.

▶ For posterior fossa aneurysms, CT often shows blood above and below the tentorium, in the ventricular system, and in association with hydrocephalus. The technique is not fully specific for the diagnosis of the site of bleeding. Magnetic resonance imaging may be more helpful in certain cases.—R.M. Crowell, M.D.

The International Cooperative Study on the Timing of Aneurysm Surgery: The North American Experience
Haley EC Jr, Kassell NF, Torner JC, and the Participants (Univ of Virginia, Charlottesville)
Stroke 23:205–214, 1992   23–4

Background.—A decade ago, the consensus in North America was that optimal results were achieved by operating on ruptured cerebral aneurysm after the patient had become clinically stable and reactive brain swelling had subsided. Some, however, argued that delaying surgery posed an unacceptable risk of rebleeding, and that early clipping would yield acceptable results.

The Study.—A total of 3,521 patients in 14 countries were enrolled from 1980 through 1983, 772 of them in North America. The patients were seen within 3 days after subarachnoid bleeding, and the outcome was assessed by a blinded evaluator after 6 months. All participants had a first major subarachnoid bleed from a saccular aneurysm.

Observations.—The overall outcome was similar with respect to mortality in patients for whom early surgery (in the first 3 days) was planned, and in those scheduled for surgery 11–32 days after rupture. Nevertheless, 71% of those operated on early and 62% of those for whom surgery was delayed had a good recovery. When surgery was planned for 7–10 days after rupture, the mortality rate was nearly twice as high as that in the other groups.

Implications.—The best outcome is achieved when surgery is planned for the first 3 days after aneurysmal rupture. Further efforts are needed to diagnose and refer these patients at an early stage to avoid the effects of rebleeding and vasospasm.

▶ This brief report provides the final flourish for the cooperative study on the timing of aneurysm surgery: in North America, patients with early surgery did somewhat better than those planned for delayed surgery. This provides further underpinning for the strategy of early surgery. Because these patients were seen in the period from 1980 through 1983, before the onset of the widespread use of hypervolemic therapy for vasospasm, it is to be expected that substantial further improvement can be made by the application of this current technique (and others) to reduce the impact of vasospasm.—R.M. Crowell, M.D.

Management of Intraoperative Rupture of Aneurysm Without Hypotension
Giannotta SL, Oppenheimer JH, Levy ML, Zelman V (Univ of Southern California, Los Angeles)
Neurosurgery 28:531–536, 1991   23–5

Perioperative and Intraoperative Aneurysm Ruptures

Parameter	Before 1986 (no.)	After 1986 (no.)
Operations	168	108
Aneurysms	185	132
Ruptures	25 (14.8)	16 (14.8)
Permanent deficit	6	0
Death	8	0

(Courtesy of Giannotta SL, Oppenheimer JH, Levy ML, et al: *Neurosurgery* 28:531–536, 1991.)

Objective.—Intraoperative rupture of intracranial aneurysm is associated with a high mortality rate. A total of 276 consecutive surgical procedures for 317 intracranial aneurysms were performed from July 1980 to October 1988. These procedures were reviewed retrospectively to determine factors that may influence outcome of intraoperative rupture of intracranial aneurysms.

Data Analysis.—There were 41 intraoperative or perioperative ruptures of aneurysm, for an incidence rate of 14.8% per operation and 12.9% per aneurysm. Of these, 5 were preexposure ruptures, including 3 that occurred during anesthetic induction. Only 1 patient made a good recovery. For the remaining 36 patients, neurologic outcome was correlated with 3 hemostatic modalities. The use of tamponade or temporary clips did not influence outcome, whereas the use of these adjuncts with induced hypotension was associated with poorer outcome. Overall, hypotension was associated with a 38% favorable recovery compared with 87% without its use. Before 1986, 168 operations were performed for 185 aneurysms with the use of induced hypotension. From 1986 to 1988, 108 operations for 132 aneurysms were performed without the use of induced hypotension. Although the percentage of intraoperative ruptures of aneurysms increased slightly, but insignificantly, from 11.9% in 1986 to 14.8% in 1988, all 16 patients with intraoperative rupture after 1986 had favorable recovery (table). In contrast, before 1986, only half the 20 patients with intraoperative rupture had favorable recovery. Another factor that influenced outcome was the location of the aneurysm; basilar aneuryms and middle cerebral aneurysms were associated with unfavorable recovery from perioperative rupture.

Conclusion.—Induced hypotension may not be a necessary adjunct to the management of intraoperative rupture of intracranial aneurysms. This study shows that timing, location of the aneurysm, and adjunctive hemostatic modalities can affect outcome of perioperative rupture of intracranial aneurysms.

▶ This study of intraoperative rupture in 276 operative cases provides important information. The authors note that simple tamponade and temporary clipping both yielded excellent patient outcome (87%), whereas concomitant hypotension was associated with only a 38% favorable outcome. The actual incidence of intraoperative bleeding was not different after induced hypertension cases were excluded from the operative routine for aneurysm dissection. In addition, it was noted that there was a high incidence of hemorrhage from anterior communicating and distal basilar aneurysms. Even modest hemorrhage in these sites dramatically heightens the risk of poor outcome. It is to be noted that the practice effect could play a role in this series extending over 8 years. Moreoover, the use of prophylactic cerebral protection agents is probably warranted in these cases to minimize the deleterious effects of temporary clipping should it be necessary.—R.M. Crowell, M.D.

Temporary Clipping in Aneurysm Surgery: Technique and Results
Charbel FT, Ausman JI, Diaz FG, Malik GM, Dujovny M, Sanders J (Henry Ford Neurosurgical Inst, Detroit)
Surg Neurol 36:83–90, 1991   23–6

Background.—The use of temporary clipping in aneurysm surgery has become an established practice. The associated operative protocols and results were studied.

Patients and Outcomes.—Sixty-two patients treated consecutively between 1982 and 1987 were studied. All underwent temporary vascular occlusion during aneurysm surgery. A total of 35% had unruptured aneurysms; 24% had grade I aneurysms; 25% had grade II, 8% had grade III; and 7% had grade IV. In 29 patients, the aneurysms were located in the middle cerebral artery. In 13 patients, they were found in the anterior communicating artery. Seventeen percent had new, persistent deficit after surgery. However, temporary clipping was believed to be responsible for the deficit in only 1 case, or 2%. In another 3 cases, the effect of temporary clipping could not be ruled out, but it was believed to be unlikely. Overall, 92% of the patients had a good or excellent outcome. The mortality was 3%, and the morbidity was 5%.

Conclusion.—Temporary clipping in aneurysm surgery reduced morbidity and mortality at one center. It has, therefore, become a standard technique in the attempt to improve the outcomes of patients undergoing craniotomy and clipping of cerebral aneurysms.

▶ This extensive experience with temporary clipping for aneurysm surgery (from the experienced group at Henry Ford Hospital) indicates some of the advantages and problems associated with this approach. Amongst 62 consecutive patients, the authors were able to achieve a 92% good-to-excellent result, with 3% mortality and 5% morbidity. The use of normotension with pentothal (3–5 mg/kg, given every 15–20 minutes) resulted in new deficits in 17% of the patients. Temporary clipping was implicated in only 1 case (2%), although it possibly was involved in 5%. The authors believe that temporary occlusion was associated with 2 lasting occlusions in this series. The complications appeared to be unpredictable in terms of time of occlusion— temporary clipping seemed safe for as long as 24 minutes for the middle cerebral artery and for as long as 16 minutes for the bilateral A1.

In this series, the mean clip times were 14 minutes for the middle cerebral artery and 16 minutes for the anterior communicating artery, i.e., rather brief clipping times were used. It seems likely that the temporary clipping approach permitted a more rapid surgical obliteration. The frequency of intraoperative rupture in this series is not recorded but, presumably, it was reduced by the temporary clipping maneuver.

Our experience at Massachusetts General Hospital has suggested that, with mannitol protection, clipping times of as much as 1 hour may be used with safety in the middle cerebral, anterior cerebral, and basilar arteries. We have found that temporary occlusion of this sort almost eliminates the problem of intraoperative rupture and its attendant risks.

Temporary clipping for aneurysm surgery seems well established as a important adjunct in the reduction of intraoperative rupture and poor outcomes. It may also be said that, in most cases, this approach obviates the need for cardiopulmonary bypass for profound hyperthermia, although it may be important when adequate control of the parent vessels cannot be obtained.—R.M. Crowell, M.D.

Deep Hypothermic Circulatory Arrest for the Management of Complex Anterior and Posterior Circulation Aneurysms
Solomon RA, Smith CR, Raps EC, Young WL, Stone JG, Fink ME (Columbia Univ College of Physicians and Surgeons, New York)
Neurosurgery 29:732–738, 1991   23-7

Introduction.—Surgery on giant intracranial aneurysms continues to be a technical challenge, but it is aided by using techniques of deep hypothermic circulatory arrest that were developed for use in cardiac surgery. Fourteen patients with giant aneurysms were operated on using total circulatory arrest under deep hypothermia with barbiturate anesthesia (table).

Methods.—Thiopental loading was done before cooling began. Anesthesia was induced, and cardiopulmonary bypass was instituted with cooling until the brain temperature reached 16°–18°C and the axillary temperature was less than 28°C. Defibrillation was performed during rewarming. The patients received autologous platelet-rich plasma as well as red cells.

Results.—The time of circulatory arrest ranged from 6 to 51 minutes. A majority of patients had the aneurysm directly clipped and successfully obliterated. Two patients had proximal ligation and 2 had trapping. The cardiopulmonary bypass time averaged approximately 2 hours. There were no operative deaths. Seven patients had an excellent outcome, returning to work with normal neurologic findings. Five others had moder-

Clinical Data and Parameters of Cardiopulmonary Bypass and Deep Hypothermic Arrest

Patient Number	Sex/Age (yr)	Diagnosis	Presentation	Bypass Time (min)	Circulatory Arrest time (min)	Temperature at Start of Circulatory Arrest (°C)	
						Core	Brain
1	M/60	Giant basilar	Subarachnoid hemorrhage	137	26	18	
2	M/28	Giant ophthalmic	Optic nerve compression	186	38	20	
3	M/41	Giant middle cerebral artery	Chronic headache	120	23	16	
4	F/17	Giant vertebral	Brain stem compression	131	41	16	16
5	F/69	Giant basilar	Subarachnoid hemorrhage	112	12	16	15
6	M/59	Giant basilar	Chiasmal syndrome	137	17	15	
7	M/61	Giant basilar	Brain stem compression	116	20	19.5	17.5
8	F/46	Giant internal carotid artery	Subarachnoid hemorrhage	110	17	19	15.5
9	F/49	Giant basilar	Subarachnoid hemorrhage	127	10	15.5	15
10	M/24	Giant basilar	Brain stem compression	91	17	19	16
11	F/34	Giant basilar	Chronic headache	110	8	22.5	17.5
12	M/41	Giant anterior communicating	Subarachnoid hemorrhage	85	6	21	18
13	M/41	Giant anterior communicating	Optic nerve compression	91	51	22.5	18
14	F/65	Giant vertebral	Brain stem compression	109	18	16	18

(Courtesy of Solomon RA, Smith CR, Raps EC, et al: *Neurosurgery* 29:732–738, 1991.)

ate-to-severe deficits postoperatively, but they were improved at 3 months; 3 were living independently. One patient had intraoperative subcortical infarction but was living independently. Another had a thalamic infarction and pulmonary embolism and was left with hemiparesis and aphasia. Five patients had less serious complications.

Conclusion.—This limited experience suggests that patients requiring surgery for giant or complex intracranial aneurysms may benefit from deep hypothermic circulatory arrest.

Aneurysms Arising From the Proximal (A₁) Segment of the Anterior Cerebral Artery: A Study of 38 Cases

Suzuki M, Onuma T, Sakurai Y, Mizoi K, Ogawa A, Yoshimoto T (Tohoku Univ; Sendai City Hosp; Sendai Natl Hosp, Sendai, Japan)
J Neurosurg 76:455–458, 1992   23–8

Background.—Aneurysms of the anterior cerebral circulation usually occur on the anterior communicating artery or the peripheral portion (A_2) of the anterior cerebral artery (ACA). Infrequently, they occur on the proximal segment (A_1) of the ACA. An experience with a series of patients with A_1 aneurysms prompted an investigation of the clinical, angiographic, and CT features of these aneurysms.

Patients and Findings.—A total of 38 patients were studied. There were 37 saccular aneurysms and 1 fusiform aneurysm. The incidence of A_1 aneurysms among a total of 4,295 cases was .88%. Seventeen of the 38 patients, or 44.7%, had multiple aneurysms. In 58.8%, bleeding from the A_1 aneurysm was noted. The aneurysms were classified into 5 categories based on mode of origin in relation to the A_1 segment. In 21 cases, the aneurysms originated from the junction of the A_1 segment and a perforating artery. In 8, they originated from the A_1 segment directly. In 6, the aneurysms originated from the proximal end of the A_1 fenestration, and in 2, from the junction of the A_1 segment and cortical branch. Computed tomography showed bleeding extending to the septum pellucidum comparable to that of aneurysms of the anterior communicating artery.

Conclusion.—In this series, the incidence of A_1 aneurysms among all cases of aneurysms was less than 1%. When performing radical surgery in such cases, the surgeon must recognize the characteristics of A_1 aneurysms, including their multiplicity, high incidence of vascular anomalies, and similarity to anterior communicating artery aneurysms on CT scans.

▶ This review of a substantial number of cases (38) indicates that, although they are rare (approximately 1%), A_1 cerebral artery aneurysms have a typical radiographic appearance and often involve fenestrations of the vessel and multiple aneurysms, thus assisting the surgeon in surgical obliteration of these lesions.—R.M. Crowell, M.D.

Cerebral Arterial Fenestrations Associated With Intracranial Saccular Aneurysms

San-Galli F, Leman C, Kien P, Khazaal J, Phillips SD, Guérin J (Hôpital Pellegrin, Bordeaux, France)

Neurosurgery 30:279–283, 1992   23–9

Introduction.—Fenestrations of cerebral vessels other than the anterior communicating artery are rare congenital anomalies. They are most often seen in the vertebral or basilar site, but they also may involve the middle cerebral or internal carotid arteries. These fenestrations often are asymptomatic, but saccular aneurysms are not infrequent.

Methods.—Data were reviewed on 4 patients who had fenestrations of cerebral vessels associated with intracranial aneurysms. In 2 patients, there were basilar artery fenestrations; 1 patient had aneurysmal dilatation at 1 end of a short fenestration of the anterior cerebral artery, and the other had a vertebral artery fenestration associated with an aneurysm of the supraclinoid part of the ipsilateral carotid artery.

Conclusion.—Those patients with a fenestration and associated aneurysm often have subarachnoid bleeding, but cerebral infarction has been described. A variety of angiographic projections may be necessary to make the diagnosis. Magnetic resonance imaging may be helpful.

Transoral Transclival Clipping of Anterior Inferior Cerebellar Artery Aneurysm Using New Rotating Applier: Technical Note

Crockard HA, Koksel T, Watkin N (Natl Hosps for Neurology and Neurosurgery, London)

J Neurosurg 75:483–485, 1991   23–10

Background.—Surgical access to midbasilar aneurysms is difficult. The midline transclival approach theoretically should provide the best access, because the vessel and aneurysm are directly on the dura, way from the cranial nerves. In the past, this route was largely abandoned because of technical difficulties with the application and release of the clip and with wound care. The incidence of postoperative meningitis also was too high. However, new techniques have helped to alleviate the risks associated with some of these problems. A large aneurysm at the anterior inferior cerebellar artery (AICA)/basilar junction was successfully occluded in 1 man.

Case Report.—Man, 23, was seen at another hospital with a subarachnoid hemorrhage and sudden onset of left fourth and sixth nerve palsies. The patient was transferred with a persisting nerve palsy. Because the aneurysm appeared to be buried in the substance of the pons and was not accessible through conventional posterolateral routes, transclival transdural surgery was planned. A midline hard and soft palatal split was added to a standard Le Fort maxillotomy, hinging laterally on the palatine vessels and nerves in each half of the palate, which allowed exposure of whole clivus and craniocervical junction to C-2. The midportion of the clivus was removed using a high-speed air drill. The aneurysm was found deep in the brain substance on the left, its neck posterolateral to the origin of a very dominant AICA. The sixth nerve arising from its nucleus was on the brain surface, distorted and damaged by the aneurysm. The aneurysm neck was occluded with a curved variangle McFadden clip, using a rotating pistol-grip aneurysm clip applier designed especially for transoral vascular surgery. Several clips were applied and removed until occlusion was satisfactory, with preservation of the AICA. The spring of the clip was entirely epidural. The dural defect was repaired with fascia lata, fat, and thrombin fibrin glue, and the nasopharyngeal mucosa was closed using interrupted Vicryl sutures. The maxilla and hard palate were reconstituted, and CSF was drained for 5 days through a lumbar drain. No CSF leaked, nor did meningitis develop. The patient was discharged from the hospital 8 days after aneurysm occlusion. Angiography confirmed that the aneurysm was excluded from the circulation. Two months after surgery, the patient's sixth nerve weakness had almost completely disappeared.

Conclusion.—The transoral approach is recommended for aneurysms originating in the middle and lower thirds of the basilar artery, especially for those buried in the brain substance. When care is taken with dural closure, the route is not unduly hazardous. The prototype pistol grip applier is useful for treating these difficult aneurysms. The instrument and steering technique used should also be considered for anterior circle aneurysms.

▶ Crockard and Connolly have popularized the transoral approach to lesions of the clivus. Crockard and colleagues now extend this methodology to the treatment of basilar trunk aneurysms. In this report, an extensive maxillotomy and splitting of the palate were carried out to approach the lesion. Although the patient did well, experience with palate-splitting procedures in other patients has suggested a substantial number of postoperative swallowing and speech difficulties. The successful use of a new rotating clip applier is described for the application of clips at right angles to the axis of vision in this narrow field. The authors also have been able to prevent CSF leakage by meticulous layer closure of the dura and lumbar drain. The use of fibrin glue has also been useful in this kind of situation.

At Massachusetts General Hospital, we have directly had the opportunity to treat 4 patients with midline basilar aneurysms on the clivus using a similar but different technique. To avoid the problems of palate splitting, we have chosen to work transnasally, with a nasal flap approach. The working space with this technique is typically 2 × 2 cm, which permits very satisfactory working room for the application of temporary clips for aneurysm dissection and obliteration. We have tried Dr. Crockard's clip applier and have found it to be useful; however, other standard clip appliers may also be used (such as the Sano). Closure is extremely important, and I have found that a laryngeal mucosal flap closure, together with fibrin glue, appears to offer an effective method of seal. Ventral approaches to midline clival aneurysms appear to be both safe and effective.—R.M. Crowell, M.D.

Surgical Treatment of Multiple Intracranial Aneurysms

Inagawa T (Shimane Prefectural Central Hosp, Izumo, Japan)
Acta Neurochir (Wien) 108:22–29, 1991   23–11

Background.—Opinions on the surgical indications for multiple intracranial aneurysms vary. The results of surgery on 126 patients with multiple intracranial aneuryms were analyzed retrospectively.

Patients.—A total of 46 men and 80 women (mean age, 60 years) were studied. These patients had 302 aneurysms, with 28% having 3 or more aneurysms.

Findings.—Direct operations were performed on 97 patients. Both ruptured and unruptured anerysms were treated in 69 (71%) patients, with 1-stage operations done in 48 and 2-stage operations done in 21. Only the ruptured aneuryms were treated in the remaining 28 (29%) patients. Among the 48 patients who underwent 1-stage operations for treatment of both ruptured and unruptured aneurysms, 34 were operated on by day 4 after the initial subarachnoid hemorrhage (SAH). In 12 of these patients, 13 tiny unruptured aneurysms were discovered during surgery, including 9 that were discovered during the removal of clots to reduce cerebral vasospasm. Only the ruptured aneurysms were treated in 28 patients, either because the patient was 70 years of age or older, or because there was a presence of small and physically inaccessible unruptured aneurysms (the C3 or C4 portion of the internal carotid artery). There were no operative deaths among the patients who underwent a second-stage operation for unruptured aneurysms. The operative mortality rate was 10% for patients who had a 1-stage operation for both ruptured and unruptured aneurysms and 14% for patients treated only for ruptured aneurysms. These rates were comparable to the 12% operative mortality rate among 228 patients with single aneurysms treated during the same period. None of the patients died of bleeding of the unruptured aneurysm at 1 year after the initial SAH.

Conclusion.—The surgical results for multiple intracranial aneurysms are satisfactory, even for every operation by day 4 after SAH. Nevertheless, the surgical indications for unruptured aneurysms should be considered carefully.

▶ This study indicates the difficulty in obtaining useful guidelines on the treatment of unruptured aneurysms using data derived from a single center. A retrospective study of 126 patients with 302 aneurysms gives a substantial amount of data; however, in terms of comparing the results with an alternative mode of therapy, very little may be said. Basic questions are left unanswered: What is the risk of rupture of an unruptured aneurysm in the setting of rupture of another aneurysm? What is the risk of surgical correction of this unruptured lesion during an operation for a ruptured lesion or during a staged operation after clipping of a ruptured lesion? By gathering data on thousands of lesions from many institutions, the International Cooperative Study of Unruptured Intracranial Aneurysms, headed by Weibers, will give useful information on this topic.—R.M. Crowell, M.D.

Vasospasm

Effect of AT877 on Cerebral Vasospasm After Aneurysmal Subarachnoid Hemorrhage: Results of a Prospective Placebo-Controlled Double-Blind Trial

Shibuya M, Suzuki Y, Sugita K, Saito I, Sasaki T, Takakura K, Nagata I, Kikuchi H, Takemae T, Hidaka H, Nakashima M (Nagoya Univ, Nagoya, Japan; Kyorin Univ, Mitaka, Japan; Tokyo Univ; Kyoto Univ, Kyoto, Japan; Shinshu Univ, Shinsu, Japan; et al)
J Neurosurg 76:571–577, 1992   23–12

Background.—Delayed cerebral ischemia associated with vasospasm remains the chief cause of a poor operative outcome in patients with a ruptured intracranial aneurysm. Nimodipine, a calcium antagonist, has improved outcomes, but it has not altered the severity of vasospasm. The drug AT877 is a new calcium antagonist that acts differently than calcium entry blockers such as nimodipine, inhibiting the action of free intracellular calcium and also inhibiting protein kinases.

Study Design.—A prospective multicenter trial of AT877 was undertaken in 267 patients who underwent surgery within 3 days of the onset of subarachnoid hemorrhage. The patients received either 30 mg of AT877 or a saline placebo given intravenously for a 30-minute period, 3 times daily for 2 weeks after surgery. The groups were closely matched demographically and clinically.

Outcome.—The patients given AT877 had significantly less vasospasm than did the placebo recipients, and they had smaller low-density regions associated with vasospasm on CT. The proportion of patients who had a moderate or greater disability a month after bleeding because of vasospasm was reduced from 26% to 12% with AT877. No serious adverse events occurred in patients treated with AT877. Rebleeding and hematoma formation were comparably frequent in the 2 groups, occurring in 6% of all patients.

Conclusion.—The findings confirmed the spasmolytic potency of AT877, which appears to be an effective and safe agent for use in patients with aneurysmal rupture.

▶ This report on AT-877, a new calcium antagonist, is the first placebo-controlled, double-blind trial to demonstrate a significant reduction in angiographical vasospasm after subarachnoid hemorrhage. The sizable study is impressive, and if confirmation can be obtained from other centers, this may become routine in the care of these patients.—R.M. Crowell, M.D.

Prevention of Cerebral Vasospasm by Actinomycin D

Shigeno T, Mima T, Yanagisawa M, Saito A, Goto K, Yamashita K, Takenouchi T, Matsuura N, Yamasaki Y, Yamada K, Masaki T, Takakura K (Saitama Med School, Saitama, Japan; Univ of Tokyo; Univ of Tsukuba, Japan; Research Inst of Taiho Pharmaceuticals, Tokushima, Japan; Kyowa Hakko Kogyo, Tokyo)
J Neurosurg 74:940–943, 1991   23–13

Background.—In delayed vasospasm after a subarachnoid bleed, the arterial smooth muscle contracts strongly and there is abnormal proliferation and necrosis of the arterial wall. Endogenous vasoactive factors (e.g., endothelin) have been implicated in this process. Because endothelin synthesis is regulated at the level of messenger RNA transcription, the effect of actinomycin D, an inhibitor of RNA synthesis, was examined in relation to the development of vasospasm in dogs with subarachnoid hemorrhage.

Methods.—Arterial blood was injected into the cisterna magna of beagle dogs, and the injection was repeated 2 days later (as basilar artery caliber was monitored). Some animals received intravenous actinomycin D, 10 μg/kg/day, for 4 days after hemorrhage was induced.

Findings.—The basilar artery became progressively constricted after induction of subarachnoid hemorrhage. All but 1 of the animals that received actinomycin D had a complete resolution of vasospasm within a week (Fig 23–2). Endothelin immunoreactivity was much more evident after subarachnoid hemorrhage, and administration of actinomycin D tended to suppress reactivity.

Conclusion.—This approach may prove to be a helpful adjuvant measure for patients with subarachnoid hemorrhage. In addition, it may help clarify the pathogenesis of cerebral vasospasm.

▶ This interesting study indicates that actinomycin D, which inhibits RNA synthesis, can prevent cerebrovascular vasospasm. Although the drug is too toxic to recommend it for clinical use, the data suggest that other suppressants of metabolic activity (and possibly inflammatory activity) might be useful in the treatment of vasospasm. Studies using cyclosporine in our institution have been promising in this regard.—R.M. Crowell, M.D.

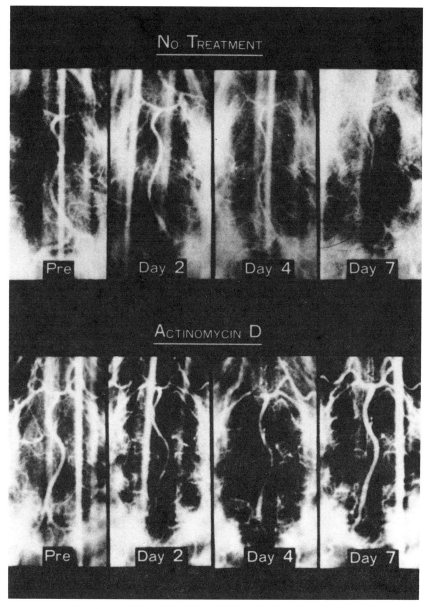

Fig 23–2.—Typical examples of basilar artery angiograms in dogs with subarachnoid hemorrhage. **Upper,** angiograms from a dog in the vehicle-treated control group showing progressive basilar artery constriction. **Lower,** angiograms from a dog treated with actinomycin D showing inhibition of arterial constriction by actinomycin D. (Courtesy of Shigeno T, Mima T, Yanagisawa M, et al: *J Neurosurg* 74:940–943, 1991.)

Cerebral Vasospasm and Vasoconstriction Caused by Endothelin

Kobayashi H, Hayashi M, Kobayashi S, Kabuto M, Handa Y, Kawano H, Ide H (Fukui Med School; Yoyama Med and Pharmaceutical Univ, Toyama, Japan)
Neurosurgery 28:673–679, 1991   23–14

Introduction.—Cerebral vasospasm is a significant cause of cerebral ischemia after subarachnoid bleeding, but its pathogenesis is not well understood. Endothelin (ET) is a vasoconstrictor peptide that has been implicated in cerebral vasospasm. It is capable of constricting cerebral arteries for sustained periods through a calcium-mediated process.

Methods.—A miniosmotic pump was implanted in the neck of adult dogs for administering either water or synthetic endothelin-1 (ET-1) into the cisterna magna for 7 days. Other animals had vasospasm induced by 2 injections of autologous cisternal blood given 48 hours apart.

Results.—The basilar artery was 35% constricted after 1 week of ET-1 administration and it was 43% constricted after blood injections. The vessel exhibited degenerative changes of both the endothelial cells and the smooth-muscle cells in both groups. Endothelin was demonstrated immunohistochemically only in the endothelial cells of ET-treated animals.

Conclusion.—Endothelin may have an important role in the development of cerebral vasospasm after subarachnoid hemorrhage.

▶ Kobayashi et al. studied dogs after continuous intracisternal injection of endothelin-1 or double injection of cisternal blood. Follow-up angiographic and histologic studies were carried out to assess the basilar artery. This is the first direct evidence that intracisternal endothelin-1 can cause angiographic-persisting vasospasm.

Many other agents associated with angiographic and histologic vasospasm have not turned out to be of major clinical significance. Thus, further investigation of endothelin-1 will be needed before it can be accepted as an important cause of vasospasm. It would be interesting to know whether calcium channel blockage can prevent the vasoconstrictive effects of the agent. Other studies might be directed toward the determination of the effect of the concentration of endothelin required to produce vasoconstriction. The fate of intracisternal endothelin-1 might also be studied with radiolabelled peptide. In short, although this is tantalizing information, follow-up studies will be needed to confirm its significance.—R.M. Crowell, M.D.

Preventive Effect of Synthetic Serine Protease Inhibitor, FUT-175, on Cerebral Vasospasm in Rabbits

Yanamoto H, Kikuchi H, Okamoto S, Nozaki K (Kyoto Univ, Japan)
Neurosurgery 30:351–357, 1992   23–15

Purpose.—Some research suggests that the arterial narrowing that occurs after subarachnoid hemorrhage (SAH) represents a vasculopathy or an inflammatory reaction in the vascular wall rather than a simple physiologic constriction. Other studies have emphasized the immune system's role in the origin of cerebral vasospasm in the subarachnoid space. A study was performed in rabbits using the potent complement system inhibitor FUT-175 to explore the possibility that this system is involved in the pathogenesis of cerebral vasospasm after SAH.

Methods.—An SAH was simulated in 40 anesthetized rabbits by a single injection of autologous arterial blood into the cisterna magna. Over the next 7 days, angiography was used to investigate the caliber of each basilar artery. Animals were randomized to receive no treatment, 10 animals, FUT-175 in 3 intravenous doses of 1 mg, 9 animals; 2 mg, 13 animals; or 3 mg, 5 animals. Another 3 rabbits received 6 mg of FUT-175 intravenously on day 2 when arterial narrowing was at its peak.

Results.—On day 2, arterial narrowing was 35% in the untreated animals vs. 21% in animals that received 3 mg of FUT-175, 5% in those that received 6 mg, and 14% in those that received 9%. Differences were significant between controls and the low-dose group on days 1 and 2 and between controls and the 2 higher-dose groups on days 1–4. In the animals treated on day 2, FUT-175 had no vasodilatory effect.

Conclusions.—Intravenous administration of FUT-175 at an early stage of SAH appears to prevent vasospasm in a rabbit model. No vasodilatory effect is seen after narrowing reaches its full development. Thus vasospasm can be prevented by inhibition of the plasma serine protease cascades at an early stage of SAH. Delayed pathologic arterial narrowing could result from the inflammation caused by activation of plasma protease cascades.

▶ This report demonstrates that FUT 175, an inhibitor of the complement system, is a safe and effective treatment of cerebral vasospasm in rabbits. The fact that this agent interferes with the complement system again brings into discussion the role of inflammation in the development of vasospasm.—R.M. Crowell, M.D.

Direct Evidence for a Key Role of Protein Kinase C in the Development of Vasospasm After Subarachnoid Hemorrhage

Nishizawa S, Nezu N, Uemura K (Hamamatsu Univ, Hamamatsu, Japan)

J Neurosurg 76:635–639, 1992   23–16

Background.—How vasospasm develops after subarachnoid hemorrhage (SAH) remains uncertain. Some signal is required to induce a contractile response, and protein kinase C may have a critical role in the process. Therefore, direct measurements of protein kinase C activity were made in the basilar arteries of dogs with subarachnoid hemorrhage.

Methods.—Three millimeters of autologous blood was injected into the cisterna magna on 2 occasions 3 days apart, and the animals were killed on day 7. Protein kinase C was assayed by measuring the incorporation of ^{32}P from $(\gamma\text{-}^{32}P)$ adenosine triphosphate (ATP) into substrate-peptide.

Results.—Protein kinase C activity was much greater in membranes from dogs with SAH than in control samples. The proportion of membrane activity to total activity was significantly greater in SAH vessels than in control vessels, whereas the proportion of cytosol activity was reduced.

Conclusion.—Activation of protein kinase C appears to have an important role in the development of vasospasm after SAH.

▶ In canine experimental SAH, protein kinase C activity is remarkably enhanced compared with such activity in a control group. Because protein kinase C plays a crucial role in activating contractile proteins of smooth muscle, the findings provide direct evidence for a role of protein kinase C in the development of vasospasm. Also, because this is a step far along in the development of muscular vascular contraction, the trigger for this reaction could be a number of stimuli. Nonetheless, this provides another clue in the mystery of cerebrovascular vasospasm after SAH.—R.M. Crowell, M.D.

Arteriovenous Malformations

Comparison of Magnetic Resonance Angiography, Magnetic Resonance Imaging and Conventional Angiography in Cerebral Arteriovenous Malformation

Nüssel F, Wegmüller H, Huber P (Inselspital, Bern, Switzerland)
Neuroradiology 33:56–61, 1991   23–17

Background.—Although MRI provides excellent visualization of the nidus and the involved brain areas, it fails to give sufficient information on the detailed vascular supply and hemodynamics of cerebral arteriovenous malformation (AVM). New MRI techniques, based on 3-dimensional phase contrast methods, provide angiographic images without injection of contrast agents. The role of magnetic resonance angiography (MRA) in the evaluation of cerebral AVM was studied in relation to that of conventional cerebral angiography (CCA) and MRI.

Methods.—Ten patients with an AVM of the brain were examined by MRI, MRA, and CCA. Six patients had medium- to large-sized AVMs (3–7 cm), and 4 had small AVMs (less than 2 cm).

Results.—With MRA, important information about the vascular supply was evident in 7 patients, but it could only be suspected in 3, all of whom had small AVMs. In contrast, CCA showed the vascularization of the AVMs in all patients and showed additional hemodynamic aspects better than MRA (Fig 23–3). With MRI, the size and location of the nidus and the involved brain structures could be well visualized, better than by MRA and CCA; however, only the involvement of the main cerebral vessels was evident.

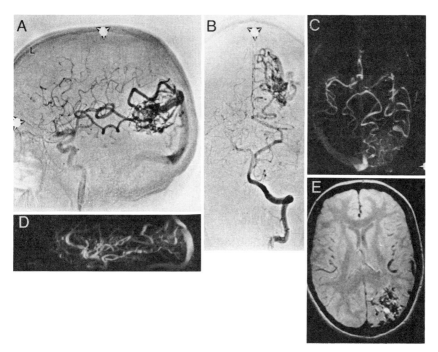

Fig 23–3.—Patient with a left parietal AVM nearly equally supplied by branches of the left MCA and PCA. **A,** CCA—left carotid angiogram, lateral view shows the arterial supply by the angular and posterior temporal artery of the left MCA and the early venous drainage into the SSS. **B,** CCA—left vertebral angiogram, Towne's view demonstrates parieto-occipital branches of the left PCA as feeders of the AVM. **C,** MRA—axial collapsed view visualizes the involvement of posterior temporal and angular branches of the MCA and the parieto-occipital branches of the PCA. The nidus appears as a cloud-shaped grey area. **D,** MRA—lateral rotation demonstrates supply by the angular artery and the parieto-occipital branches of the left PCA as well as the venous drainage to the SSS. **E,** MRI-SE, proton-weighted (TR 2000, TE 30) axial planes showing the nidus as an area with punctate and tortuous structures of increased and decreased signal intensity and dilated feeder branches of the MCA. (Courtesy of Nüssel F, Wegmüller H, Huber P: *Neuroradiology* 33:56-61, 1991.)

Conclusion.—Conventional angiography still remains the method of choice to obtain the best information about the vascular anatomy and hemodynamics of AVMs. Although MRA can be used in combination with MRI to obtain information about the vascular supply of AVM, it appears to be of limited value in small AVMs.

► This comparison of MRA, MRI, and conventional angiography provides results that are close to what you'd expect: MRA adds something beyond MRI data, but the most precise cerebrovascular dynamics are provided only by cerebral angiography. Thus, in critical surgical decision making for AVMs, MRA cannot supplant conventional angiography. On the other hand, in certain cases, one could make a decision not to perform cerebral angiography on the basis of MRI plus MRA. For example, a patient with a 7-cm AVM with multiple feeders, deep venous drainage, and advanced age would be at such high risk that conservative treatment without intervention would be suggested solely on the basis of MRI and MRA.—R.M. Crowell, M.D.

An Analysis of the Venous Drainage System as a Factor in Hemorrhage From Arteriovenous Malformations

Miyasaka Y, Yada K, Ohwada T, Kitahara T, Kurata A, Irikura K (Kitasato Univ, Sagamihara, Kanagawa, Japan)
J Neurosurg 76:239–243, 1992   23–18

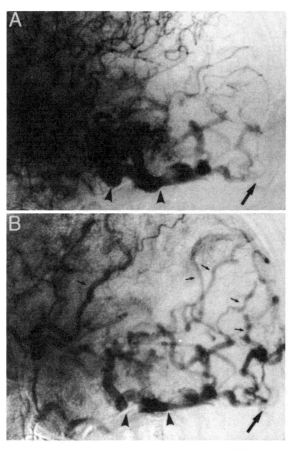

Fig 23–4.—Left carotid angiograms, lateral views, in a man, 45, with a left temporal hematoma. The late arterial phase (**A**) and late venous phase (**B**) show a temporal lobe arteriovenous malformation (AVM). Drainage of the AVM is through the inferior cerebral vein (*arrowheads*), which is obstructed at the junction of the transverse sinus (*large arrows*). Note the absence of opacification of the transverse sinus and the numerous collateral venous pathways through the superior cerebral veins (*small arrows*). (Courtesy of Miyasaka Y, Yada K, Ohwada T, et al: *J Neurosurg* 76:239-243, 1992.)

Background.—The indications for surgical intervention in patients with arteriovenous malformations (AVMs) are controversial because of the lack of understanding about the risk of bleeding from these lesions. No one has done a critical analysis of the venous drainage system and its pathologic changes in such patients. Detailed observations of the draining veins in 108 cerebral AVMs were reported, along with a statistical assessment of the effect of the venous drainage system on the rate of hemorrhage.

Methods and Findings.—The proportion of AVMs bleeding, or the hemorrhage rate, was calculated in relation to the number of draining veins, the presence or absence of impairment in venous drainage, and the location of draining veins. Arteriovenous malformations with certain characteristics were found to have a high risk of hemorrhage. The hemorrhagic rate was 89% in 54 patients with 1 draining vein, 94% in 18 patients with severely impaired venous drainage, and 94% in 32 patients with deep venous drainage alone. Segmental stenosis in the venous drainage system with more than a 50% reduction in diameter was regarded as abnormal (Fig 23-4).

Conclusion.—The venous drainage system of AVMs appears to be significantly related to the risk of hemorrhage in these lesions. Arteriovenous malformations characterized by 1 draining vein, severely impaired venous drainage, and deep venous drainage alone carried a high risk of hemorrhage. Careful preoperative angiographic assessment of the venous drainage system is, therefore, essential for decision making in the treatment of AVMs.

▶ This important contribution documents clearly that there is a high bleeding rate in cases with 1 draining vein, severe overflow obstruction, or deep venous drainage only. This will enable preoperative evaluation to identify those patients with especially high risk of intracranial bleeding, and thus set the stage for appropriate management. Needless to say, the venous obstruction may also make treatment of the lesion more difficult, because treatment must avoid occlusion of the venous outflow to be successful.—R.M. Crowell, M.D.

Intranidal Aneurysms in Cerebral Arteriovenous Malformations: Evaluation and Endovascular Treatment

Marks MP, Lane B, Steinberg GK, Snipes GJ (Stanford Univ, Calif)
Radiology 183:355–360, 1992   23–19

Background.—Patients with cerebral arteriovenous malformations (AVMs) and an intranidal aneurysm are at increased risk of hemorrhage. The radiologic and pathologic features and endovascular treatment of 15 intranidal aneurysms were evaluated.

Methods.—Angiograms from 125 patients with cerebral AVMs were analyzed. Fifteen patients, or 12%, had intranidal aneurysms. All 15 had a history of hemorrhage. Five patients had particulate or liquid embolization before surgical excision or radiation therapy. All aneurysms were thrombosed when embolization was done. Radiosurgery alone was done in 10 cases, and angiographic follow-up was done in 8 of those 10 patients at a mean of 33 months.

Findings.—Seven of the 10 patients who were followed angiographically had complete obliteration of the AVM without residual aneurysm. Histologic assessment demonstrated intranidal aneurysms that were thin-walled, vascular structures—the likely site for AVM hemorrhage.

Conclusion.—Intranidal aneurysms are highly correlated with bleeding in patients with AVMs. These aneurysms are thin-walled structures rather than pseudoaneurysms from previous bleeding. They appear to be exposed to arterial pressures and may represent an important site of hemorrhage in an AVM. Embolization is an effective way to achieve thrombosis in these aneurysms. Embolization with thrombosis of intranidal aneurysms may be beneficial in patients undergoing radiation therapy, because there is a latency period between irradiation and thrombosis of AVM.

▶ The Stanford group has drawn attention to intranidal aneurysms in AVMs as a predictor of increased risk of hemorrhage. They have also demonstrated that endovascular treatment can obliterate these components. At Massachusetts General Hospital, we have a similar experience as regards these extremely dangerous components of AVMs. In some instances, when total obliteration of a lesion appears extremely hazardous, then obliteration of the intranidal aneurysm alone may provide some benefit for the patient by way of reducing risk of bleeding.—R.M. Crowell, M.D.

Unruptured Intracranial Aneurysms and Arteriovenous Malformations: Frequency of Intracranial Hemorrhage and Relationship of Lesions
Brown RD Jr, Wiebers DO, Forbes GS (Mayo Clinic and Found, Rochester, Minn)
J Neurosurg 73:859–863, 1990   23–20

Objective.—The frequency of intracranial aneurysms associated with arteriovenous malformations (AVM) ranges from 3.7% to 8.7% of patients with AVM. The cerebral angiograms of all patients seen between 1974 and 1985 with intracranial AVM and co-existing aneurysms diagnosed before clinically evident intracranial hemorrhage were reviewed to define the relationship between these 2 lesions and the pathogenesis of intracranial saccular aneurysms.

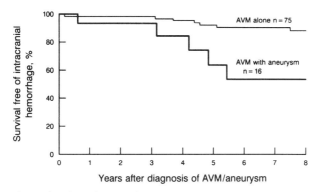

Fig 23–5.—Actuarial analysis of survival free of intracranial hemorrhage, comparing patients with arteriovenous malformations (AVM) alone (75 cases) and patients with AVM co-existing with saccular aneurysms (16 cases). (Courtesy of Brown RD Jr, Wiebers DO, Forbes GS: *J Neurosurg* 73:859–863, 1990.)

Data Analysis.—Of the 91 patients with unruptured intracranial AVMs, 16 (18%) had 26 unruptured intracranial saccular aneurysms. During a mean follow-up period of 4.5 years, intracranial hemorrhage occurred in 6 (38%) of these patients. Actuarial analysis showed that the risk of intracranial hemorrhage in patients with co-existing AVM and aneurysm was 7% per year at 5 years, compared with 1.7% per year among patients with AVM alone (Fig 23–5). The difference in length of survival free of intracranial hemorrhage was significant. The frequency of aneurysms was similar among patients with small, medium, or large AVMs. Twenty-five aneurysms were located on arteries feeding the AVM, usually on enlarged feeding arteries. Eleven aneurysms were atypical and 15 were typical in location, and both occurred with relatively similar frequency on a range of arterial size ratios. All aneurysms at atypical sites originated from primary or secondary branch feeders to the malformation. All aneurysms in typical locations were associated with high-flow/high-shunt AVMs, whereas aneurysms at atypical locations were associated with high-flow, low-flow, and high-shunt, and low-shunt AVMs. The relative sizes of the aneurysmal parent arteries closely approximated those of the overall group of AVM feeders, and there was no linear correlation between the size of the feeding artery and the presence of an aneurysm. Aneurysms with medium and large AVMs developed most commonly at an arterial bifurcation, whereas none of the aneurysms with a small AVM formed at an arterial bifurcation.

Conclusion.—These findings suggest that the hemodynamic abnormalities in the arteries feeding to an AVM may predispose to aneurysm formation, and that the mechanism is not solely based on the high-flow or high-shunt characteristics in these systems.

▶ This interesting study of 16 patients with AVM and aneurysm demonstrates that, in AVMs with aneurysm formation on the feeding system, there is an especially high risk of hemorrhage (7% per year).—R.M. Crowell, M.D.

Stereotactic Craniotomy in the Resection of Small Arteriovenous Malformations

Sisti MB, Solomon RA, Stein BM (Columbia Univ, New York)
J Neurosurg 75:40–44, 1991   23–21

Introduction.—Delineation of an arteriovenous malformation (AVM) by angiography or CT ensures accurate intraoperative location of the AVM using conventional stereotactic methods.

Technique.—The stereotactic frame is applied after anesthesia, and the entry point of the surgical trajectory is defined by the phantom method. Mannitol and spinal drainage are avoided until the nidus of the AVM is localized. A direct orthogonal approach is taken to cortical and subcortical lesions. Deeper or paraventricular AVMs are approached via the anterior frontal lobe, temporal lobe, or superior parietal lobule. The craniotomy flap usually is less than 6 cm in diameter. An operating micrscope is used to follow the ventricular catheter to the AVM.

Experience.—Stereotactically guided resection was carried out in 10 patients with small AVMs that were difficult to locate and had caused intracerebral bleeding. In 6 patients, the nidus of a small AVM was well defined preoperatively. All lesions were totally removed microsurgically. One patient had temporary worsening of hemiparesis in the postoperative period. The others were neurologically intact when followed up 6–24 months after the procedure.

Conclusion.—Stereotactically guided craniotomy is a means of resecting small AVMs with minimal injury of surrounding areas of the brain.

▶ This study describing 10 small-size AVMs resected by stereotactic craniotomy indicates the usefulness of this approach in certain selected areas. In our institution, we have had similar encouraging experience in 6 deep-seated AVMs or cavernomas.—R.M. Crowell, M.D.

Intracranial Venous Hypertension and the Effects of Venous Outflow Obstruction in a Rat Model of Arteriovenous Fistula

Bederson JB, Wiestler OD, Brüstle O, Roth P, Frick R, Yasargil MG (Montefiore Med Ctr, Bronx, NY; Univ Hosp of Zürich, Switzerland)
Neurosurgery 29:341–350, 1991   23–22

Background.—The roles of venous hypertension and venous outflow obstruction in arteriovenous fistulas are not clear. More information is needed about the mechanisms by which venous hypertension and outflow obstruction contribute to altered cerebral hemodynamics adjacent to arteriovenous malformations (AVMs) and arteriovenous fistulas (AVFs).

Methods and Findings.—A model of rat AVF, created with a proximal common carotid artery to distal external jugular vein anastomosis, was studied. Anatomical dissection showed that the external jugular vein is the primary vessel that drains intracranial venous blood. Opening the AVF increased torcular pressure from 6.5 to 13.5 mm Hg and reduced the mean arterial pressure from 82.7 to 62.8 mm Hg. Cerebral perfusion pressure was decreased from 76.2 to 49.3 mm Hg, and the middle cerebral artery blood flow velocity was reduced from 6.8 to 4.2 cm/sec. Occlusion of venous outflow in rats with an AVF increased torcular pressure to 34.8 mm Hg. The middle cerebral artery blood flow velocity decreased to 1.8 cm/sec, and severe ischemic changes occurred. In those conditions, torcular pressure and systemic arterial pressure had a positive linear relationship. In control rats, torcular pressure and arterial pressure were unrelated. Restoring cerebral perfusion pressure by releasing venous outflow occlusion and AVF closure transiently increased the middle cerebral artery flow velocity to 69% above baseline values. One week after permanent venous outflow occlusion, histologic assessment revealed venous infarction, subarachnoid hemorrhage, and severe brain edema in rats with an AVF; it did not do so in those without an AVF.

Conclusion.—This model of AVF reproduces the hemodynamic and hemorrhagic complications of human AVMs and AVFs. The findings stress the importance of venous hypertension and venous outflow obstruction in the pathophysiology of these lesions. Venous pressure is linearly related to systemic arterial pressure in AVFs associated with venous outflow obstruction.

▶ This is an interesting study of a rat AVF that appears to mimic cerebrovascular steal with venous hypertension, as seen in human intracranial AVF. It adds to the growing power of data emphasizing the importance of venous outflow obstruction. Such obstruction appears to cause spontaneous rupture of intracranial AVM and bleeding occurring during embolization or surgical procedures.—R.M. Crowell, M.D.

Cavernous Angiomas

Natural History of the Cavernous Angioma
Robinson JR, Awad IA, Little JR (Cleveland Clinic Found, Ohio)
J Neurosurg 75:709–714, 1991   23–23

Background.—It may be very difficult to diagnose and follow cavernous angioma before surgical excision, because it is not well imaged by either cerebral angiography or CT. For this reason, little is known about its incidence and natural history. Magnetic resonance imaging (MRI) was used to explore the clinical findings and natural history of this lesion.

Patients.—During a 5-year period, 66 of 14,305 patients consecutively undergoing MRI had a total of 76 lesions with an appearance typical of presumed cavernous angioma. Thirty-six were males and 30 were fe-

Outcome in 57 Symptomatic Cases of Cavernous
Angioma Correlated With Hemorrhage and Treatment

Hemorrhage	Surgical Treatment	Outcome		
		Good	Fair	Poor
yes (7 cases)	yes	4	0	0
	no	2	0	1
no (50 cases)	yes	10	0	0
	no	32	8	0

Outcome definitions: good = minor impairment, occasional symptoms, no limitation of activities; fair = recurrent impairment, several symptomatic occurrences per week, limitation of activities; poor = frequent symptoms, an invalid.

(Courtesy of Robinson JR, Awad IA, Little JR: *J Neurosurg* 75:709–714, 1991.)

males; the mean patient age was 34.6 years. A total of 86% of the patients were followed up clinically for a mean of 26 months, resulting in a total of 143 lesion-years of clinical survey.

Findings.—The most common sites were the frontal and temporal lobes, and the most common findings at presentation were seizure, focal neurologic deficit, and headache. Magnetic resonance imaging showed evidence of occult bleeding in most cases; however, only 7 of 57 symptomatic patients had overt hemorrhage, and only 1 patient had overt hemorrhage during follow-up (table). The bleeding rate was thus .7% per year per lesion. The risk of overt hemorrhage was significantly greater in females. Fourteen patients underwent surgery, most for intractable seizures; the diagnosis was confirmed in every case. No deaths were directly attributable to cavernous angioma.

Conclusion.—Magnetic resonance imaging is valuable in the diagnosis and follow-up of cavernous angioma. It also allows study of the natural history of this lesion, assisting in treatment planning and prognosis. Further studies, including the identification of features predisposing to an aggressive course, are underway.

Microsurgery of Deep-Seated Cavernous Angiomas: Report of 26 Cases
Bertalanffy H, Gilsbach JM, Eggert H-R, Seeger W (Univ of Freiburg i Br, Germany)
Acta Neurochir (Wien) 108:91–99, 1991   23–24

Introduction.—Surgery on deep-seated cerebral cavernous angiomas may be associated with substantial morbidity and mortality. In a retrospective study, the results of microsurgery for deep-seated cavernous angiomas were reviewed in 26 patients.

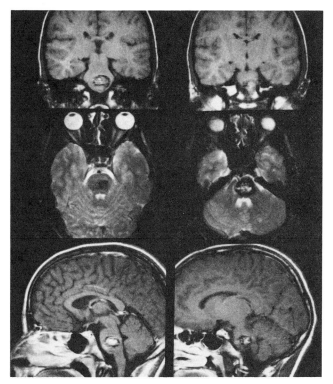

Fig 23–6.—T1-weighted (*top and bottom*) and T2-weighted MRI (*center*) demonstrating a well-circumscribed dishomogeneous mass in the pons. The central increased signal intensity is caused by methemoglobin and the rim of decreased signal intensity by hemosiderin. (Courtesy of Bertalanffy H, Gilsbach JM, Eggert H-R, et al: *Acta Neurochir (Wien)* 108:91–99, 1991.)

Clinical Features.—The study included 16 men and 10 women, aged 5–63 years (mean age, 37 years). On CT and/or MRI, the angiomas were evident in the insula and basal ganglia in 10 patients; in the thalamus in 2; in the midbrain in 5, in the pons in 8 (Fig 23-6); and in the brachium pontis in 1. The main indication for surgery was progressive neurologic disorder. The mean follow-up period was 1.8 years (range, 6 months–4.5 years).

Outcome.—There was no surgical mortality. Total excision of the angioma was achieved without additional neurologic deficits in 11 patients, and the preoperative neurologic deficits improved in all. In 7 patients, transient neurologic deterioration and/or new deficits occurred postoperatively. The remaining 8 patients had severe complications caused by bleeding from residual parts of the malformation in 2 patients; from damage to the internal capsule by direct manipulation in 2; from vascular injury during dissection in 3; and from paradoxical air embolism in 1.

Conclusion.—Radical excision of deep-seated cavenous angiomas is technically feasible, but it carries the price of significant permanent morbidity. Further improvement and experience are necessary to obtain the satisfactory surgical results, with particular attention to the operative approach; to careful dissection and complete removal of the malformation; to perforating arteries; and to anomalous venous drainage. Magnetic resonance imaging with axial, coronal, and sagittal sections provides excellent visualization of the malformation and sufficient information for adequate planning.

▶ This interesting study gives results after resection of deep cavernous angiomas in 26 patients. In 11 patients there was no new deficit, and in 7, recovery was slow. In the remaining 8 patients, there was increased neurologic deficit; 3 of the 8 were severely disabled, 2 were mildly disabled, and the others were only slightly afflicted. Note that all cases had neurologic deficits before surgery. Whereas 81% of the cases had slight or no new neurologic deficit in relation to surgery, the 3 severely disabled patients had lesions in the basal ganglion and dorsal pons. When progressive neurologic symptoms relate to cavernous angioma, the results favor surgical removal, even in deep locations.—R.M. Crowell, M.D.

Cavernous Malformations of the Brain Stem
Zimmerman RS, Spetzler RF, Lee KS, Zabramski JM, Hargraves RW (Barrow Neurological Inst, Phoenix, Ariz)
J Neurosurg 75:32–39, 1991   23–25

Background.—Cavernous malformations of the brain stem apparently can be distinguished by their unique clinical presentation and course af-

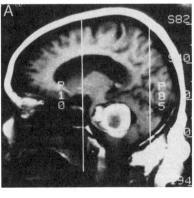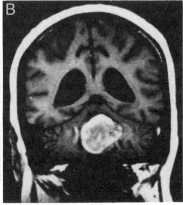

Fig 23–7.—A, sagittal T1-weighted MRI showing massive hemorrhage from a pontine cavernous malformation of the brain stem. Note expansion of floor of the fourth ventricle by the hematoma, but no hemorrhage disrupting the pial surface to enter the fourth ventricle. **B,** coronal T1-weighted MRI showing the massive hematoma causing obstructive hydrocephalus. (Courtesy of Zimmerman RS, Spetzler RF, Lee KS, et al: *J Neurosurg* 75:32–39, 1991.)

ter they have produced a neurologic deficit. The treatment and outcome of a group of patients with symptomatic cavernous malformations of the brain stem were analyzed.

Methods.—Twenty-four patients with long-tract and/or cranial nerve findings from their cavernous malformations of the brain stem were treated either surgically or conservatively. The decision to operate was based on the patient's neurologic status, the proximity of the malformation to the pial surface of the brain stem, and the number of symptomatic episodes.

Outcomes.—Of the 16 patients who underwent definitive surgery directed at malformation excision, associated venous malformations influenced the surgical approach in 4. The recognition of these associated malformations enabled the surgeons to avoid inappropriate excision. Some of the 16 patients had transient, immediate, postoperative worsening of their neurologic deficits. However, in all but 1 patient, the outcome was the same or improved. One patient had recurrent symptoms. In this case, a new deficit occurring $2\frac{1}{2}$ years later required reoperation after cavernous malformation regrowth. One patient died 6 months after surgery of a shunt infection and sepsis. Of the 8 patients treated conservatively, 7 had minor intermittent or no symptoms. The eighth patient died of a hemorrhage 1 year after initial presentation. Conservative treatment consisted of annual MRI studies (Fig 23-7).

Conclusion.—Surgical extirpation of symptomatic cavernous malformations of the brain stems seems to be the treatment of choice in symptomatic patients when the lesion is superficially located and an operative approach can spare eloquent tissue. When these malformations can be excised completely, the cure appears to be permanent.

▶ This communication regarding 24 patients with brain stem cavernous malformations and negative angiography provides some interesting lessons. Sixteen cases were treated by definitive surgical excision, avoiding removal of an associated venous malformation in 4 patients. Of the 16 patients, only 1 had a lasting postoperative increase in deficit. Only 1 patient had recurrent symptoms that required reoperation. One patient died of shunt sepsis 6 months after surgery. All the other patients were stable after excision of their lesions.

Note that, in this group of symptomatic brain stem cavernous angiomas, surgical excision was able to accomplish cure in all but one, with an acceptable low morbidity. For patients with deep cavernous angiomas that do not come to the surface, conservative management seems appropriate in the absence of symptoms. When there is progressive symptomatology, however, one may consider surgery in this group as well.—R.M. Crowell, M.D.

Other

The Natural History of Intracranial Venous Angiomas

Garner TB, Curling OD Jr, Kelly DL Jr, Laster DW (Wake Forest Univ, Winston-Salem, NC)
J Neurosurg 75:715–722, 1991   23–26

Introduction.—Venous angiomas are among the most common intracranial vascular malformations. It is widely believed that these congenital anomalies carry a high risk of bleeding and neurologic dysfunction, but recent imaging studies suggest that many venous angiomas are asymptomatic.

Series.—The findings were reviewed for 100 patients with radiographically identified intracranial venous angiomas who were treated in a 14-year period. Frontal angiomas occurred most frequently and the parietal region and cerebellum were the next most common sites of involvement. Eighteen patients had significant intracranial lesions other than the venous angioma.

Course.—Headache was a common presenting feature. Eight patients had a transient focal deficit, 5 had seizures, and 1 had hemorrhage. Fifteen patients remained free of neurologic signs and symptoms. None of the patients have undergone surgery. The mean time from diagnosis to last follow-up was $2^{1}/_{2}$ years.

Diagnosis.—Dilated medullary veins are found converging on a large central vein in the late venous phase of angiography. Contrast CT shows a linear enhancing density entering the deep venous system, a major dural sinus, or a cortical vein. Magnetic resonance imaging demonstrated a tubular area of reduced signal intensity in the white matter on T1-weighted images, and a hypointense or hyperintense signal on T2-weighted images.

Conclusion.—The occurrence of venous infarction after removal of a venous angioma supports a role for venous drainage in these malformations. Significant complications are infrequent. Resection of these lesions is rarely indicated.

▶ This important study, emanating from Bowman Gray College of Medicine at Wake Forest University, focuses on patients with intracranial venous angioma diagnosed by angiography, CT, and MRI. A total of 100 patients were studied. Headache was common, seizures and focal deficits were occasional, and hemorrhage was rare (1 in 100 cases). Careful study of the patient with the hemorrhage indicates only a venous angioma on angiography, CT, and MRI, but it is possible that Figure 6 in the original article (panel D) may demonstrate an associated cavernous angioma. In all events, hemorrhage occurred extremely rarely (1 hemorrhage per 4,498 person-years of follow-up; .22%/year). Resection of venous angiomas has been associated with fatal venous infarction; therefore, the best treatment of venous angioma appears to be careful follow-up, with removal of hematomas in the extremely rare instance of intracerebral hemorrhage.

Other studies have suggested that when hemorrhage does occur in relation to venous angioma, an associated angioma is responsible. There is a body of literature indicating that venous angioma is better thought of as venous anomaly, a normal variant of venous anatomy.—R.M. Crowell, M.D.

Surgical Risk of Hemorrhage in Cerebral Amyloid Angiopathy
Matkovic Z, Davis S, Gonzales M, Kalnins R, Masters CL (Royal Melbourne Hosp; Univ of Melbourne; Austin Hosp, Melbourne)
Stroke 22:456–461 1991   23–27

Purpose.—Cerebral amyloid angiopathy (CAA) is recognized as a common cause of sporadic, recurrent, and multiple nontraumatic lobar intracerebral hemorrhages (ICH) in normotensive elderly patients. Neurosurgical intervention to evacuate intracerebral hematomas is hazardous, with a high risk of precipitated hemorrhage. To determine the risk of hemorrhage precipitated by neurosurgery, 16 patients were reviewed retrospectively.

Method.—A retrospective review of medical records identified 16 sporadic cases of histologically proven CAA. Fifteen neurosurgical procedures were performed in 8 patients for 8 clot evacuations, 3 abscess drainage procedures, 2 ventriculoperitoneal shunts, 1 biopsy, and 1 lobectomy. Eight nonoperated patients were controls.

Results.—Neurosurgical intervention was deemed to have precipitated further clinically significant bleeding in only 1 of 4 patients with recurrent postoperative cerebral hemorrhage. Recurrent hemorrhage occurred in 2 of the 8 nonoperated cases.

Conclusion.—Recurrent cerebral hemorrhage is characteristic of cerebral amyloid angiopathy, but neurosurgical intervention to evacuate intracerebral hematomas has been deemed hazardous. In this retrospective review of 16 cases, neurosurgical intervention precipitated hemorrhage in only 1 case. Neurosurgical intervention in cerebral amyloid angiopathy is not associated with a major risk of precipitated hemorrhage.

▶ This interesting communication suggests that surgery can be performed safely for hemorrhage from cerebral amyloid angiopathy. Sixteen overall cases and 8 surgical cases were presented, but hemorrhage was thought to be precipitated by surgery in only a single case. Another study from Iowa had a similar experience. It is worth noting that the original impression of adverse hemorrhagic effects from surgery in amyloid angiopathy was based on a very small number of patients. Finally, at present, it is reasonable to consider surgical treatment in these cases if progressive neurologic deficit warrants.—R.M. Crowell, M.D.

Nonaneurysmal Perimesencephalic Subarachnoid Hemorrhage: CT and MR Patterns That Differ From Aneurysmal Rupture

Rinkel GJE, Wijdicks EFM, Vermeulen M, Ramos LMP, Tanghe HLJ, Hasan D, Meiners LC, van Gijn J (Univ of Utrecht, The Netherlands; Univ of Rotterdam)
AJR 157:1325–1330, 1991   23–28

Background.—Patients with perimesencephalic hemorrhage and a normal angiogram should have an uncomplicated clinical course and an excellent prognosis. The clinical picture of these patients argues against an undetected aneurysm and contrasts with the aneurysmal type of subarachnoid hemorrhage. Whether imaging methods could be used to distinguish nonaneurysmal perimesencephalic hemorrhage from aneurysmal subarachnoid hemorrhage was investigated in 52 patients with a mean age of 53 years.

Methods.—All patients had signs and symptoms of subarachnoid hemorrhage, a normal 4-vessel angiogram, and a CT study performed within 72 hours of the first clinical symptoms that showed a subarachnoid hemorrhage located predominantly in the posterior portion of the basal cisterns. The results of these and additional CT scans were shown separately to 2 experienced neuroradiologists.

Results.—All patients had a sudden onset of headache and a normal level of consciousness at admission. Neurologic examinations were normal (WFNS grade 1), except for neck stiffness. The amount of cisternal blood varied considerably. Blood distribution in these patients was compared with the pattern charcteristic of patients with subarachnoid hemorrhage from a ruptured basilar artery aneurysm. The center of bleeding in the majority (87%) of patients was located immediately anterior to the midbrain and pons. In the remaining patients, bleeding extended from the interpeduncular cistern to the left ambient cistern. The only site of hemorrhage in 2 patients was a prepontine clot. Ten patients with a posterior hemorrhage were thought by observers to have an aneurysm when they did not.

Conclusion.—Examination of CT scans yielded excellent interobserver agreement and a high predictive value for the perimesencephalic pattern of hemorrhage. It is important for clinicians to recognize the pattern, for patients with this subset of subarachnoid hemorrhage have a favorable prognosis.

▶ These Dutch investigators describe studies of 52 patients with nonaneurysmal subarachnoid hemorrhage with normal angiography. A symmetric perimesencephalic pattern of blood was identified with extension to adjacent cisterns but absence of ventricular blood in 221 CT scans of patients with subarachnoid hemorrhage and negative angiography. The studies were reviewed by 2 neuroradiologists. Only 1 patient with a basilar aneurysm received an incorrect diagnosis of having the nonaneurysmal perimesencephalic pattern of hemorrhage based on CT.

I agree that cerebral angiography should be performed on patients with proven subarachnoid hemorrhage, because an occasional aneurysm could be missed, despite the apparent nonaneurysmal pattern of perimesencephalic blood.—R.M. Crowell, M.D.

Lobar Intracerebral Hemorrhage: A Clinical, Radiographic, and Pathological Study of 29 Consecutive Operated Cases With Negative Angiography
Wakai S, Kumakura N, Nagai M (Dokkyo Univ, Tochigi, Japan)
J Neurosurg 76:231–238, 1992   23–29

Background.—Lobar intracerebral hemorrhage (ICH) can be caused by vascular malformations, microaneurysms, cerebral amyloid angiopathy, and brain tumors. The treatment options for patients with small- or medium-sized hematomas and negative angiography are still debated, primarily because no one has identified the definitive clinicoradiographic features that indicate its underlying cause. The findings of a clinical, radiographic, and pathologic study of operated patients with negative angiography were examined.

Methods.—Fifty patients with lobar ICH underwent surgery between 1986 and 1990. The correlations between the underlying causes and the clinicoradiographic features were studied in 15 male and 14 female patients, aged 7–76 years, with no angiographic vascular abnormalities.

Findings.—The histologic diagnosis of the surgical specimens included vascular malformation in 9 patients, microaneurysm in 11, cerebral amyloid angiopathy in 6, and brain tumor in 2. The cause could not be verified histologically in 1 patient. The underlying cause was established in 96.5% of the patients. The mean patient age was lowest among those with cavernous malformations, at 27 years. The mean age for those with arteriovenous malformation (AVM) was 45.8 years; with microaneurysm, 59.8 years; and with cerebral amyloid angiopathy, 70 years. Four patients with vascular malformation had had previous bleeding episodes at the same site. None of those with microaneurysms or cerebral amyloid angiopathy had such episodes. Computed tomography (CT) showed a round or oval hematoma related to the presence of an AVM or cavernous malformation in contrast to microaneurysms and cerebral amyloid angiopathy. On contrast material infusion, variable enhancement was seen in 5 of the 9 vascular malformations, whereas no enhancement was seen in patients with microaneurysm or cerebral amyloid angiopathy at the acute state. Subarachnoid extension of the hematoma was related to cerebral amyloid angiopathy significantly more often than it was related to AVMs and microaneurysms (Fig 23–8).

Conclusion.—Patients with vascular malformation, microaneurysm, and cerebral amyloid angiopathy and negative angiography have very different clinicoradiographic pictures. The underlying cause of a given lobar ICH with negative angiography may be predicted by a combination of

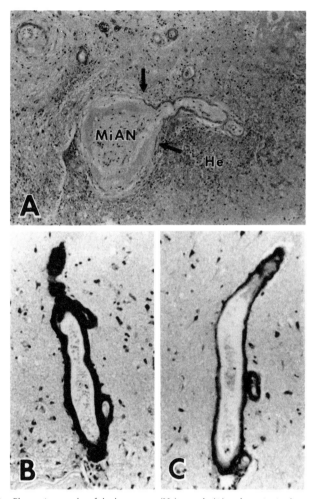

Fig 23–8.—Photomicrographs of the hematoma (*He*) capsule (**A**) and arteries in the cortex overlying the hematoma (**B** and **C**) removed from a 72-year-old woman 14 days after hemorrhage. **A,** a microaneurysm (*MiAN*) about 500 μ in diameter is seen in the center of the figure. The wall of the parent artery is strongly positive for Congo red stain, but the wall at its orifice to the microaneurysm (*arrows*) has lost its ability to stain. Congo red, × 50. **B** and **C,** photomicrographs of specimens that have been incubated for monoclonal antibodies against β-protein (**B**) and cystatin (**C**). The arterial wall contains dense reaction products to both. Peroxidase-antiperoxidase method for amyloid proteins, × 160. (Courtesy of Wakai S, Kumakura N, Nagai M: *J Neurosurg* 76:231–238, 1992.)

patient age, history of bleeding at the same site, hematoma shape, and subarachnoid extension of the hematoma on CT scans.

▶ This important and careful study indicates that meticulous radiologic search and microsurgical evaluation of intracerebral hemorrhage, combined with meticulous histopathologic evaluation, can identify the cause of bleeding in many of these cases, despite negative angiography. The authors have found the underlying cause of bleeding in more than 90% of the patients. On the basis of this experience, they firmly urge surgical excision of oval hematomas suggesting AVM in accessible locations. Elderly patients with dementia and suspicion of amyloid angiopathy are not recommended for routine evacuation.—R.M. Crowell, M.D.

24 Trauma

Traumatic Brain Injuries: Predictive Usefulness of CT
Kido DK, Cox C, Hamill RW, Rothenberg BM, Woolf PD (Univ of Rochester, NY)
Radiology 182:777–781, 1992   24–1

Background.—The initial assessment of patients with acute head trauma routinely involves emergency imaging studies to determine whether a surgically correctable lesion is present. Computed tomographic (CT) scans from 72 patients with traumatic brain injury were analyzed to determine whether a specific type, location, or size of lesion is associated with changes in neurologic function and other parameters.

Methods.—The Glasgow Coma Scale (GCS) was used to assess neurologic function, and the Glasgow Outcome Scale (GOS) was used to determine patient outcome. The catecholamine levels were also examined, and lesions were categorized as focal or diffuse.

Findings.—In 48 patients with focal hemorrhage, GOS changed as a function of lesion size, regardless of whether the lesions were intra- or extra-axial. Those patients with lesions greater than 4,100 mm³) had a twofold higher risk of poor outcomes than those with smaller lesions. Patients with normal CT studies were significantly more likely to have mild or no neurologic dysfunction than those with abnormal scans. Lesion location, skull fracture, and pineal shift did not significantly predict GCS or GOS scores. Lesion size was positively related to both plasma norepinephrine and epinephrine levels. There also was a significant relationship between lesion size and GCS score.

Conclusion.—These findings support and extend previous observations that suggest that CT scans may provide important prognostic data on neurologic status and outcome in victims of head trauma. A clear relationship was found between the amount of intra- or extra-axial bleeding and outcomes.

▶ This interesting study shows a clear-cut correlation of the GCS and GOS after head injury with CT lesion size. The study team, which did not include a neurosurgeon, did not investigate further features known to be of value as predictors, such as increased intracranial pressure and hypotension. It seems likely that quantitative CT features such as lesion size, when coupled with other predictors such as GCS, increased intracranial pressure. It also seems likely that hypotension may be helpful in improving the ability to predict outcome after a traumatic brain injury.—R.M. Crowell, M.D.

Continuous Monitoring of Jugular Venous Oxygen Saturation in Head-Injured Patients

Sheinberg M, Kanter MJ, Robertson CS, Contant CF, Narayan RK, Grossman RG (Baylor College of Medicine, Houston)

J Neurosurg 76:212–217, 1992   24–2

Purpose.—Research has established the adverse effects of cerebral ischemia and hypoxia superimposed on severe head injury. A sensitive clinical method of detecting cerebral ischemia is needed to identify decreased cerebral oxygen delivery before neurologic injury occurs. Continuous measurement of jugular venous oxygen saturation ($SjvO_2$) was evaluated for this purpose.

Methods.—A total of 45 patients with severe head injury were studied. The average patient age was 31 years, with most patients having closed head injuries. All were admitted in coma. The patients underwent continuous and simultaneous monitoring of $SjvO_2$ by fiberoptic catheter, as well as monitoring of intracranial pressure, arterial oxygen saturation, and end-tidal CO_2. In addition, cerebral blood flow, cerebral oxygen and lactate metabolic rates, arterial and jugular venous blood gas levels, and hemoglobin were measured every 8 hours. A standard protocol was used to confirm desaturation and identify the cause whenever $SjvO_2$ decreased to less than 50%.

Results.—After in vivo calibration with adequate light intensity at the catheter tip, there was excellent correlation of $SjvO_2$ values obtained in 2 ways—through the catheter and through direct measurement of O_2 saturation by a co-oximeter or venous blood drawn through the catheter. The patients had 60 episodes of jugular venous oxygen desaturation, confirmed by the co-oximeter in 20 patients. This group had 33 episodes of desaturation,m which resulted from intracranial hypertension in 12 cases, hypocarbia in 10, arterial hypoxia in 6, combinations of these in 3, and systemic hypotension and cerebral vasospasm in 1 each.

Conclusion.—In patients with head injury, continuous $SjvO_2$ measurement appears to have clinical value. Episodes of jugular venous oxygen desaturation appear to be common in severely head-injured patients, even with intensive care and advanced cardiovascular and intracranial monitoring.

▶ This study describes experience with fiberoptic measurement of venous oxygen saturation in 45 patients. The patients with desaturation of jugular venous blood showed a higher mortality. Frequent changes in jugular venous O_2 were noted, some as a result of artifact, possibly with movement of the catheter tip.

Fiberoptic catheter measurement of jugular venous O_2 is a promising method for the monitoring of critically ill neurosurgical patients; however, the techniques require modification to avoid artifacts.—R.M. Crowell, M.D.

Serial Multimodality-Evoked Potentials in Severely Head-Injured Patients: Diagnostic and Prognostic Implications

Barelli A, Valente MR, Clemente A, Bozza P, Proietti R, Della Corte F (Catholic Univ School of Medicine Hosp, Rome)

Crit Care Med 19:1374–1381, 1991   24–3

Purpose.—In patients with head injury, it is difficult to evaluate functional abnormalities by neuroimaging modalities. Clinical neurologic examination is more useful, except in patients who are comatose, sedated, or paralyzed. The prognostic reliability of multimodality-evoked potentials, including their diagnostic usefulness and limitations were evaluated.

Patients and Procedure.—A total of 73 patients with severe head injury were studied. They ranged in age from 10 to 75 years. All had a Glasgow Coma Score of 8 or less, and the average delay before assessment was 6 hours. Beginning 24 hours after admission and for 21 days thereafter, the brain stem auditory-evoked and somatosensory-evoked potentials were recorded. These findings were compared with the patients' clinical outcomes.

Findings.—Single recordings were accurate in predicting a poor outcome only when brain stem auditory-evoked potentials were severely abnormal. Serial brain stem auditory-evoked and simultaneous brain stem auditory-evoked and somatosensory-evoked potentials were accurate in predicting a favorable outcome. All patients who had grade 1 for both potentials survived. Brain stem reflexes and pupil asymmetries showed good correlation with brain stem auditory-evoked potentials, but Glasgow Coma Scores did not.

Conclusion.—Serial multimodality-evoked potentials appear to be the best prognostic tool for patients with severe head injury. Brain stem auditory-evoked potentials may be able to dected brain stem compression before pupil abnormalities develop and to monitor brain stem function in patients receiving high doses of barbiturates. Peripheral acoustic damage, electromagnetic artifacts in the intensive care unit, and use of ototoxic drugs limit the usefulness of these techniques.

▶ This study offers further data supporting the notion that multimodality-evoked potentials in severely head-injured patients can offer some diagnostic and prognostic benefit. Specifically, serial brain stem auditory-evoked potentials and somatosensory-evoked potentials offer a good prognostic index for a favorable outcome. This is particularly useful in cases in which barbiturate coma has been used. The physician should be aware of problems secondary to peripheral acoustic damage, electromagnetic sources of artifact, and the effects of ototoxic drugs.—R.M. Crowell, M.D.

Impact of ICP Instability and Hypotension on Outcome in Patients With Severe Head Trauma

Marmarou A, Anderson RL, Ward JD, Choi SC, Young HF, Eisenberg HM, Foulkes MA, Marshall LF, Jane JA (Med College of Virginia, Richmond; Univ of Texas, Galveston; Natl Inst of Neurological Disorders and Stroke, Bethesda, Md; Univ of California, San Diego)

J Neurosurg 75:S59–S66, 1991   24–4

Background.—The putative effect of increased intracranial pressure (ICP) and ischemia on outcomes in patients with severe head trauma is difficult to measure directly, because many other factors are involved. The relationship between increased ICP, hypotension, and outcome in such patients was further explored.

Methods.—The data were derived from the Traumatic Coma Data Bank, from which the ICP records of 1,030 patients were available. A total of 428 patients met minimum monitoring duration criteria for study inclusion. The outcomes were determined by Glasgow Outcome Scale scores 6 months after injury. One hundred eighty-seven candidate summary descriptors were considered. The subset of descriptors that best explained 6-month outcome was chosen by a stepwise ordinal logistic regression model.

Findings.—Age, admission motor score, and abnormal pupils were each highly significant in accounting for outcomes. The proportion of hourly ICP readings higher than 20 mm Hg was selected next, and it was also highly significant. A cutoff point of 20 mm Hg was selected next and was also highly significant. A cut off point of 20 mm Hg was selected (in addition to the ICP factor) as being most indicative of outcome. The next factor chosen was the proportion of hourly blood pressure readings less than 80 mm Hg. This was also a highly significant outcome indicator. The blood pressure cutoff of 80 mm Hg was chosen as best indicating outcomes.

Conclusion.—Mortality and morbidity from severe head trauma are strongly related to increased ICP and hypotension as measured during ICP management. These factors are better indicators of outcome than central perfusion pressure or treatment intensity.

▶ These important data from the Traumatic Coma Data Bank demonstrate that mortality and morbidity after severe head injury are strongly related to increased ICP and hypotension. These data provide strong support for the routine use of ICP and blood pressure monitoring and control for patients with severe head injury.—R.M. Crowell, M.D.

Effect of Head Elevation on Intracranial Pressure, Cerebral Perfusion Pressure, and Cerebral Blood Flow in Head-Injured Patients

Feldman Z, Kanter MJ, Robertson CS, Contant CF, Hayes C, Sheinberg MA,

Villareal CA, Narayan RK, Grossman RG (Baylor College of Medicine, Houston)
J Neurosurg 76:207–211, 1992   24–5

Background.—It is common to elevate the head of the bed for patients with increased intracranial pressure (ICP), but the cerebral perfusion pressure (CPP) also may decrease. Maintenance of adequate cerebral blood flow (CBF) is the chief reason for maintaining the CPP in patients with increased ICP.

Methods.—The effects of a horizontal position and 30-degree head evaluation were examined in 22 head-injured patients with a mean age of 35 years. The most common diagnoses were subdural hematoma and cerebral contusion. The Glasgow Coma Scale after resuscitation ranged from 3 to 12. Cerebral blood flow was measured by the nitrous oxide technique.

Findings.—The mean carotid artery pressure was significantly lower with the head elevated, as was the mean ICP (14 mm Hg vs. 20 mm Hg). There were no significant positional differences in CPP, CBF, cerebral metabolic rate of oxygen, arteriovenous lactate difference, or cerebrovascular resistance.

Implication.—Elevating the head to 30 degrees seems to lower ICP in most head-injured patients, without simultaneously reducing CPP or CBF. It remains possible that regional CBFs decrease in the presence of normal global flow values.

▶ This detailed physiologic study provides clear evidence that elevation of the head to 30 degrees significantly reduces the ICP in head-injured patients without reducing cerebral blood flow or perfusion. This study provides worthwhile confirmation of a useful maneuver in the intensive care unit; however, this information does not obviate the need for careful monitoring of patients after head injury, as regards physiologic parameters including intracranial pressure.—R.M. Crowell, M.D.

Adverse Effects of Prolonged Hyperventilation in Patients With Severe Head Injury: A Randomized Clinical Trial

Muizelaar JP, Marmarou A, Ward JD, Kontos HA, Choi SC, Becker DP, Gruemer H, Young HF (Med College of Virginia, Richmond)
J Neurosurg 75:731–739, 1991   24–6

Introduction.—Many physicians recommend hyperventilation to reduce the $PaCO_2$ in patients with traumatic coma, but considerable debate continues regarding whether it is helpful to induce controlled hyperventilation in this setting. Theoretically, hyperventilation can help control intracranial pressure and reverse CSF acidosis, but the consequent cerebral vasoconstriction may induce ischemia. In addition, the effect on the pH of CSF may be transitory, but this might be overcome by administering the buffer tromethamine (THAM).

Methods.—A total of 113 patients (age, 3 years or older) with severe closed head injury were enrolled in a study comparing hyperventilation, both alone and with THAM, to normal ventilation. The patients had a Glasgow Coma Scale score of 8 or less after aggressive resuscitation and treatment of acute mass lesions. Hyperventilation was intended to decrease the $PaCO_2$ to 25 mm Hg. The dose of THAM was based on the amount needed to increase the arterial pH to 7.6.

Results.—Good outcomes 3 and 6 months after injury for patients with motor score of 4 or 5 were significantly fewer in hyperventilated patients than in either the control or hyperventilation/THAM groups; however, no such difference was evident 1 year after injury. Hyperventilation alone did not sustain alkalinization of the CSF, but THAM treatment did. Cerebral ischemia did not occur in any group. The mean intracranial pressure remained well below 25 mm Hg in all groups, but pressure was most stable in the patients who were hyperventilated and given THAM.

Conclusion.—If sustained hyperventilation is necessary to control intracranial pressure in a head-injured patient, then administration of THAM may be beneficial.

▶ This extremely important study from the University of Virginia regards hyperventilation in patients with severe head injury. Although it is complex in its design and execution, the study clearly demonstrates a deleterious effect from hyperventilation in head-injured patients with motor scores of 4–5. While confirmation from other investigators is awaited, hyperventilation in this group of patients probably should be avoided.

Secondary observations are improvements of intracranial pressure stabilization in the group treated with hyperventilation and THAM buffer. Hyperventilation does not sustain alkalinization in the CSF, although THAM can.—R.M. Crowell, M.D.

Treatment of Postconcussional Symptoms With CDP-Choline
Levin HS (Univ of Texas, Galveston)
J Neurol Sci 103:S39–S42, 1991   24–7

Background.—A few case studies in the literature suggest that using precursors of cytidine diphosphoryl (CDP)-choline may be helpful in facilitating recovery from mild-to-moderate head injury. However, these were not placebo-controlled or double-blinded studies, the effects of CDP-choline in head-injured patients were further explored.

Methods.—Fourteen young men were enrolled in the preliminary, double-blind placebo-controlled trial. The patients had been admitted to the neurosurgery service after having mild-to-moderate closed head inju-

	Neuropsychological Findings at Baseline (BL) and Follow-Up (FU)					
	CDP-choline			Placebo		
	BL	FU	% Change	BL	FU	% Change
Memory						
Recall of words	76	111	147	117	106	8
Recall of locations	67	94	40	95	95	−1
Recall of designs	25	38	104 *	40	45	29 *
Fluency						
Verbal (words)	22	41	8	35	37	13
Designs-free	18	16	−9	13	20	25
Designs-fixed	14	11 *	0	13	19 *	77
Attention						
CPT (msec)	1527	1225	−9	1444	1108	−15
PASAT (correct/time)	0.315	0.344	25	0.398	0.479	27

*P < .05.
(Courtesy of Levin HS: *J Neurol Sci* 103:S39–S42, 1991.)

ries. They were randomly assigned to receive orally administered CDP-choline or placebo. The groups were matched for age, education, and severity of impaired consciousness. The baseline and 1-month examinations consisted of neuropsychological tests and a structured postconcussional symptoms interview.

Findings.—According to the Wilcoxon test, CDP-choline resulted in a greater reduction of postconcussional symptoms than placebo. Analysis of the neuropsychological findings showed a significantly greater improvement in recognition memory for designs in the CDP-choline-treated patients. Other changes in test performance did not differ between the groups (table).

Conclusion.—Cytidine diphosphoryl-choline may be useful in the treatment of sequelae of mild-to-moderate closed head injuries. Larger trials are now needed.

▶ This interesting study suggests that CDP-choline may be effective in treating sequelae of mild-to-moderate closed head injury. Further results are needed.—R.M. Crowell, M.D.

Prognosis in Contre-Coup Intracranial Haematomas—A Clinical and Radiological Study of 63 Patients

Jayakumar PN, Sastry Kolluri VR, Basavakumar DG, Subbakrishna DK, Arya BYT, Das BS, Narayana Reddy GN (Natl Inst of Mental Health and Neuro Sciences, Bangalore, India)
Acta Neurochir (Wien) 108:30–33, 1991   24–8

Objective.—The clinical features and CT scans of 63 patients (11–80 years of age) with contrecoup intracranial hematoma were analyzed to define the prognosis.

Patients.—Forty-four patients had pure contrecoup hemorrhage, and 19 had associated coup hematomas. The frontal and temporal regions were the common sites of contrecoup hematoma.

Results.—The overall mortality rate was 53%. The mortality rate in patients with contrecoup hemorrhage alone was 40%, which was significantly lower than the rate in patients with associated coup hematomas (80%). However, the mortality rates were higher in patients with contrecoup hematomas in the frontal and temporal regions, and in those with hematomas with maximum linear dimension of 4 cm or more. Poor outcome was also associated with advanced age of the patients. Glasgow Coma Score ≤ 8 on admission, severe degree of midline shift, and obliteration of the basal cisterns.

Conclusion.—The adverse prognosis of contrecoup head injury is further worsened in the presence of associated coup injury. Other prognostic factors include age, GCS on admission, and CT findings such as location and size of the contrecoup injury, cisternal obliteration, and degree of shift of midline structures.

▶ This study has a remarkably high rate of overall mortality (80% for coup hematoma and 40% for contrecoup hemorrhage alone). It is interesting that the contrecoup lesion alone had the lower mortality.—R.M. Crowell, M.D.

The Relationship Between Intelligence and Memory Following Minor or Mild Closed Head Injury: Greater Impairment in Memory Than Intelligence

Hall S, Bornstein RA (Ohio State Univ, Columbus)
J Neurosurg 75:378–381, 1991   24–9

Background.—Both intellectual ability and memory function are impaired after closed head injury, but the relationship between these deficits remain unclear. It has proved difficult to make direct comparisons between scores on measures of intellect and of memory, but the Wechsler Memory Scale-Revised (WMS-R) makes such comparisons possible.

Study Design.—Twenty-two patients with closed head injury were matched with normal individuals for age, gender, and educational level. The patients were studied for a mean of 13 months after injury. Both the WMS-R and the Wechsler Adult Intelligence Scale-Revised (WAIS-R) were administered.

Findings.—The control individuals had significantly higher scores than the head-injured patients on all WAIS-R and WMS-R indices. The patients had greater impairment in delayed memory relative to intellectual performance than did the control individuals, regardless of the interval between injury and assessment.

Implications.—Memory is evidently affected more than intellectual function is in patients with less severe closed head injury, as well as in those with marked injury. None of the patients had retrograde amnesia for longer than 24 hours. It remains to be learned whether the disproportionate memory deficit persists.

▶ This contribution provides detailed studies of intelligence and memory after minor closed head injury. The main finding is that the deficit in head injury is greater in the sphere of memory than in that of intelligence. It would be of value to know the extent of the head injury as indicated by the Glasgow Coma Scale at the outset and the eventual Glasgow Outcome Scale. Correlation with MRI findings also would be valuable, in that the head injuries might have preferentially damaged areas affiliated with memory. Nonetheless, the findings are of value to those who deal with patients with minor head injury.—R.M. Crowell, M.D.

Vegetative State After Closed-Head Injury: A Traumatic Coma Data Bank Report

Levin HS, Saydjari C, Eisenberg HM, Foulkes M, Marshall LF, Ruff RM, Jane JA, Marmarou A (Univ of Texas, Galveston; Natl Insts of Health, Bethesda, Md; Univ of California, San Diego; Univ of Virginia, Charlottesville; Med College of Virginia, Richmond)
Arch Neurol 48:580–585, 1991   24–10

Background.—Few recent studies have addressed the persistent vegetative state (PVS), especially in patients with head injury. The clinical course of the vegetative state after severe closed head injury was studied.

Methods.—The Traumatic Coma Data Bank was consulted to determine the outcomes both at the time of discharge from the hospital and at follow-up as long as 3 years after injury. A total of 650 patients with closed head injuries were available for the analysis. Ninety-three, or 14%, were discharged in a vegetative state. These patients were compared with those discharged in a conscious state.

Findings.—Patients in a vegetative state sustained more severe closed-head injuries, as reflected by the Glasgow Coma Scale scores, than did the conscious patients. Patients in a vegetative state also had diffuse injury complicated by swelling or shift in midline structures more frequently than did conscious patients. Of 84 patients in a vegetative state for whom follow-up data were available, 41% became conscious by 6 months, 52% regained consciousness by 1 year, and 58% regained consciousness by 3 years. No predictors of recovery could be identified in a logistic regression analysis.

Conclusion.—These and previous longitudinal findings suggest that recovery from PVS is most likely to occur in the first year after injury. More than half the patients in this study regained consciousness by 1 year. A physiologic measure (e.g., the regional cerebral metabolic rate for glucose and cerebral blood flow) may be more useful in predicting vegetative state outcome.

▶ This remarkable study shows that nearly half the patients discharged in a vegetative state after closed head injury will eventually regain consciousness in the first year. This fact and the lack of effective predictors of outcome demand an aggressive treatment program, especially in the young.—R.M. Crowell, M.D.

Plateau-Wave Phenomenon (II): Occurrence of Brain Herniation in Patients With and Without Plateau Waves

Hayashi M, Kobayashi H, Handa Y, Kawano H, Hirose S, Ishii H (Fukui Med School, Fukui, Japan)
Brain 114:2693–2699, 1991   24–11

Background.—Brain herniation is the most serious complication in patients with intracranial hypertension. The occurrence of brain herniation was studied in patients with and without plateau waves in continuous intracranial pressure recordings.

Methods.—Brain herniation developed in 15 patients from 1980 to 1989 as a result of aneurysmal rebleeding, uncontrollable brain swelling, and/or edema despite attempts to treat increased intracranial pressure (ICP). The relationship between the ICP level at which herniation occurred and the ICP fluctuation patterns in continuous recordings made before herniation developed was analyzed. The patients were assigned to 2 groups on the basis of the presence or absence of plateau wave of Lundberg: in group 1, 8 patients had no plateau wave and a high ICP, and in group 2, 7 patients had both plateau waves and a high ICP.

Observations.—Herniation resulted from aneurysmal rebleeding or brain swelling after subarachnoid hemorrhage in group 1 patients. In group 2 patients, herniation resulted from brain tumor, meningitis carcinomatosa, and superior sagittal sinus thrombosis. In group 1, herniation developed at a mean ICP of 70–98 mm Hg. In group 2, it occurred at a mean level of 120–150 mm Hg.

Conclusion.—Patients with a plateau-wave phenomenon in continuous ICP recordings have a marked impairment of CSF absorption and a delayed CSF flow. In this series, group 2 patients may have had an impairment of CSF absorption and very sluggish CSF flow, a condition producing a large accumulation of CSF in the cranial or spinal canal cavities. This may create a critically taut condition in which pressure gradients can no longer be permitted in these cavities and can act as a defense mechanism against the herniation, despite markedly increased ICP.

▶ This clever study presents data clearly indicating that patients with plateau waves of Lundberg herniate at a lower mean ICP (70–98 mm Hg) compared with patients without plateau waves (120–150 mm Hg). Interestingly, all the patients with the plateau waves had subarachnoid hemorrhage, and those without plateau waves had brain tumor or other intracranial pathology. The authors' suggestion that the difference is related to an abnormality of CSF physiology in the former group seems reasonable because subarachnoid hemorrhage often causes such abnormalities. The observation also suggests that ventricular drainage might be helpful in the patients with plateau waves.—R.M. Crowell, M.D.

25 Spine

Lumbar

Lumbar Disc Surgery: Results of the Prospective Lumbar Discectomy Study of the Joint Section on Disorders of the Spine and Peripheral Nerves of the American Association of Neurological Surgeons and the Congress of Neurological Surgeons
Abramovitz JN, Neff SR (New England Med Ctr, Boston, Mass)
Neurosurgery 29:301–308, 1991   25–1

Introduction.—Most studies of the results of lumbar disk surgery come from a single center using a small number of patients. This prospective, multiphysician, multicenter consecutive-patient study evaluates current indications for and applications of lumbar disk surgery.

Methods.—Of the 840 patients enrolled who had undergone lumbar disk surgery, 533 were available for 3-month follow-up, and 450 were available for 12-month follow-up. The factors that were predictive of outcome were assessed, and unsatisfactory outcomes were analyzed.

Results.—The independent predictors of good surgical outcome included reflex asymmetry, absence of back pain on straight leg-raise exam, correspondence of leg pain to typical radicular patterns, and leg pain on straight leg-raise exam. Within subgroups, use of the operating microscope, sensory deficit, central disk bulge, and free disk fragment were correlated with outcome. An increased risk of radicular failure was associated with preoperative motor deficit, and an increased likelihood of mechanical back pain failure was associated with facetectomy and preoperative sensory deficit. Age, motor deficit, and obesity were not associated with outcome.

Discussion.—The predictive value of collected clinical data was assessed by nonparametric, multivariate techniques. The study results support currently used clinical practice and generally accepted indications for lumbar disk surgery.

▶ The data firmly support the contention that patients with unremitting radiculopathy do better after discectomy than those with back pain. Abnormal sensory findings and radiologic evidence suggesting a free-fragment were associated with an increased likelihood of good outcome. Those patients with less evidence of root compression and only a radiological "bulge" tended to have less satisfactory outcomes.

As a surgical response to such procedures as chemonucleolysis and percutaneous discectomy, this study provides a useful confirmation that the results are generally excellent with surgery when the proper selection criteria and approach are used.—R.M. Crowell, M.D.

The Outcome of Decompressive Laminectomy for Degenerative Lumbar Stenosis

Katz JN, Lipson SJ, Larson MG, McInnes JM, Fossel AH, Liang MH (Brigham and Women's Hosp, Boston; Robert B Brigham Multipurpose Arthritis Ctr; Harvard Univ, Boston)
J Bone Joint Surg 73A:809–816, 1991   25–2

Introduction.—Many patients with degenerative lumbar stenosis will not respond to conservative treatment and are candidates for decompressive laminectomy, with or without arthrodesis. Despite the frequency of laminectomies for lumbar stenosis, little data are available on the indications for the procedure or its long-term outcome. These questions were addressed in a study of 88 patients, 8 of whom had a concomitant arthrodesis.

Methods.—The patients were treated between 1983 and 1986. Subjects younger than 55 years of age were excluded to rule out congenital or developmental causes of lumbar stenosis, and those patients who had previously undergone laminectomy and/or spinal arthrodesis for spinal stenosis also were excluded. The mean patient age at the time of the operation was 69.3 years. The variables examined at baseline and postoperatively included pain, walking ability, and co-morbid illnesses.

Results.—Seventy patients who were available for outcome analysis were followed up for a median of 4.2 years. Of the original 88 patients, 8 had undergone a repeat operation, 5 in the first postoperative year. Of the 70 patients who completed questionnaires in 1989, 21 had very severe or severe pain, 32 were unable to walk at least 2 blocks, and 15 could not walk a distance of 50 feet. However, almost half the patients (48%) reported being very satisfied with the results of laminectomy. The predictors of poor outcome were the co-morbidity score, the duration of follow-up, and an initial laminectomy involving a single interspace.

Conclusion.—The therapeutic benefits of laminectomy for degenerative lumbar stenosis tend to deteriorate with time. The operation appears to be most successful in patients without substantial co-morbidity, such as cardiovascular disease and/or arthritic conditions.

▶ Decompressive laminectomy has long been thought to be a highly effective treatment for degenerative lumbar stenosis (1). This communication from an orthopedic group provides information on 88 patients who underwent surgery between 1982 and 1986. By 1989, 17% of the patients had reparation and 30% had severe pain. The authors noted a variety of factors associated with long-term poor results, including co-existing illnesses and initial laminectomy limited to one interspace.

The results are somewhat surprising. Other factors that could play a role include a lack of quantitative data regarding radiographic criteria for operation, technique of surgical decompression, and use of postoperative radiographic confirmation of adequacy of decompression. Despite this study, wide laminectomy is indicated for patients with clinical and radiographic features of lumbar stenosis.—R.M. Crowell, M.D.

Reference

1. Weir B, DeLeo R: *J Neurol Sci* 8:295, 1981.

Failed Back Surgery Syndrome: 5-Year Follow-Up in 102 Patients Undergoing Repeated Operation
North RB, Campbell JN, James CS, Conover-Walker MK, Wang H, Piantadosi S, Rybock JD, Long DM (Johns Hopkins Univ, Baltimore, Md)
Neurosurgery 28:685–691, 1991   25–3

Background.—The indications for repeated surgery in patients with persistent or recurrent pain after lumbosacral spine operations have not been well delineated. There are few studies of the long-term results, and follow-up beyond 3 years has never been reported. A 5-year follow-up in a large patient series undergoing repeated operations was evaluated.

Methods.—A total of 102 patients with failed back surgery syndrome were studied. The patients had had an average of 2.4 previous operations. All underwent a repeated operation for lumbosacral decompression and/or stabilization. At a mean of 5 years after surgery, the patients were interviewed. Patient characteristics and treatment mode were assessed as predictors of long-term outcome.

Outcomes.—Of the patients, 34% had a successful outcome, which was defined as at least 50% sustained relief of pain for 2 years or at last follow-up, and patient satisfaction with the result. Twenty-one patients who were disabled before surgery were able to return to work after surgery; 15 who were working before surgery became disabled or retired after surgery. Overall, there were improvements in activities of daily living as often as there were decrements. The patients had loss of neurologic function more often than improvement. Most patients had either reduced or eliminated their intake of analgesic. According to a statistical analysis of patient characteristics as prognostic factors, young patients and women had significant advantages. Favorable outcome was also associated with a history of good results from previous surgery, the absence of epidural scar necessitating surgical lysis, preoperative employment, and predominance of radicular pain.

Conclusion.—The selection criteria for repeated surgery on the lumbosacral spine are in need of further refinement. Critical analysis of treatment outcome also needs to be improved. Alternative approaches to failed back surgery syndrome should be considered.

▶ This paper on failed back surgery syndrome indicates a dismal success for repeated operation. However, the study was not performed with the use of modern studies such as MRI, and this might have helped in terms of the selection of patients for surgical intervention. The major problem is the overwhelming number of people who are subjected to ill-advised surgery and other procedures leading to this syndrome. Most of the patients probably should never have had surgery in the first place. Moreover, secondary surgery will not be successful, except in the case of a retained disk fragment or recurrent extrusion. These can be identified by MRI with and without gadolinium.—R.M. Crowell, M.D.

Failed Back Surgery Syndrome: 5-Year Follow-Up After Spinal Cord Stimulator Implantation

North RB, Ewend MG, Lawton MT, Kidd DH, Piantadosi S (Johns Hopkins Univ, Baltimore, Md)
Neurosurgery 28:692–699, 1991   25–4

Background.—Spinal cord stimulation has been in use for more than 20 years. It has evolved into an easily implemented technique, with percutaneous methods for electrode placement. This technique for treating "failed back surgery syndrome" was studied.

Methods.—Fifty patients who had undergone an average of 3.1 previous operations were treated with spinal cord stimulator implantation. The patients were interviewed at mean follow-up intervals of 2.2 years and 5 years. Successful outcome was defined as at least 50% sustained pain relief and patient satisfaction with the result.

Outcomes.—A total of 53% of the patients had successful outcomes at 2.2 years, and 47% had successful outcomes at 5 years postoperatively. Ten of 40 patients who were disabled before treatment were able to return to work. Most of the patients had improvements in most activities of daily living. The loss of function was rare. Analgesic intake was reduced or eliminated in most cases. According to a statistical analysis of patient characteristics as prognostic factors, female patients and those with programmable multicontact implanted devices had significant advantages.

Conclusion.—These results in patients with postoperative lumbar arachnoid and epidural fibrosis without surgically remediable lesions compare well with results in 2 other series of patients with failed back surgery syndrome: 1 with diagnosed surgical lesions and repeated surgery done, and 1 with diagnosed monoradicular pain syndromes and dorsal root ganglionectomies done. There is a need for further evaluation of selection criteria, critical analysis of treatment outcome, and postoperative study of spinal cord stimulation and alternative approaches to failed back surgery syndrome.

▶ This report from a respected unit demonstrates an almost 50% successful outcome, as graded by the patients, at 2 years. This certainly is impressive in this difficult group of patients.—R.M. Crowell, M.D.

Percutaneous Posterolateral Lumbar Discectomy and Decompression With a 6.9-Millimeter Cannula: Analysis of Operative Failures and Complications

Schaffer JL, Kambin P (Univ of Pennsylvania, Philadelphia)
J Bone Joint Surg 73A:822–831, 1991   25–5

Introduction.—Protrusion of a lumbar disk with associated persistent radiculopathy can be treated by several operative means. Posterolateral diskectomy, accomplished through a 7-mm incision, spares patients the pain and morbidity of an open operative procedure and permits rapid rehabilitation. Whether percutaneous posterolateral diskectomy compares favorably with laminectomy in the rate of operative failures and complications was determined.

Methods.—The 100 patients who were eligible for posterolateral lumbar diskectomy had failed conservative treatment and had neurologic impairment and positive tension signs. The operative procedure was performed using local anesthesia, and it involved a sheath with an internal diameter of 4.9 mm. All patients were followed up for at least 2 years (Fig 25–1).

Results.—Four patients could not be located, and 3 had died during the follow-up period. The cause of death in these patients was unrelated to the diskectomy; all 3 were judged to have had excellent results at a minimum of 15 months postoperatively. Of the 93 patients available for review, 81 (83 herniated disks) had a successful result. There were no major complications or instances of postoperative neurologic or muscular deficits. Relief of pain was immediate in 61 patients; 71 patients returned to work. Eleven of the 12 failures underwent a subsequent laminectomy, which was successful in 8 cases. The causes of failure included lateral-recess stenosis and a history of multiple unsuccessful operations.

Conclusion.—The technique examined is effective and safe for treatment of a herniated disk in selected patients. Operative failures are few, and they can be improved by a subsequent laminectomy. Use of a modified arthroscopic instrument and intermittent uniportal diskscopic control are recommended.

▶ The authors report a 12% failure rate and a 3% transient morbidity in 100 patients treated with this novel technique. This is an interesting approach that has the advantage of a reduced amount of invasive treatment.

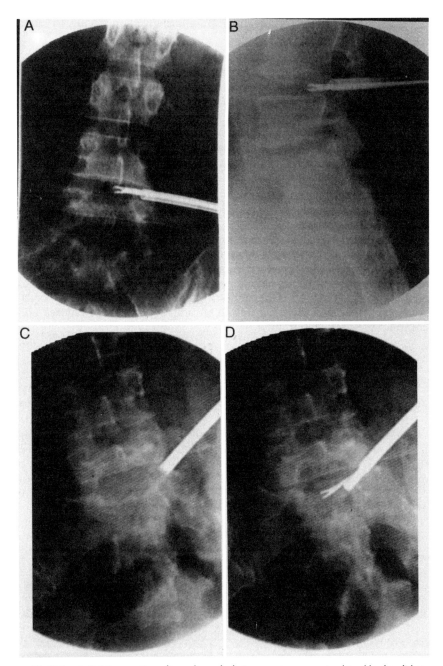

Fig 25–1.—A–D, intraoperative radiographs made during percutaneous posterolateral lumbar diskectomy and decompression. **A,** anteroposterior radiograph showing the 6.9-mm cannula and forceps in the disk space between the fourth and fifth lumbar vertebrae. **B,** corresponding lateral radiograph. **C,** the 6.9-mm cannula in the disk between the fifth lumbar and first sacral vertebrae. **D,** deflector tube and flexible forceps inserted into the disk space between the fifth lumbar and first sacral vertebrae. (Courtesy of Schaffer JL, Kambin P: *J Bone Joint Surg* 73A:822–831, 1991.)

On the other hand, surgeons who are familiar with disk surgery are understandably concerned about the possibility for inadequate disk removal or trauma to nearby neural elements.

The results appear to answer some of these concerns; however, the precise indications for surgery have not been provided. Likewise, the extent of pathology has not been indicated. In addition, one cannot judge the relative effectiveness and safety of the method as compared with standard discectomy—or even with automatic percutaneous disc removal as described by Onik. Further results will be needed before this novel treatment technique can be accepted.—R.M. Crowell, M.D.

Cauda Equina Syndrome Secondary to an Improperly Placed Nucleotome Probe
Onik G, Maroon JC, Jackson R (Allegheny Gen Hosp, Pittsburgh, Pa; St Paul Med Ctr, Dallas, Tex)
Neurosurgery 30:412–415, 1992   25–6

Introduction.—Experience in more than 3,300 cases has established that automated percutaneous lumbar diskectomy is effective and safe, but it remains possible that erroneous placement of the instrument within the thecal sac will cause serious damage.

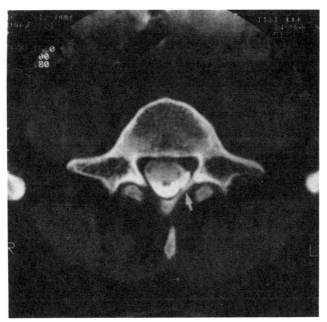

Fig 25-2.—CT scan at the L5-S1 level showing a pseudomeningocele on the left (*arrow*) with a paucity of nerve roots within the thecal sac. (Courtesy of Onik G, Maroon JC, Jackson R: *Neurosurgery* 30:412-415, 1992.)

Case Report.—Woman, 37, with a left L5-S1 herniated disk syndrome, underwent percutaneous lumbar diskectomy with local anesthesia after failing to respond to conservative measures. The Nucleotome was inserted with some difficulty. Crushing headache developed when it was activated, but the patient was heavily sedated and the procedure was completed. Perineal numbness and urinary incontinence occurred on recovery, and both spinal headache and left-sided sciatica persisted. Bowel incontinence also was present. There was anesthesia in the S2-S5 region, and rectal tone was absent. Imaging, including CT myelography (Fig 25-2), demonstrated a herniated disk, pseudomeningoceles at L5 and S1 on the left, and arachnoid adhesions. Two dorsal holes and 1 ventral hole were noted in the dura at L5 laminectomy, emitting CSF into the epidural space. There also was a small intradural hematoma with arachnoidal adhesions. Several nerve roots were transected and retracted cephalad. The patient improved after diskectomy and repair of the dorsal dural openings, but she continued to have S2-S5 anesthesia as well as bowel and bladder incontinence.

Discussion.—Proper training and a respect for fluoroscopic landmarks are necessary to insure that the Nucleotome will be used safely. This patient might have been spared major damage to the cauda equina if her headache had been ascribed to aspiration of CSF.

▶ A case of cauda equina syndrome, with loss of bowel and bladder control, is reported secondary to use of Nucleotome probe in the treatment of a herniated intervertebral disc at L5-S1. This illustrates the fact that his procedure may have catastrophic consequences.

The source of the complication is suggested to be improper use of the nucleotome. The frequency of such complications is not known. This indicates that absolute adherence to the technical details of proper performance are essential if one is to avoid complications. It also raises the question as to whether this method or open surgery is more appropriate for many patients with herniated intervertebral disk. Only the accrual of substantial data on both sides of this fence will help define indications more precisely.—R.M. Crowell, M.D.

A Controlled Trial of Corticosteroid Injections Into Facet Joints for Chronic Low Back Pain

Carette S, Marcoux S, Truchon R, Grondin C, Gagnon J, Allard Y, Latulippe M (Laval Univ, Quebec City, PQ)
N Engl J Med 325:1002–1007, 1991   25–7

Background.—Chronic low back pain is a common problem. Many treatments exist for this condition, few of which have been assessed rigorously. The efficacy of corticosteroid injected into the facet joints to treat chronic low back pain was evaluated in a randomized, placebo-controlled trial.

Methods.—Ninety-seven patients were enrolled in the trial. All had chronic low back pain and immediate relief of the pain after injections of local anesthetic into the facet joints between the fourth and fifth lumbar vertebrae and the fifth lumbar and first sacral vertebrae. By random assignment, 49 patients received injections of methylprednisolone acetate, 20 mg, and 48 received injections of isotonic saline in the same facet joints. The injections were done under fluoroscopic guidance. Ninety-five patients were followed up for 6 months.

Results.—At 1 month, there were no clinical or statistical differences between the groups in any of the outcome measures assessing pain, functional status, and back flexion. A total of 42% of those in the treatment group and 33% in the placebo group had marked or very marked improvement. At 3 months, the result were similar. At 6 months, patients treated with methylprednisolone had more improvement, less pain on the visual-analogue scale, and less physical disability. However, the between-group differences were reduced when concurrent interventions were considered. Moreover, only 22% of those in the treatment group and 10% in the placebo group had sustained improvement from the first to the sixth month.

Conclusion.—Injection of methylprednisolone into the facet joints appears to be of little benefit in the treatment of chronic low back pain. Even though the patients in this series were selected for their positive response to facet-joint injections with a local anesthetic, only 1 in 5 had sustained improvement 6 months after the steroid injection compared with 1 in 10 after placebo injection.

▶ This carefully controlled trial of injection of steroids into the facet joints demonstrated no clear value for patients with chronic low back pain. Thus, this widespread and costly approach should be discarded.—R.M. Crowell, M.D.

Neural Foraminal Ligaments of the Lumbar Spine: Appearance at CT and MR Imaging
Nowicki BH, Haughton VM (Froedtert Mem Lutheran Hosp, Milwaukee, Wis)
Radiology 183:257–264, 1992   25–8

Rationale.—The ligaments traversing the neural foramen limit the space available for the nerve roots and may even contribute to root entrapment. Therefore, it may be helpful to identify these ligaments on CT and MRI studies.

Methods.—Axial and parasagittal CT scans and MR images were examined along with corresponding microtome sections in 18 human cadavers. Computed tomography was used to examine 114 neural foramina at 57 spinal levels, and 27 foramina were studied by MRI.

Findings.—The ligaments were seen originating from the posterolateral margin of the intervertebral disk and attaching to the inferior pedicle, superior articular process, transverse process, or ligamentum flavum. Computed tomography demonstrated linear structures with higher attenuation coefficients than the adjacent fat and areolar tissue. Magnetic resonance images demonstrated the ligaments as linear structures with lower signal intensities than adjacent tissues in the neural foramina. In both CT and MR images, the ligaments were closely related anatomically to the spinal nerves.

Conclusion.—Both CT scanning and MRI effectively demonstrate the ligaments in the neural foramina of the spine.

▶ Spinal surgeons are familiar with ligaments within the neural foramina of the lumbar spine. The ligaments are viewed as dispensable as one attempts to assure satisfactory decompression of the nerve root exiting the foramen. There is also a widely held impression that hypertrophy of the ligamentum flavum within the foramen may contribute to root compression and symptomatology. However, both preoperatively and intraoperatively, the surgeon is hampered by insufficient precision in the anatomical understanding of the contribution of ligaments to nerve root compression within the foramen.

Nowicki and Haughton offer a useful contribution to the understanding of this problem by providing microtome cadaver comparisons with CT and MR images. Their results show that foraminal ligaments can be imaged very nicely by both CT and MR techniques. With this background, the stage is set for correlation of clinical syndromes and pathoanatomical data on foraminal ligaments in patients with sciatica. The overall effort should help in the diagnosis and management of patients with back and sciatic pain.—R.M. Crowell, M.D.

Thoracic

Circumferential Decompression of Upper Thoracic Spinal Stenosis Through a Posterior Approach
Osamu K, Tomoya S, Yasuro N, Masatoshi S (Natl Kobe Hosp, Kobe, Japan)
J West Pacific Orthop Assoc 27:131–138, 1990   25–9

Introduction.—For anatomical reasons, an adequate decompression of the upper thoracic spinal cord (for lesions such as ossification of the posterior longitudinal ligament [OPLL]) is difficult to perform. A posterior laminectomy or sternum-split approach will not adequately treat a continuous lesion extending upward or downward beyond T3. Circumferential decompression of the spinal cord via a posterior approach was used to treat 4 cases of severe thoracic myelopathy resulting from OPLL located on the upper thoracic level.

Technique.—Circumferential decompression from the back may be tailored according to the pathology encountered. (Fig 25–3). Posterior elements of the spine are exposed bilaterally as lateral and as wide to the

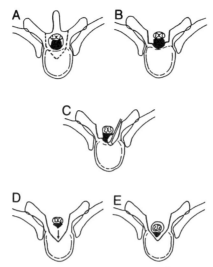

Fig 25–3.—Schematic drawing of anterior decompression of spinal cord through a posterior approach. (Courtesy of Osamu K, Tomoya S, Yasuro N, et al: *J West Pacific Orthop Assoc* 27:131-138, 1990.)

transverse process. A wide laminectomy must be performed laterally to the medial one third of the pedicles and medial two thirds of facet joints. The posterior part of the vertebral body with a part of OPLL is scraped from the posterolateral side of the dura using an air drill with a diamond burr. When the anterior part of the OPLL is resected or the posterior part of vertebral body with accompanying OPLL is removed, the posteriorly compressed spinal cord moves anteriorly into the scraped groove with or without accompanying OPLL.

Conclusion.—A circumferential decompression of the spinal cord via the posterior approach is a new procedure that can adequately treat OPLL of the upper thoracic level. This approach allows treatment of a continuous lesion extending upward or downward beyond T3. There was significant recovery in 4 cases described. The primary disadvantages of circumferential decompression via a posterior approach are the length of the surgery and the significant blood loss.

▶ This communication describes the interesting circumdecompression of the thoracic spinal cord by bilateral posterolateral drilling technique. Four cases are reported, with good results in all. Further experience will be needed to confirm this interesting suggestion.—R.M. Crowell, M.D.

Surgical Approaches to Thoracic Disc Herniations

El-Kalliny M, Tew JM Jr, van Loveren H, Dunsker S (Univ of Cincinnati, Ohio)
Acta Neurochir (Wien) 111:22–32, 1991   25–10

Background.—The advent of MRI has resulted in earlier diagnosis of thoracic disk herniations. Early diagnosis combined with a surgical approach that will ensure adequate decompression without excessive cord and root manipulation will yield the best results. More lateral and anterior approaches to the thoracic spine appear to be needed to attain this goal. Three surgical approaches to thoracic disk herniation were evaluated.

Patients and Methods.—Fourteen women and 7 men were treated from 1985 to 1990. The mean patient age was 47 years. Thirteen patients had a history of spinal trauma, which was mild in 12. Magnetic resonance imaging was used to establish the diagnosis in 19 cases. Myelography and postmyelography CT were diagnostic in 2 patients and confirmatory in 6. Sixteen patients had single disk herniation, and 5 had multiple herniation. The transpedicular-transfacetal approach was used in 8 patients, the posterolateral-extrapleural approach was used in 5, and the transthoracic-transpleural approach was used in 8. The latter procedure was chosen for patients with central and centrolateral herniations, especially those with calcified disks. The posterolateral-extrapleural approach was used in patients with centrolateral herniations.

Outcomes.—Eleven patients had significant improvement in their back and radicular pain immediately after surgery. After 3 months to 4 years of follow-up, 38% of the patients were asymptomatic, showing marked improvement of their neurologic deficit. Another 43% were significantly improved in symptoms and neurologic deficits; 14% were unchanged. Five percent worsened.

Conclusion.—The total improvement rate in this series was 81%. Although nonsurgical treatment can still be used initially in thoracic disk herniation, many patients will eventually require surgery. To determine which surgical approach is most appropriate, surgeons must consider the anatomy of the herniation as seen on MRI and/or CT, the ability of the patients to undergo a major operation, the presence of co-existing spinal diseases (e.g., thoracic stenosis or Scheuermann's disease), and his or her own level of expertise. Through this comprehensive approach, gratifying surgical results with minimal postoperative complications can be expected.

▶ This study outlines the other recommended approach to thoracic disk herniation dependent on the details of the herniation. The impression results are reported, and the study appears to be a benchmark for those doing this kind of surgery.—R.M. Crowell, M.D.

Texas Scottish Rite Hospital Rod Instrumentation for Thoracic and Lumbar Spine Trauma

Benzel EC, Kesterson L, Marchand EP (Univ of New Mexico, Albuquerque)
J Neurosurg 75:382–387, 1991   25–11

Patients.—Twenty-eight patients with unstable thoracic or lumbar spinal fractures were stabilized intraoperatively using the Texas Scottish Rite Hospital universal instrumentation system. All but 3 of the patients underwent surgery within 2 weeks of injury.

Procedures.—The procedure involved either lateral extracavitary decompression and fusion, or posterolateral (transpedicular) dural sac decompression with posterior fusion. The former patients had anterior interbody fusion after instrumentation. The indication for a posterior procedure was definite evidence of complete spinal cord disruption with a complete myelopathy. Initially, sublaminar hooks were used in conjunction with longer rods; but later, such hooks were placed in the region of the spinal cord without long rods. The compression mode of rod placement was used when there was a need to maintain reduction of the spinal segments (Fig 25–4). Distraction was used when spinal compression might have led to neural impingement or spinal deformity.

Results.—No instability or pseudoarthrosis was found during an average follow-up of 9 months. No instrumentation failure occurred, regardless of the number of spinal levels fused or the number instrumented. Three patients had superficial wound separation after repeated periods of prolonged pressure on the incision.

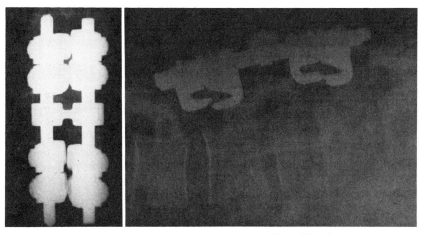

Fig 25–4.—Postoperative radiographs, anteroposterior (**left**) and lateral (**right**) views in patient 26, demonstrating the application of the "short-rod 2-claw" technique in a patient with an L-2 fracture and an incomplete myelopathy. Anterior column stabilization was obtained with the placement of an anterior interbody fusion by the lateral extracavitary approach. (Courtesy of Benzel EC, Kesterson L, Marchand EP: *J Neurosurg* 75:382–387, 1991.)

Conclusion.—The Texas Scottish Rite Hospital universal instrumentation system is an alternative to the Cotrel-Dubousset system for stabilizing the injured thoracolumbar spine. The use of multiple hooks and shorter rods can provide secure fixation while immobilizing fewer motion segments.

► This report describes an experience with 28 patients with unstable thoracic and lumbar spine fractures treated with the Texas Scottish Rite Hospital (TSRH) instrumentation system. This system uses both compression and distraction elements fixed to axial rods. The unique feature is a cross link between para-axial rods in an attempt to limit rotational forces. Overall, the experience seems rather satisfactory, and the concept seems encouraging. Further experience will be needed to determine whether this novel methodology is really worthwhile.—R.M. Crowell, M.D.

Cervical

Neurologic Complications of Surgery for Cervical Compression Myelopathy
Yonenobu K, Hosono N, Iwasaki M, Asano M, Ono K (Osaka Univ, Japan)
Spine 16:1277–1282, 1991   25–12

Background.—Few specific reports of neurologic complications after surgery for cervical compression myelopathy have been published. The manifestations, causes, and treatment results of such complications are studied.

Methods.—A total of 384 cases were examined. The surgical procedures performed included anterior interbody fusions in 134 patients, subtotal corpectomies with strut bone graft in 70, laminectomies in 85, and laminoplasties in 95.

Findings.—Twenty-one patients, or 5.5%, had surgery-related neurologic deterioration. Two types of deterioration were identified based on the neurologic signs: spinal-cord function and nerve-root function. Spinal-cord function deterioration had varying manifestations, from hand weakness to tetraparesis. Deltoid and biceps brachii muscle paralysis occurred exclusively in nerve-root function deterioration. The causes of paralysis included malalignment of the spine related to graft complications and a tethering effect on the nerve root. Function deterioration included spinal-cord injury during the operation, malalignment of the spine associated with graft complication, and epidural hematoma (table).

Conclusion.—Optimal results rely on the prevention or early detection of neurologic deterioration after surgery for cervical compression myelopathy. Surgeons must be fully aware of the potential complications associated with each procedure. Patients should be checked carefully in the immediate postoperative period for signs and symptoms of impending or progressing neurologic deterioration.

Deterioration of Nerve-Root Function

Case (Age, yr)	Disease	Procedure	Level of Surgery	Onset	Side	Deterioration		
						Motor	Sensory	Pain
1 (52)	CSM	AIF (RS)	4/5-6/7	3 dy	L	+	+	−
2 (47)	CSM	SCS	4/5-6/7	30 dy	R	+	+	−
3 (62)	CSM	SCS	3/4-5/6	14 dy	R	+	−	−
4 (66)	CSM	LP	2/3-7/1	6 hr	R	−	+	+
5 (53)	CSM	SCS	3/4-4/5	24 hr	R	+	+	+
6 (64)	CSM	SCS	3/4-5/6	15 hr	R	+	+	+
7 (61)	CSM	SCS	3/4-6/7	2 dy	R	+	+	+
8 (38)	OPLL	SCS	2/3-6/7	6 dy	R	+	+	+
9 (75)	OPLL	SCS	3/4-6/7	6 hr	L	−	+	+
10 (48)	OPLL	L	1/2-7/1	3 dy	L	−	−	+
11 (64)	CSM	LP	2/3-7/1	24 hr	R	+	+	+
12 (68)	CSM	LP	2/3-7/1	3 dy	R	+	+	+
13 (51)	OPLL	LP	2/3-7/1	36 hr	R	+	+	+

(continued)

Table *(continued)*

| | | Severity of Myelopathy* | | Results (MMT) | |
Cause	Treatment	Preop	Postop	Deltoid	Biceps
Deepening of graft	Revision	8	14	4	4
Fracture of graft	Halovest	8	15	4	5
Fracture of graft	Halovest	5	13	4	4
Hyperextension	Realignment	11	13	5	5
Unknown	Halter traction	9	14	4	4
Unknown	Halovest	8	12	4	4
Unknown	Halter traction	7	11	4	4
Unknown	Exploration	7	11	4	4
Unknown	Halovest	4	9	4	4
Unknown	Halter traction	8	15	5	5
Unknown	Observation	9	12	4	4
Unknown	Observation	10	13	3	4
Unknown	Observation	6	9	3	4

* Assessed by the assessment scale for cervical myelopathy proposed by the Japanese Orthopaedic Association.
Abbreviations: CSM, cervical spondylotic myelopathy; AIF, anterior interbody fusion; RS, Robinson-Smith method; SCS, subtotal corpectomy with strut graft; LP, laminoplasty; OPLL, ossification of the posterior longitudinal ligament; L, laminectomy; MMT Manual Muscle Testing for 6 grades (0 = no muscle construction, 5 = normal).
(Courtesy of Yonenobu K, Hosono N, Iwasaki M, et al: *Spine* 16:1277–1282, 1991.)

▶ This extensive study of 384 patients who underwent surgery in 1970–1988 gives evidence of sustained neurologic deterioration after surgery in 5.5%. Because of changing technology over the interval of study, it is difficult to make hard conclusions. Nonetheless, one notes that myelopathies were caused by intraoperative injury, graft displacement, epidural hematoma, or hyperextension. Nerve root deterioration was often unexplained, although graft displacement and hyperextension might have been a fact. There may be a correlation between the aggressive nature of the procedures and a higher risk factor.—R.M. Crowell, M.D.

Cervical Stability After Foraminotomy: A Biomechanical *In Vitro* Analysis
Zdeblick TA, Zou D, Warden KE, McCabe R, Kunz D, Vanderby R (Univ of Wisconsin, Madison)
J Bone Joint Surg (Am) 74A:22–27, 1992   25–13

Introduction.—It may be necessary to perform laminectomy or facetectomy on the cervical spine to decompress the cord or nerve roots. These procedures may render the spine unstable, creating a risk of progressive kyphosis and neurologic deterioration.

Methods.—Acute cervical spinal stability was tested after laminectomy and staged foraminotomy in specimens from 12 cadavers aged 32–60 years. Biomechanical tests were performed with the application of axial loads, flexion and extension moments, and a torsional moment. Each specimen was tested after laminectomy of C5 and after incremental foraminotomy of the sixth cervical root.

Results.—Torsional stiffness decreased markedly after removal of more than half the facet. A 50% facetectomy led to a 2.5% increase in posterior strain, whereas 75% or 100% facetectomy led to a 25% increase in posterior strain compared with intact specimens. The spine appeared to subluxate during flexion testing after 75% or 100% facetectomy.

Recommendations.—If cervical foraminotomy is required, facet resection and stripping of the capsule should be limited to less than half the facet. If more of the facet must be removed to achieve adequate decompression, then stabilization is indicated to prevent segmental hypermobility of the cervical spine.

▶ This interesting report from the University of Wisconsin shows that cervical stability is maintained after foraminotomy if 50% of the facet surface can be maintained. This is of obvious use to the surgeon who is about to perform such an operation.

The importance of maintaining the facet depends on several factors, including the number of facets to be operated on, the age of the patient (and thereby the likelihood of hypermobility vs. autofusion), and the presence of effective fusion at other levels. In the older patient, a total facetectomy at one level on one side is extremely rarely the cause of spinal instability. The incidence of swan neck deformity is probably higher in the younger age group with this type of procedure, and it is in this group that the recommendation of a limited facetectomy is particularly appropriate.—R.M. Crowell, M.D.

Surgical Stabilization of Cervical Spinal Fractures Using Methyl Methacrylate: Technical Considerations and Long-Term Results in 52 Patients

Duff TA, Khan A, Corbett JE (Univ of Wisconsin, Madison)
J Neurosurg 76:440–443, 1992   25–14

Objective.—The long-term results of posterior surgical stabilization using cement but not bone grafting were examined in 52 consecutively treated patients having acute cervical spinal fracture-dislocation.

Patients.—Two thirds of the group were less than 30 years of age whereas 10% were older than 60 years. A typical range of accidents was responsible for the injuries. A majority of patients exhibited instability on neutral radiographs of the neck. Three patients had nerve root injuries, 12 had partial cord injuries, and 13 were paraplegic.

Management.—Methyl methacrylate was used to stabilize the injuries. In some cases, stainless steel wire was looped around the screws on either side before acrylic was applied. In repairing fractures of the upper cervical spine, the upper screws were inserted obliquely.

Results.—Acrylic failure occurred twice in this series. No patient had progressive neurologic impairment during follow-up for 6 months to 9 years. There was a single wound infection, which did not prevent fracture healing.

Conclusion.—Methyl methacrylate can provide long-term stability in patients with traumatic cervical spinal fractures, but the risk of infection must be kept in mind.

▶ This study reviews 52 patients treated with posterior cervical stabilization using methyl methacrylate without bone grafting. Follow-up from 6 months to 9 years showed 2 failures early in the series, no increase in neurologic impairment, and 1 serious wound infection. The authors emphasize that (1) the acrylic inlay must be provided with an anchor to bone that cannot easily erode; (2) the wire must be completely encased; and (3) substantial cross-sectional area is important for satisfactory stabilization (1.5 cm in depth and width). In this study, methyl methacrylate posterior cervical stabilization appears to be both effective and safe.—R.M. Crowell, M.D.

Injury

Recovery of Motor Function After Spinal-Cord Injury: A Randomized, Placebo-Controlled Trial With GM-1 Ganglioside

Geisler FH, Dorsey FC, Coleman WP (Maryland Inst for Emergency Med Services Systems, Baltimore; Fidia Pharmaceutical Corp, Washington, DC)
N Engl J Med 324:1829–1838, 1991   25–15

Background.—Although the treatment of spinal cord injuries in specialized centers has decreased morbidity and mortality, only a minority of patients have major neurologic recovery, and recovery is rarely complete. In recent animal studies, monosialotetrahexosylganglioside (GM-1) ganglioside enhanced the functional recovery of damaged neurons. Gangliosides, complex acidic glycolipids present in high concentrations in CNS cells, form a major component of the cell membrane. Their function is unknown, but experimental evidence shows that they augment neurite outgrowth in vitro, induce regeneration and sprouting of neurons, and restore neuronal function after injury in vivo. The GM-1 ganglioside was studied to determine whether it altered recovery in humans after a spinal-cord injury.

Methods.—In a prospective, randomized, placebo-controlled, double-blind drug trial of GM-1, 34 of 37 eligible patients completed the study. The criteria for entry were written informed consent, the absence of contraindications to the use of GM-1, sterility or postmenopausal status in female patients, an age of at least 18 years, and the presence of a spinal cord injury with a major motor deficit in the hands or legs. Patients in the study group, which was comprised of 23 patients with cervical injuries and 11 with thoracic injuries, were randomly assigned to either a treatment (16 patients) or placebo (18 patients) group. In both groups, the 2-hour median injury-to-emergency-room time allowed for prompt spinal cord decompression and resuscitation. Nine GM-1 treatment patients and nine patients in the placebo treatment group underwent surgery within 72 hours after the injury. Medical mangement for all patients included 250 mg of methylprednisolone sodium succinate administered intravenously on admission, followed by 125 mg given intravenously every 6 hours for 72 hours. The Frankel scale and the American Spinal Injury Association (ASIA) motor score used to measure the severity of spinal cord injury and its subsequent recovery were administered at the time of first contact in the emergency room, at entry into the study, twice per week for the first 4 weeks, and after 2, 3, 6, and 12 months.

Results.—The GM-1 treated patients' Frankel grades improved more than the placebo-treated patients' grades. Among the 28 patients who could have improved by 2 or more Frankel grades, 7 of 14 in the GM-1-treated group improved compared with 1 of 14 of the patients in the placebo group. The overall number of patients (8 of 34) whose scores improved by 2 or more Frankel grades was larger than historical data would have predicted. Seven of the 8 patients with this considerable neurologic recovery were in the GM-1 group. In the placebo group, the recovery of 1 of 18 patients was similar to that predicted on the basis of historical data. Despite randomization, the ASIA motor scores at entry were imbalanced, with 25.9 in the GM-1-treated group and 39.8 in the placebo group. The mean motor recovery from entry score to the score after 1 year for the GM-1-treated patients was 36.9 points compared with 21.6 points for the placebo-treated patients.

Conclusion.—The drug effect of GM-1 dramatically increased neurologic function, with a majority of the small study group changing from paralyzed to ambulatory status. The effect of GM-1 appears to occur by the conversion of motor groups that were initially paralyzed into those with useful motor function after 1 year. It is suggested that GM-1 is safe to administer in spinal cord injury, and that it enhances the recovery of neurologic function after 1 year; however, a larger study is needed to confirm its clinical benefit and safety.

▶ This prospective, randomized, double-blind study of spinal cord injuries pitted GM-1 ganglioside against placebo for treatment. A very extensive and carefully quantitative study has been provided for 37 patients entered into the study. By motor score evaluation, a statistically significant degree of improvement was documented in the GM-1 group. In addition, the majority of patients with improvement in the GM-1 group advanced to ambulatory status. Although the study is small and further studies are required for confirmation, a dramatic helpful response was seen, and further careful follow-up is indicated.—R.M. Crowell, M.D.

The Effects of Removal of Bullet Fragments Retained in the Spinal Canal: A Collaborative Study by the National Spinal Cord Injury Model Systems

Waters RL, Adkins RH (Rancho Los Amigos Med Ctr, Downey, Calif)
Spine 16:934–939, 1991   25–16

Background.—Gunshot wounds are a major cause of spinal cord injury in the United States. The effects of the removal of bullet fragments retained in the spinal canal were determined.

Methods.—Ninety patients with bullet fragments lodged in their spinal canal underwent serial motor and sensory assessments. Sixty-six patients had annual follow-up examinations. Seventy were paraplegic and 20 were quadriplegic. There were 81 men and 9 women, (average age, 30 years).

Outcomes.—No infections occurred after fragment removal, even though the bullets had perforated the alimentary canal in approximately 20% of the cases. According to statistical analyses, bullet fragment removal made no significant difference in pain reduction or recovery of

ASIA Motor Index Score for T1–T10 Injuries (Mean ± SD)

All Thoracic Injuries (T1–T10)

	Initial	Annual	Difference	N
Removed	45.4 ± 7.6	53.8 ± 14.4	8.8 ± 9.2	8
Not removed	47.9 ± 8.4	51.7 ± 13.0	3.8 ± 8.1	24
				32

Complete Thoracic Injuries (T1–T10)

	Initial	Annual	Difference	N
Removed	43.0 ± 6.5	46.0 ± 4.2	3.0 ± 4.2	5
Not removed	45.7 ± 5.0	47.2 ± 4.7	1.5 ± 3.7	21
				26

Incomplete Thoracic Injuries (T1–T10)

	Initial	Annual	Difference	N
Removed	49.3 ± 9.0	66.7 ± 17.0	17.3 ± 8.1	3
Not removed	63.7 ± 11.9	83.3 ± 2.9	19.7 ± 13.9	3
				6

(Courtesy of Waters RL, Adkins RH: *Spine* 16:934–939, 1991.)

sensation. However, bullet removal did affect motor recovery, depending on the level of the lesion. In patients with lesions between vertebral levels T12 and L4, those with bullet removal had significantly greater motor recovery than those without bullet removal. Bullet removal from the canal between T1 and T11 did not significantly influence motor recovery (table).

Conclusion.—Bullet fragment removal from the spinal canal influences neurologic outcome in some patients. However, bullet removal did not affect secondary complications, including CSF leak, pain, meningitis, and lead toxicity.

▶ In patients with lesions between T12 and L4, motor recovery was better when the bullet was removed. By contrast, bullet removal between T1 and T11 had no significant effect on motor recovery. This seems explicable in terms of the differences between spinal cord and nerve roots.—R.M. Crowell, M.D.

26 Infection

Intracranial Infection After Missile Injuries to the Brain: Report of 30 Cases From the Lebanese Conflict
Taha JM, Haddad FS, Brown JA (Univ of Cincinnati, Ohio; American Univ of Beirut Med Ctr, Beirut, Lebanon; Medical College of Ohio, Toledo)
Neurosurgery 29:864–868, 1991   26–1

Background.—The last large series of patients with brain abscesses developing after penetrating craniocerebral injuries was reported in 1981. Since then, CT and modern coma care have become available. Thirty intracranial infections developing after missile injuries to the brain occurring during the Lebanese conflict were evaluated.

Patients and Outcomes.—The 30 infections complicated a total of 600 injuries treated between 1981 and 1988. The patients were followed up for 1 month to 7 years, with a mean of 2$\frac{1}{2}$ years. Brain abscess occurred in 16 patients, cerebritis occurred in 9, infected intracerebral hematoma occurred in 2, and meningitis occurred in 5. The infections occurred 4 days to 7 years after the initial débridement. Infecting organisms were Gram positive in 36%, Gram negative in 40%, and a combination in 7%. Eighty percent had wound dehiscence or CSF leakage when the infection appeared. A 76% correlation was seen between the organisms cultured from the dehisced scalp wound and brain. Intracranial bone retention occurred in 23 patients. Infection developed around the bone fragments in 16 patients, around a metallic fragment in 4, around absorbable gelatin sponge in 2, and along the missile tract in 3. Two patients had an infected intracerebral hematoma, and 3 had meningitis. Each patient had at least 1 risk factor, including extensive brain injury, coma, trajectory through an air sinus, CSF fistula, inadequate initial débridement, or incomplete dural closure. The incidence of intracranial infection in pa-

Incidence of Intracranial Infection in Relation to Cerebrospinal Fluid Fistula and Retained Bone Fragments

Bone Fragments	Cerebrospinal Fluid Fistula (%)	
	Absent	Present
Absent	0.6	21.1
Present	4.0	84.6

(Courtesy of Taha JM, Haddad FS, Brown JA: *Neurosurgery* 29:864–868, 1991.)

tients with postoperative retention of bone was 4% in the absence of scalp wound dehiscence and 84.6% when wound dehiscence was seen. A total of 43% of the patients still retained a bone fragment of less than 1 cm after excision of a brain abscess or treatment for cerebritis or meningitis. No one had recurrent infection (table).

Conclusion.—A retained bone fragment that is still seen after treatment of an intracranial infection caused by a missile injury to the brain alone does not necessarily mean that the patient is at an increased risk of infection. When other major risk factors (e.g., wound dehiscence or CSF leakage), do not occur, the surgeon may decide that such a fragment need not be removed.

▶ The authors obtained a low overall rate of infection. They conclude that retained bone fragments that are smaller than a centimeter need not be removed when there is no wound dehiscence or CSF leakage. However, their data indicate that retained bone fragments substantially increase the risk of subsequent intracranial infection. That the risk of infection is still low (approximately 4%) leaves room for judgment as to whether the risk of aggressive débridement to remove the retained fragment exceeds the risk of subsequent infection. This judgment would depend on many factors, such as overall health status, the location of the retained fragment, etc. It may not be wise to attempt a fixed policy regarding the removal of retained foreign bodies. Information such as that provided by the authors allows rational decision-making based on balancing risk and benefit.—R.M. Crowell, M.D.

The Role of Stereotactic Biopsy in the Management of HIV-Related Focal Brain Lesions
Chappell ET, Guthrie BL, Orenstein J (George Washington Univ, Washington, DC)
Neurosurgery 30:825–829, 1992   26–2

Introduction.—Encephalitis is considered the most common cause of neurologic symptoms in patients with AIDS. Focal lesions may, however, result from cytomegalovirus infection, bacterial infections (e.g. mycobacterial disease), and various fungal infections. In addition, patients with AIDS may have the same focal cerebral diseases as other patients.

Patients.—Twenty-five patients with AIDS and focal cerebral lesions underwent stereotactic biopsy in 1988–1990. All the patients had lesions identified on CT scans. Those with enhancing lesions had failed to improve on a trial of pyrimethamine and sulfadiazine or intravenously administered clindamycin.

Findings.—Biopsy led to a diagnosis of lymphoma in 36% of the patients, progressive multifocal leukoencephalopathy in 24%, and toxoplasmosis in 8%. One patient each had low-grade glioma, herpetic cere-

Appearance of Lesion on CT Scan vs. the Impact of Biopsy on
Subsequent Treatment

Impact on Treatment	Appearance of Lesion	
	Contrast-enhancing	Non-enhancing
Changed treatment	11	0
Confirmed treatment in progress	3	0
No help with treatment	2 (12.5%)	9 (100%)

(Courtesy of Chappell ET, Guthrie BL, Orenstein J: *Neurosurgery* 30:825–829, 1992.)

britis, and cryptococcal abscess. Five biopsy specimens were abnormal but nondiagnostic. Whether a lesion was enhanced was well correlated with whether biopsy enhanced patient management (table). The biopsy findings did not influence management in any of the patients with nonenhancing lesions. The only significant complication of biopsy was a small hematoma with significant edema which produced transient somnolence.

Conclusion.—Patients positive for HIV who have an enhancing cerebral lesion should receive antitoxoplasmosis treatment empirically. Those who have such lesions late in the course of AIDS, however, should have immediate biopsy because of the high risk of lymphoma. Biopsy specimens may provide prognostic data for patients with nonenhancing lesions, and they may qualify some patients for participation in experimental treatment programs.

▶ This interesting study provides data on the question of whether stereotactic biopsy should be used in the management of HIV-related focal brain lesions. The authors presents 25 cases with a variety of AIDS-related lesions treated during a 2-year period. Those patients who harbored enhancing lesions were treated first with an antitoxoplasmosis program. Biopsy was considered only in those patients who did not respond. In the patients with enhancing lesions, 87.5% of biopsies done with stereotactic technique were diagnostic.

The authors concluded that the diagnosis contributed to the patient's treatment; therefore, they recommend that this approach be used for all patients with contrast-enhancing lesions. However, there is a different way in which one can interpret the data. If we look at all the patients treated, we find that only 1 patient, the patient with a low-grade glioma, had a diagnosis that altered treatment and led to expected survival of more than 8 weeks. In the 9 lymphomas and several other lesions, the mean survival was between 1 and 8 weeks. Thus, although the biopsy may have led to a diagnosis, it had no substantial impact on outcome. One can argue that biopsy is only rarely justified by having a positive impact on the outcome of the patient harboring such a lesion. This is particularly true because there is a risk to both the patient and the surgeon in performing this biopsy.—R.M. Crowell, M.D.

Primary Central Nervous System Lymphoma in Acquired Immune Deficiency Syndrome: A Clinical and Pathologic Study With Results of Treatment with Radiation
Goldstein JD, Dickson DW, Moser FG, Hirschfeld AD, Freeman K, Llena JF, Kaplan B, Davis L (Montefiore Med Ctr/Albert Einstein College of Medicine, Bronx, NY)
Cancer 67:2756–2765, 1991   26–3

Introduction.—An increased incidence of primary CNS lymphoma has been described in patients with AIDS, but the optimal management of lymphoma in these patients is uncertain. Life expectancy remains brief. Seventeen patients with AIDS who received radiotherapy for primary CNS lymphoma were studied. Most patients received cobalt radiotherapy to the whole brain.

Clinical Findings.—The average age at diagnosis was 35 years. Three patients were women infected by their spouses. Fifteen patients had other AIDS-related illness before lymphoma was diagnosed, and most of them were severely debilitated. Central nervous system symptoms were seen for an average of less than 2 months before a diagnosis was made. Seizures and paresis/paralysis occurred most frequently. Most patients had a high-grade, large-cell undifferentiated lymphoma. The mean overall survival was only 72 days.

CT Findings.—No single CT appearance was characteristic of lymphoma, but all patients had low-density, contrast-enhancing mass lesions. Posttreatment scans typically showed diffuse cerebral atrophy and lucency at the sites of tumor. The CT appearances correlated with the anatomical sites of tumor. The 3 distinct patterns of contrast enhance-

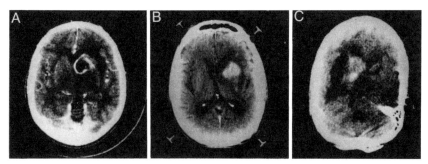

Fig 26–1.—A, CT scan shows ring-enhancing lesion in basal ganglia. Patient also has several other small ring-enhancing lesions. Central nonenhancing regions correspond to areas of central necrosis. **B,** CT shows uniform enhancement in basal ganglia mass. This tumor is thought to contain very little necrosis. **C,** CT scan shows patchy enhancement that corresponds to lymphoma interspersed with necrotic tissue. (Courtesy of Goldstein JD, Dickson DW, Moser FG, et al: *Cancer* 67:2756–2765, 1991.)

ment observed are shown in Figure 26-1. Radiation effects on the CNS were identified in 4 cases.

Conclusion.—Primary CNS lymphoma in patients with AIDS is responsive to irradiation, but a tumor response does not always mean longer survival; many patients die of opportunistic infection in a short time.

▶ This study indicates that the approach of biopsy and radiation for primary CNS lymphoma in AIDS can often lead to clinical improvement (10 of 17 cases). On the other hand, patients typically progress to or die of other aspects of the AIDS-related illnesses. Moreover, biopsy is not necessarily warranted initially in many of the patients seen with CNS manifestations, because many of these lesions turn out to be infectious (typically, toxoplasmosis). Patients with appropriate CT scan profiles may be initially treated with appropriate antimicrobial agents and treated with radiation therapy only if there is deterioration related to lymphoma.—R.M. Crowell, M.D.

27 Pediatrics

Multidrug Resistance Gene Expression in Pediatric Primitive Neuro-ectodermal Tumors of the Central Nervous System
Tishler DM, Weinberg KI, Sender LS, Nolta JA, Raffel C (Childrens Hosp of Los Angeles, Calif)
J Neurosurg 76:507–512, 1992   27–1

Background.—Primitive neuroectodermal tumor (PNET) is a malignancy of the pediatric CNS that frequently recurs, despite aggressive surgery, radiotherapy, and chemotherapy. The poor outcome may be partly a result of drug-resistant tumor cells. The multidrug resistance gene MDR1 encodes a membrane-associated glycoprotein, P-glycoprotein, which acts as a drug efflux pump to reduce the intracellular levels of cytotoxic drug to sublethal concentrations.

Patient Data in 15 Instances of Pediatric Primitive Neuroectodermal Tumor

Case No.	Sex, Age (yrs)	Tumor Location	Initial Tumor	Recurrent Tumor	P-Glyco-protein Expression	MDR1 mRNA Expression
3	M, 3½	pf	X		−	−
6	F, 2	po	X		−	0
9	F, 1	pf	X		+	+
10	M, 3½	pf	X		−	−
12	M, 5½	pf	X		−	−
14	M, 9	pf	X		−	−
21	M, 8½	pf		X	+	+
24	F, 5	pf	X		−	+
41	M, 6½	pf		X	−	0
42	F, 9	pf	X		−	+
43	M, 5½	pf	X		−	+
45	F, 4	fp	X		−	−
		fp		X	−	+
49	M, 6½	pf		X	−	0
51	F, 16½	pf	X		−	−

* P-glycoprotein expression tested by Western blot analysis; multidrug resistance gene 1 (MDR1) messenger RNA (*mRNA*) expression tested by RNA polymerase chain reaction.
    Abbreviations; pf, posterior fossa; *po,* parieto-occipital; *fp,* frontoparietal; −, negative test; +, positive test; 0, not tested.
    (Courtesy of Tishler DM, Weinberg KI, Sender LS, et al: *J Neurosurg* 76:507–512, 1992.)

Objective and Methods.—The role of MDR1 was examined in 16 pediatric patients with PNET (table); Western blot analysis was used to detect the expression of P-glycoprotein messenger RNA. The polymerase chain reaction technique served to detect the expression of MDR1 messenger RNA. Gene amplification was assessed by Southern blot analysis.

Findings.—Two of 15 analyzed tumors expressed detectable levels of P-glycoprotein. Six of 12 tumors, including both recurrent tumors, expressed MDR1 messenger RNA. Southern blot analysis of DNA from all 16 PNETs gave no evidence of MDR1 amplification in any of the tumors.

Implication.—Therapeutic strategies designed to overcome MDR1 drug resistance in patients with non-CNS tumors also may prove useful in treating pediatric PNET.

▶ This report identifies the expression of MDR1 and its protein product (P-glycoprotein) in cases of pediatric PNET. The studies failed to show evidence of MDR1 amplification in any tumor. Resistance to chemotherapeutic agents may be related to MDR1 and P-glycoprotein. This article offers the first evidence of both of these moieties within PNETs. Further studies aimed at overcoming MDR1 resistance may play an important role in the treatment of pediatric PNET.—R.M. Crowell, M.D.

Arteriovenous Malformations of the Brain in Children: A Forty Year Experience
Kondziolka D, Humphreys RP, Hoffman HJ, Hendrick EB, Drake JM (Hosp for Sick Children, Toronto)
Can J Neurol Sci 19:40–45, 1992   27–2

Background.—A child's brain has a great capacity for recovery after stroke. However, the morbidity and mortality in children harboring an arteriovenous malformation (AVM) continue to be high.

Methods.—The clinical data and management of 132 children with brain AVMs were studied. The patients were treated between 1949 and 1989. All were 18 years of age or younger.

Outcomes.—The tendency for a childhood AVM to occur with hemorrhage (79%) remained constant throughout the study period. However, the associated morbidity and mortality of hemorrhage changed. Death resulting from hemorrhage occurred in 25% of the entire series, decreasing from 39% to 16% after the introduction of CT. Death resulting from AVM bleeding since 1975 depended on location: 57% of those with a cerebellar AVM died of bleeding compared with 4.5% of those with a cerebral hemisphere AVM. Twelve percent of the children were seen with a chronic seizure disorder. In 73% of this group, surgical excision of the malformation resulted in complete seizure control off anticonvulsant medication. A total of 21% were treated nonsurgically, many of whom had terminal poor-grade bleeding. Of the 79% who had surgery, total AVM excision was achieved in 53.1%. In 67%, complete AVM resection produced a normal neurologic outcome. Most partial excisions and feeding artery clippings were done in the early years and did not provide protection from rebleeding.

Conclusion.—Treatment of an AVM in a child should involve 1 or more techniques to eliminate the risk of intracranial bleeding in the succeeding decades. The goal of treatment of those with sustained prior hemorrhage should be rapid extirpation of the malformation. In most cases, this can be done safely with open microsurgical excision. Although children who survive hemorrhage and undergo surgery can have excellent outcomes, the death rates associated with hemorrhage remain high.

▶ This report of 132 patients from the Toronto Group indicates that essentially all children with AVMs should be treated to eliminate the risk of bleeding. This is in accord with other centers' conclusions on this topic.—R.M. Crowell, M.D.

Diffuse Brain Swelling in Severely Head-Injured Children: A Report From the NIH Traumatic Coma Data Bank

Aldrich EF, Eisenberg HM, Saydjari C, Luerssen TG, Foulkes MA, Jane JA, Marshall LF, Marmarou A, Young HF (Univ of Texas Medical Branch, Galveston; James Whitcomb Riley Hosp, Indianapolis, Ind; Natl Inst of Neurological Disorders and Stroke, Bethesda, Md; Univ of Virginia, Charlottesville; Univ of California, San Diego; et al)
J Neurosurg 76:450–454, 1992   27–3

Objective.—Diffuse brain swelling, which reportedly is frequent in children with severe head injury, is a common cause of delayed neurologic deterioration in these patients. Evidence of diffuse brain swelling and its prognostic implications were studied in a prospective series of 111 children and 642 adults with severe head injury.

Patients.—In all cases, the Glasgow Coma Scale (GCS) score was 8 or less after nonoperative resuscitation, or it decreased to that level within 48 hours of injury. Evidence of diffuse brain swelling, with or without small parenchymal hemorrhages, was present on CT in 138 patients.

Findings.—A total of 24% of the children and 17% of the adults had diffuse brain swelling (group I). Seventy-five of the 138 patients with this change lacked small parenchymal hemorrhages (PH). Only 7 group I adults and 1 child deteriorated to a GCS score less than 8. Early hypoxia was more frequent in patients with diffuse brain swelling. Nearly half the children with diffuse brain swelling died within 6 days, compared with 15% of other children and 30% of group I adults (Fig 27–1).

Implications.—The most striking finding is a mortality rate of 53% in children seen after severe head injury with diffuse brain swelling. The

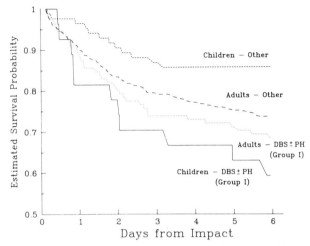

Fig 27–1.—Life-table analysis for survival of patients with diffuse brain swelling with or without small parenchymal hemorrhage (*DBS ± PH*) vs. all other patients, considering adults and children separately. (Courtesy of Aldrich EF, Eisenberg HM, Saydjari C, et al: *J Neurosurg* 76:450-454, 1992.)

presence or absence of small parenchymal hemorrhages did not substantially alter this finding.

▶ This report demonstrates the power of a cooperative study group—in this case, the National Institutes of Health Traumatic Coma Data Bank. By combining evidence from 753 patients (111 children and 642 adults), diffuse brain swelling was found to occur nearly twice as often in children as in adults. Diffuse brain swelling was described primarily in terms of the absence of perimesencephalic cisterns in the presence of small or normal ventricular size on CT scan. There were 138 patients in the group with diffuse brain swelling. For the children in this group (27), the mortality rate was found to be 3 times that found in children without diffuse brain swelling. The mortality was unchanged when the group with diffuse brain swelling group had small parenchymal hemorrhages as well. These data are valuable in terms of the prognosis and treatment of patients with these conditions.—R.M. Crowell, M.D.

Pediatric Spinal Cord and Vertebral Column Injury
Osenbach RK, Menezes AH (Univ of Iowa Hosps and Clinics, Iowa City)
Neurosurgery 30:385–390, 1992   27–4

Introduction.—Injuries to the spinal cord and/or vertebral column occur relatively infrequently in the pediatric population. A total of 179 children aged 16 years and younger who were treated for such injuries in 1970–1988 were assessed. Those with congenital spinal anomalies were excluded.

The Injuries.—Vehicular trauma caused 56% of all injuries, and 17% resulted from falls. Cervical spine injury was seen in 63% of the patients and constituted a higher proportion of injuries in younger children. Approximately half the children had neurologic dysfunction when first seen; nearly half of those had a complete transverse myelopathy. Deficit was most likely when injury involved the thoracolumbar junction, followed by thoracic and then cervical injuries. More than one third of the children had concomitant systemic injuries and one fifth had closed head injuries.

Management.—External spinal immobilization was the initial measure. At present, CT is done in a majority of patients with evidence of a fracture on plain radiography. Those with a neurologic deficit have myelography, CT-myelography or, recently, MRI. Two thirds of the children were managed nonoperatively. Injuries of the thoracolumbar junction were preferably treated surgically.

Outcome.—Nine children died of head injury. All patients who initially were neurologically intact remained so at a median follow-up of 30 months. Two thirds of the children with a complete injury were unchanged, but 5 recovered some motor function. Seven of 26 children with severe but incomplete injuries regained at least useful motor function and became ambulatory. Nine children with severe cord injuries subsequently had kyphoscoliosis. Four with cervical injuries required fusion for persistent spinal instability.

Implications.—The upper cervical spine is very vulnerable to injury in young children. Neurologic deficits (including complete myelopathy) are relatively frequent in this population. The outlook for children with complete or severe partial injuries remains unfavorable.

▶ The authors present a large series of 179 children of various ages with spinal cord injuries. They provide a compelling analysis that shows a strong correlation between initial and eventual outcome performances. The importance of the spinal cord injury without radiologic abnormality is emphasized; 4 of the cases reviewed had this problem. The type of injury differed between pre-adolescent and older children, with the younger children sustaining a greater proportion of cervical injuries, particularly at the craniovertebral junction. The possibility of late spinal deformity in patients with pediatric spinal injury also is noted.

The authors' conclusions regarding treatment are less persuasive. The approach at the University of Iowa has primarily been nonoperative, and the authors indicate that only 59 children (33%) underwent surgical intervention for irreducible or unstable injuries. The thoracolumbar junction was the most common area in which surgical treatment was preferred. Therefore, the indication for surgery was primarily of an orthopedic nature, without reference to persistent cord compression, neurologic grade, or (evidently) progression of deficit. The data do not permit secure conclusions regarding the usefulness of decompressive surgery in any of these situations. It may be argued that patients with radiographic evidence (especially CT evidence) of cord compression in a setting of incomplete deficit (progressive deficit in particular) still might benefit from reduction and, possibly, decompression.—R.M. Crowell, M.D.

Long-Term Results After Lateral Canthal Advancement for Unilateral Coronal Synostosis

Machado HR, Hoffman HJ (Hosp for Sick Children, Toronto)
J Neurosurg 76:401–407, 1992   27–5

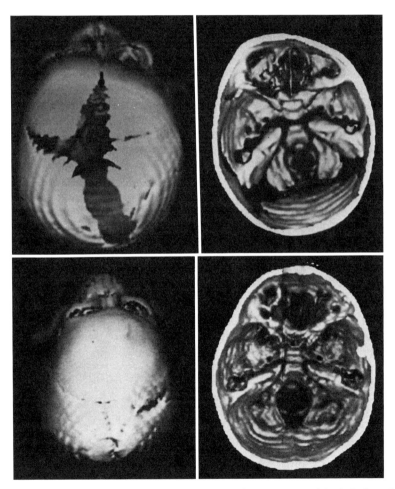

Fig 27–2.—Preoperative (*upper*) and 1-year postoperative (*lower*) CT scans of the skull of an infant with unilateral coronal synostosis. **Upper left,** preoperative vertex view showing a flattened forehead. Note the bulging of the opposite side of the forehead. **Upper right,** preoperative basal view showing the flattened forehead and decreased sphenoid-petrosal angle on the involved side. **Lower left,** postoperative vertex view 1 year after lateral canthal advancement showing a symmetrical forehead. **Lower right,** postoperative basal view showing symmetrical sphenoid-petrosal angles. (Courtesy of Machado HR, Hoffman HJ: *J Neurosurg* 76:401–407, 1992.)

Introduction.—A variety of treatments have been used for unilateral coronal synostosis. A 20-year experience with the procedure of lateral canthal advancement was evaluated.

Patients.—One surgeon treated 39 patients with unilateral coronal synostosis using lateral canthal advancement. There were 22 girls and 17 boys, 61.5% of whom were referred before 6 months of age. All had unilateral flattening of the involved forehead and a higher orbit on the affected side. Fifteen had associated problems, of which strabismus was the most common. Thirty-seven children were available at a mean follow-up of 5 years.

Outcome.—Initially excellent results were achieved in 64.9% of the patients, mild but persistent asymmetry was achieved in 16.2%, and significant asymmetry was achieved in 8.9%. All but 1 of the patients with less-than-excellent results underwent surgery before 6 months of age. Six patients who initially had mild asymmetry were eventually reclassified as having excellent results; nasal deviation also commonly improved with time. Seven patients, 2 of whom were left with poor final results, had reoperation. No serious complications were observed.

Conclusion.—With its good long-term results and minimal morbidity, lateral canthal advancement is the procedure of choice for unilateral coronal synostosis (Fig 27–2). The success of the procedure relies on the liberation of the supraorbital margin and the release of stenotic skull base sutures. Surgical indications are not restricted by the severity of the process or the age of the patient.

▶ These authors, from the Hospital for Sick Children in Toronto, present 37 cases of coronal synostosis treated with lateral canthal advancement. The technique, which is based on the concept that basal suture abnormalities are fundamental, promotes the release of compromised skull sutures, thus allowing the growing brain to reshape not only the forehead, but also the orbit and the face. Using this technique, 81% good or excellent results were obtained. Although this report does not permit precise comparison with other techniques, it *does* indicate an impressive outcome in the great majority of the cases. In addition, the age of the patient does not seem to be important in achieving a good result using this procedure.—R.M. Crowell, M.D.

Symptomatic Chiari Malformation in Adults: A New Classification Based on Magnetic Resonance Imaging With Clinical and Prognostic Significance

Pillay PK, Awad IA, Little JR, Hahn JF (Cleveland Clinic Found, Ohio)
Neurosurgery 28:639–645, 1991   27–6

Background.—Varying surgical anatomy at the craniovertebral junction has been seen in adults with Chiari malformation, with overlapping fea-

Clinical Syndrome in Relation to the Presence or Absence
of Syringomyelia

Syndrome	Syringomyelia (Type A) (n = 20)	No Syringo- myelia (Type B) (n = 15)
Foramen magnum syndrome[a]	2	8
Central cord syndrome[a]	16	0
Cerebellar dysfunction	2	4
Bulbar palsy	0	0
Paroxysmal intracranial hyper-tension	0	3
Spasticity	0	0
Total	20	15

[*] Difference statistically significant (χ^2, $P < .01$).
(Courtesy of Pillay PK, Awad IA, Little JR, et al: *Neurosurgery* 28:639–645, 1991.)

tures of both types of hindbrain pathology and a lack of association with myelo-dysplasia or hydrocephalus. A new classification based on MRI of symptomatic Chiari malformation in adults was studied.

Patients and Methods.—Thirty-five consecutive adults, aged 18–57 years, with progressive symptoms were treated at the Cleveland Clinic during a 3-year period. Magnetic resonance imaging was done before and after surgery in all cases.

Findings.—Craniovertebral junction images confirmed herniation in all patients. Two anatomically distinct categories of the Chiari malformation in this age group were defined. Twenty patients, with concomitant syringo-myelia, were classified as type A. The remaining 15 patients, with frank herniation of the brain stem below the foramen magnum but without evidence of syringomyelia, were classified as type B. Type A patients had a predominant central cord symptomatology. The patients with type B had signs and symptoms of brain stem or cerebellar compression. The main treatment consisted of decompression of the foramen magnum, opening of the fourth ventricular outlet, and plugging of the obex. Significant improvement occurred after treatment in 45% of patients who were type A and in 87% who were type B. Postoperative reduction in syrinx volume was seen in 11 patients with type A, including all 9 with excellent results (table).

Conclusion.—Magnetic resonance imaging has enabled classification of the adult Chiari malformation based on objective anatomical criteria. This classification has clinical and prognostic relevance. Patients with syringomyelia appear to respond less favorably to surgical intervention.

▶ It is appropriate that the Cleveland Clinic has emphasized the importance of the Chiari syndrome, and has offered a useful new classification of Chiari malformation in the adult, which is based on symptoms and MRI depiction.

This should be useful in evaluating the results from different centers in the future.—R.M. Crowell, M.D.

Clinical Parameters in 74 Consecutive Patients Shunt Operated for Normal Pressure Hydrocephalus
Larsson A, Wikkelsö C, Bilting M, Stephensen H (Sahlgren Hosp, Gothenburg, Sweden)
Acta Neurol Scand 84:475–482, 1991   27–7

Introduction.—Normal pressure hydrocephalus (NPH) is usually treated by diversion of cerebrospinal fluid (CSF) through a ventriculoperitoneal or ventriculoatrial shunt. Success rates as great as 80% and complication rates as great as 52% have been reported. The prevalence of the various symptoms of NPH, how the symptoms are affected by the shunt operation, and the prognostic factors, complications, and social impact of the operation were evaluated prospectively.

Methods.—During a 1½-year period, ventriculoperitoneal shunt operations were performed on 74 patients with NPH. This group consisted of 40 men and 34 women (mean age, 64 years). All underwent standardized examinations before and after surgery. This allowed creation and comparison of 6 different clinical indices to assess the effects of the operation: social functioning, neurologic signs, gait ability, continence, psychometric performance, and psychiatric condition. Mental symptoms were noted in 96%, gait disturbances in 95%, and incontinence in 75%.

Findings.—Postoperatively, 78% of patients improved and 22% deteriorated. A total of 80% had an improved psychiatric condition, and 76% had improved gait. Of the patients whose condition was caused by subarachnoid hemorrhage, 98% showed improvement vs. 73% of those with idiopathic NPH. The worst response was unrelated to old age; however, it was related to long-standing symptoms. 11% of the patients no longer required institutionalization, and the need for help in activities of daily living decreased by 36%. Half the patients had complications of their operation; the shunt-related mortality was 1%. There was a 31% rate of shunt malfunction, a 19% rate of infection, and a 9% rate of epilepsy, all appearing within 1 year postoperatively.

Conclusion.—Shunt surgery for NPH can decrease all of the classic symptoms, especially mental functioning and gait. Outcome could not be predicted by any symptom or sign, and the unfavorable factors appear to include dysphasia, incontinence, and long duration of disease. The complication rate is very high, but the social impact of treatment is important.

▶ This is yet another report of the results of ventriculoperitoneal shunting for normal pressure hydrocephalus. Substantial improvement was noted in many of the patients, with cases of subarachnoid hemorrhage improving most often (98%), and idiopathic NPH improving somewhat less often (73%). The specific features for attention include complications in 50% of the cases with a 1% mortality; shunt malfunction was the most common complication (31%), followed by infection (19%). Moreover, the preoperative evaluation cannot reliably indicate which patients will improve from treatment. Thus, this very significant complication rate cannot be reduced significantly by patient selection.—R.M. Crowell, M.D.

Characterization of Periventricular Edema in Normal-Pressure Hydrocephalus by Measurement of Water Proton Relaxation Times

Tamaki N, Shirakuni T, Ehara K, Matsumoto S (Kobe Univ School of Medicine, Kobe, Japan)
J Neurosurg 73:864–870, 1990   27–8

Introduction.—The molecular dynamics of biological water in hydrated tissues can be evaluated by use of water proton MRI, in which a direct relationship exists between the relaxation times of the water protons and the total water content of the tissues.

Study Design.—Magnetic resonance imaging was performed in 21 patients with normal pressure hydrocephalus (NPH) who underwent CSF shunting and in 17 control patients. Of the patients with NPH, 14 had good response to CSF shunting (true-NPH group), and 7 showed no response (false-NPH group). The MR longitudinal relaxation time (T_1) and the transverse relaxation time (T_2) of the water proton of the periventricular white and cortical gray matter were compared among all groups. Postshunt MRI in patients with NPH was performed at an average 51 days after surgery.

Findings.—In the true-NPH group, both the T_1 and T_2 of the periventricular white matter were significantly longer than those of the false-NPH group and the control patients. The preshunt T_1 and T_2 of the white matter were significantly longer than those of the gray matter, which was the reverse of the relationship seen in control patients. Both the T_1 and the T_2 of the white matter shortened considerably after CSF shunting. In the false-NPH group, T_1 (but not T_2) of the white matter was significantly prolonged compared with the T_1 in controls. There was no significant difference in either T_1 or T_2 between the white and gray matter in the false-NPH group, and there was no change in T_1 or T_2 after CSF shunting. Among all 3 groups, there were no significant differences in the T_1 or T_2 of the gray matter or between preshunt and postshunt measurements.

Conclusion.—True and false NPH may be distinguished by measurements of relaxation times. The difference in relaxation behavior between these 2 entities may be explained by the difference in properties of the biological water and its environment.

▶ This interesting study suggests that prolongation of T_2 in the brain is abnormal in true NPH, but not in those patients who did not respond to shunting. If confirmed, the technique might be helpful in identifying patients for shunting. The study also raises the possibility of quantitative techniques in MRI being used as a tool for understanding the pathophysiology of a variety of edema-forming conditions.—R.M. Crowell, M.D.

Benign Intrinsic Tectal "Tumors" in Children

May PL, Blaser SI, Hoffman HJ, Humphreys RP, Harwood-Nash DC (Hosp for Sick Children, Toronto)

J Neurosurg 74:867–871, 1991   27–9

Background.—Previously, children with brain stem tumors had uniformly poor prognoses; however, recent studies of aggressive surgical management in certain well-defined subgroups have been more helpful.

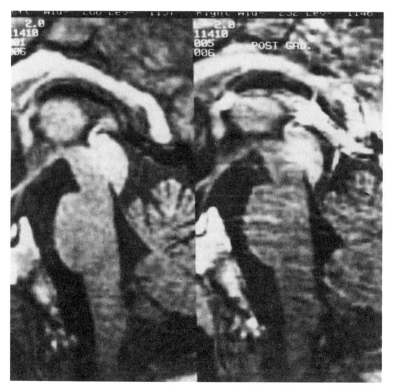

Fig 27–3.—Sagittal T1-weighted MRI before (**left**) and after (**right**) administration of Gd-DTPA. A slightly hyperintense, bulbous tectal plate is revealed with lack of contrast enhancement. (Courtesy of May PL, Blaser SI, Hoffman HJ, et al: *J Neurosurg* 74:867–871, 1991.)

Six children who belonged to a small subgroup of children with benign brain stem tumors managed with CSF diversion alone were studied.

Methods.—Computed tomography and MRI were used to identify intrinsic dorsal midbrain tumors in 5 boys and 1 girl (Fig 27–3). All patients were seen with hydrocephalus caused by obstruction of the sylvian aqueduct. No patient had brain stem signs referable to the tectal mass at presentation, and only 1 had transient Parinaud's syndrome during a period of shunt malfunction. Diversion of CSF was the only surgical procedure performed in all patients. Specific neurologic features common to all patients included: ventriculomegaly seen at diagnosis, tectal distortion by focal tectal mass, focal calcification, persistently abnormal signal on MRI, and lack of growth of lesions over time.

Results.—During follow-up of 8 months to 17 years, there was no evidence of progression in any patient. Serial scanning revealed that contrast enhancement became less prominent as the lesions became progressively more calcified. Five patients have had normal intellectual development.

Conclusion.—In contrast to most periaqueductal and tectal tumors, this group of lesions was apparently truly benign. Patients seen with these clinical and radiologic features may be managed by CSF diversion, serial CT scanning, and MRI.

▶ The results of this study support the proposition that CSF shunting and serial MRI may offer the best approach in patients with tectal lesions showing calcification or increased signal, as well as MR images with increased T_2 signal and no cyst. This is appropriate, because these lesions generally have a rather benign, indolent course.—R.M. Crowell, M.D.

28 Functional

Epilepsy

Temporal Lobectomy for Intractable Epilepsy in Patients Over Age 45 Years

McLachlan RS, Chovaz CJ, Blume WT, Girvin JP (Univ Hosp; Univ of Western Ontario, London, Ont)
Neurology 42:662–665, 1992   28–1

Objective.—Several reports have addressed the results of temporal lobectomy for the management of uncontrolled focal epilepsy in children, but little research has assessed the prognostic importance of older age. The results of temporal lobectomy in 20 patients older than 45 years of age were evaluated.

Patients.—The 20 patients had intractable seizures and were followed for more than 2 years after treatment. There were 15 men and 5 women with a mean age 51 years. All had complex partial seizures, and 13 also had secondarily generalized seizures. All but 1 had seizures recorded from the resected temporal lobe by scalp electroencephalographic telemetry, and all had interictal focal spikes recorded from the resected focus. The mean follow-up was 5 years.

Results.—At follow-up, 30% of the patients had no seizures of any kind, and 35% had a greater than 90% reduction in seizure frequency. The corresponding figures for a group of 68 younger patients with similar follow-up were 40% seizure free and 44% with greater than 90% seizure reduction; the differences were nonsignificant. The remaining 35% of the older patients had a poor outcome. A total of 85% of the patients with complex partial seizures had a good outcome, compared with only 38% of those with secondarily generalized seizures. The complications were mild and usually transient, as they were in the younger patients.

Conclusion.—The surgical management of intractable temporal lobe epilepsy appears to be an effective treatment option for older patients, with two thirds obtaining good seizure control. This is true even for patients in their 60s. Hoewver, this study and the authors' own experience suggest that surgery may be somewhat more effective in younger patients.

▶ The take-home message of this study is that temporal lobectomy for intractable epilepsy is effective in two thirds of the patients who undergo surgery after the age of 45 years. The complications of surgery are minor; therefore, the operation should not be withheld from patients on the basis of their age alone.—R.M. Crowell, M.D.

Second Operation After the Failure of Previous Resection for Epilepsy

Awad IA, Nayel MH, Lüders H (Cleveland Clinic Found, Cleveland)
Neurosurgery 28:510–518, 1991   28–2

Introduction.—In patients with recurrent intractable partial seizures after initial resection for epilepsy, seizure control may be achieved with additional resection. Patient selection and the technical aspects of remapping and second operations in these patients were reviewed.

Methods.—Fifteen patients with recurrent intractable partial seizures after resection for epilepsy underwent a second operation at a mean interval of 38 months from the time of the first operation (range, 3 months 12 years). All patients had neuroimaging studies, neurophysiological evaluation and noninvasive detailed video-electroencephalographic evaluation. Eleven patients also underwent invasive remapping using subdural electrodes before surgery.

Findings.—Recurrent epileptogenesis occurred outside the area of previous resection in 3 patients; all 3 foci were extratemporal and were located in the ipsilateral hemisphere. The other 12 patients showed persistent epileptogenicity in the area of previous extratemporal resection in 2 and previous temporal resection in 10. Both patients with extratemporal recurrences had residual unresected structural lesions. Among the patients with local temporal recurrence, recurrent epileptogenicity was demonstrated in the residual mesial structures in 6; it was demonstrated in the residual unresected lateral temporal lobes in 4. During a mean follow-up of 18 months (range, 8–82 months) after the second operation, 47% of the patients remained seizure free, and 33% achieved a reduction in seizure frequency of 90%. There was no mortality or significant morbidity.

Conclusion.—A subgroup of patients with epilepsy had failure of initial resection as a result of "failure to undergo the optimal surgical procedure," which reflected a gross mislocalization of the epileptogenic foci before the initial operation, insufficient excision of the epileptogenic brain, or incomplete resection of an epileptogenic structural lesion. Individualized second operations can be safe and effective, and they can provide selected patients with "failed cases" another chance at seizure control. The use of subdural electrodes is extremely useful and safe in the evaluation of these patients.

▶ The experience of the Cleveland Clinic group indicates that 6 of 10 patients with local temporal recurrence had proven epileptogenic potentials in residual mesial structures, and 4 had residual lateral temporal epileptogenicity. Recurrent intractable seizures usually originate in the area of previous resection, and selected patients with failure of initial resection often can benefit from a second resection of residual epileptogenesis.—R.M. Crowell, M.D.

Developmental Anterobasal Temporal Encephalocele and Temporal Lobe Epilepsy
Leblanc R, Tampieri D, Robitaille Y, Olivier A, Andermann F, Sherwin A (Montreal Neurological Inst and Hosp, Montreal; McGill Univ, PQ)
J Neurosurg 74:933–939, 1991   28–3

Background.—Surgical treatment of medically intractable seizures depends on the ability to identify epileptogenic area in an expendable region of the brain. The development of MRI has made it possible to identify previously undiagnosed structural lesions. The association between an anterobasal temporal lobe encephalocele and medically intractable temporal lobe epilepsy was examined in 3 patients who were successfully treated surgically.

Case Report.—Man, 26, had been delivered at term birth with forceps after prolonged labor. At aged 21 years, he had 2 generalized tonic-clonic seizures while sleeping. Although the generalized seizures did not recur, the patient had psychomotor seizures with complex automatisms, during which he was mute and apparently uncomprehending. Neuropsychologic assessment was consistent with dominant temporal lobe dysfunction. Epileptic activity from the mesial and anterior neocortical surfaces of the left temporal lobe was recorded. Magnetic reso-

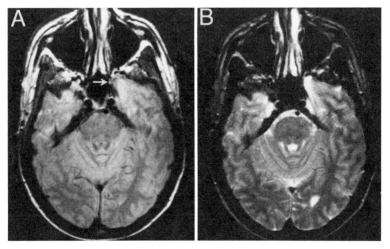

Fig 28–1.—Proton density (**A**) and T2-weighted (**B**) MR images, axial view. The meningoencephalocele (*arrow*) extends from the left temporomesial region anteriorly toward the pterygopalatine fossa. (Courtesy of Leblanc R, Tampieri D, Robitaille Y, et al: *J Neurosurg* 74:933–939, 1991.)

nance images demonstrated a meningoencephalocele extending from a defect at the base of the greater sphenoid wing and continuing into the pterygopalatine fossa (Fig 28-1). Surgery revealed that the encephalocele protruded from the middle cranial cavity through a 2-cm defect in the greater sphenoid wing in the region of the foramen rotundum. The patient remained seizure free 1 year after surgery.

Conclusion.—This case and the 2 others examined represent a condition of disordered embryogenesis in which a developmental anterobasal temporal encephalocele acts as the substrate for temporal lobe epilepsy. This lesion should be considered in the differential diagnosis of late-onset temporal lobe epilepsy. Magnetic resonance imaging can confirm the diagnosis preoperatively.

▶ The 3 cases described by the author indicate that MRI can make the diagnosis of medial temporal encephalocele, and that surgical excision (including removal of the amygdala and hippocampus) can be effective in seizure control.—R.M. Crowell, M.D.

Functional Hemispherectomy: EEG Findings, Spiking From Isolated Brain Postoperatively, and Prediction of Outcome
Smith SJM, Andermann F, Villemure J-G, Rasmussen TB, Quesney LF (McGill Univ, Montreal; Montreal Neurological Hosp and Inst, Montreal, PQ)
Neurology 41:1790–1794, 1991   28–4

Background.—In functional hemispherectomy performed for intractable epilepsy, the frontal and occipital lobes and their blood supply are left intact; however, they functionally disconnected from the rest of the brain. The prognostic significance of preoperative electroencephalographic (EEG) findings in patients undergoing functional hemispherectomy was investigated.

Patients.—All 25 patients had frequent and debilitating seizures, moderate-to-severe hemiparesis, hemianopia, and variable mental retardation. The average age at operation was 13½ years, and the mean age at seizure onset was 4 years. The patients underwent functional hemispherectomy at 1 institution during a 12-year period. Multiple preoperative and postoperative EEG examinations were performed in all cases, and most of the patients had preexcision and postexcision electrocorticography.

Findings.—Eighteen patients were seizure free postoperatively, 5 had recurrent or persistent seizures, and 2 had continued seizures. Of the 5 patients with bilateral independent epileptogenic foci, only 3 became seizure free after hemispherectomy. The outcome was good in patients with abnormal background activity over the "good" hemisphere, multifocal epileptic activity on the operative side only, or bilaterally synchronous discharges. In some patients, benign discharges occurred in the functionally isolated frontal and occipital cortex.

Discussion.—Bilateral independent epileptogenic foci usually indicate less than satisfactory outcome after functional hemispherectomy. The isolated cortex may show benign discharges postoperatively, which indicate that the cortex remains viable and continues to generate epileptogenic potentials.

▶ Functional hemispherectomy is a functionally complete but anatomically subtotal hemispherectomy, which is performed to obtain seizure control but avoid cerebral hemosiderosis. The authors note that the electrophysiologic findings may help to identify an encouraging prognosis.—R.M. Crowell, M.D.

Pain

Clinical Application of a Patient-Controlled Apparatus for Ventricular Administration of Morphine in Intractable Pain: Report of 28 Cases
Shoulong L, Jianlong W, Rongzeng W, Quan W (Naval Hosp; Naval Med Research Inst, Shanghai, People's Republic of China)
Neurosurgery 29:73–75, 1991   28–5

Purpose.—Previously, successful relief of intractable pain was achieved with injection of morphine into the ventricle through an Ommaya reservoir. A patient-controlled device, the L-224, has now been developed for patient-controlled ventricular morphine administration. It has been used in 28 patients with intractable pain.

Technique.—The L-224 consists of a drug reservoir, 1-way valve, injection pump, ventricular tube, and slit valve. A small amount of drug is delivered in response to pressing of the pump by the user. The ventricular tube is inserted into the lateral ventricle, and the scalp is undermined anterior to the hairline to make room for the reservoir. The patient is left with a slight protuberance under the scalp. One mg of morphine hydrochloride diluted with 1.5 mL normal saline is injected into the reservoir. When the patient presses the pump, approximately 50 μg of morphine, which gives nearly 20 hours of pain relief, is delivered.

Results.—The 28 patients had had intractable pain for an average of 4 months. Implantation of the L-224 was successful in 27 patients. The average initial morphine dose was 1 mg, which provided an average of 170 hours of pain relief. The average dose of morphine was 1.8 mg, and the average duration of pain relief per filling of the reservoir was 137 hours. Treatment lasted an average of 57 days, and 96% of the patients had an excellent response.

Conclusion.—The L-224 patient-controlled device for ventricular administration of morphine appears to be safe and reliable for patients with intractable pain. The effect appears best for sharp pain and neuralgias and for patients with a greater dependence on analgesics. Trained family members and family physicians may fill the reservoir for the sake of convenience.

▶ In Europe, the use of intraventricular morphine for intractable pain has become an established practice (1). This report from China documents a very satisfactory experience with patient-controlled administration of intraventricular morphine for intractable pain in 28 patients. This method should eventually become more widely available in this century for patients with intractable pain.—R.M. Crowell, M.D.

Reference

1. Weigl K, et al: *Acta Neurochir Suppl (Wien)* 39:163, 1987.

Treatment of Chronic Pain by Epidural Spinal Cord Stimulation: A 10-Year Experience
Kumar K, Nath R, Wyant GM (Univ of Saskatchewan, Regina; Univ Hosp, Saskatoon, Saskatchewan, Canada)
J Neurosurg 75:402–407, 1991   28–6

Objective.—The usefulness of long-term epidural stimulation for relief of chronic organic pain of nonmalignant origin was studied.

Treatment.—A total of 121 patients with chronic pain of benign organic etiology that was unresponsive to conventional pain control were treated by epidural spinal cord stimulation. Electrodes were implanted, either percutaneously or through a small laminotomy, at varying sites as dictated by the location of pain. Of the 140 epidural implants used, 76 were unipolar, 46 were Resume electrodes, 12 were bipolar, and 6 were quadripolar. Most (96%) of the patients had pain in the back and lower extremities, including 56 with the failed-back syndrome. The causes of pain are summarized in the table. Pain relief was based on subjective reports and on the visual analogue scale and modified McGill Pain Questionnaire.

Results.—During a mean follow-up period of 40 months (range, 6 months–10 years), 40% achieved excellent pain relief by neurostimulation alone, whereas another 12% required analgesic supplements to achieve 50% or more relief in addition to the regular stimulation program. Those patients with pain secondary to arachnoiditis or perineural fibrosis after multiple intervertebral disk operations, lower-extremity pain caused by multiple sclerosis, and pain resulting from advanced peripheral vascular disease had uniformly good results. Patients who responded to preliminary transcutaneous electric nerve stimulation generally did well with electrode implants. The patients with pain caused by cauda equina injury, paraplegic pain, phantom-limb pain, pure midline

Initial and Long-Term Results of Spinal Cord Stimulation

Etiology of Pain	No. of Cases	Initial Results		Results With Permanent Implantation	
		Success	Failure	Success	Failure
low-back & leg pain	66	57	9	37	20
multiple sclerosis	9	9	0	7	2
peripheral vascular disease	5	4	1	4	0
intercostal neuralgia	7	5	2	4	1
spinal cord tumor	2	1	1	1	0
facet syndrome	5	4	1	3	1
causalgia	3	2	1	1	1
bone & joint disease	3	1	2	1	0
cauda equina syndrome	6	4	2	1	3
brachial plexus/peripheral nerve injury	5	4	1	2	2
perianal pain	3	1	2	1	—
phantom-limb pain	2	0	2	—	—
peripheral neuropathy	2	1	1	0	1
post-herpetic neuralgia	1	0	1	—	—
spinal cord trauma	2	1	1	0	1
total cases	121	94	27	62	32

Note: Success = good or excellent pain relief; initial failure = system not internalized; subsequent failure = initial pain relief but late loss of pain relief.
(Courtesy of Kumar K, Nath R, Wyant GM: *J Neurosurg* 75:402–407, 1991.)

back pain without radiculopathy, or pain resulting from primary bone or joint disease did not appear to respond as well. Complications included wound infection, electrode displacement or fracturing, and fibrosis at the stimulating tip of the electrode. Tolerance to the analgesia developed in two thirds of the failures, particularly during the first 2 years of treatment. Three patients died of unrelated causes.

Conclusion.—Epidural spinal cord stimulation is an effective and safe means of controling chronic pain in a selected group of patients. Treatment success depends mostly on the proper selection of patients.

▶ Posterior column stimulation is enjoying a rebirth. This report details a 10-year experience with posterior column neural stimulation for benign pain. Approximately 50% of the patients had significant relief. The bulk of the cases were failed back syndromes. This method should not be forgotten in the treatment of chronic pain.—R.M. Crowell, M.D.

Microcompression of the Trigeminal Ganglion for Trigeminal Neuralgia: Experience With 70 Patients

Peragut JC, Gondin-Oliveira J, Fabrizi A, Sethian M (Hôpital de la Timone, Marseille, France; Instituto de Neurologia, Fortaleza, Brazil)
Neurochirurgie 37:111–114, 1991   28–7

Background.—Percutaneous microcompression of the trigeminal ganglion in the treatment of trigeminal neuralgia was first introduced in 1983. This surgical technique involves the percutaneous placement and inflation of a Fogarty balloon under radiographic guidance. An experience with this technique was reviewed.

Study Design.—Since 1985, 90 patients with trigeminal neuralgia have undergone percutaneous balloon microcompression of the trigeminal ganglion, 70 of whom were evaluable. There were 45 women and 25 men, aged 30–84 years, of whom 61 had typical facial neuralgia and 9 had symptomatic facial neuralgia secondary to other diseases. All patients had failed to respond to previous medical treatment with carbamazepine, dihydantoin, clonazepam, or baclofen. Thirteen patients previously had undergone unsuccessful thermocoagulation. All patients underwent preoperative CT with iodide contrast medium. The procedure was performed using general anesthesia of short duration. The patients remained hospitalized for 3 days. Follow-up ranged from 6 months to 5 years, and the average follow-up was 16.7 months.

Results.—Sixty-eight (97.5%) of the 70 patients had immediate postoperative relief of facial pain. Two operations failed completely. Fourteen patients (20.5%) had a recurrence 1–24 months after the initial procedure. Nine patients underwent repeat microcompression, with excellent results in 8 patients and failure in 1. Thus, 62 patients (88.5%) were free of pain at follow-up, 54 of them after a single procedure. Five patients obtained pain relief by other means, and 3 patients failed to respond to any treatment. Postoperative facial hypoesthesia occurred in 14.3% of the patients, loss of the corneal reflex without keratitis occurred in 11.4%, and dysesthesias without anesthesia dolorosa was noted in 11.4% of the patients.

Conclusion.—In the treatment of trigeminal neuralgia, percutaneous microcompression of the trigeminal ganglion is a safe and effective procedure that should be considered a first-line therapy. The procedure is particularly suitable for elderly and uncooperative patients, or for patients who are in poor physical health. In case of recurrence, the procedure may be repeated.

▶ The results of percutaneous balloon compression were excellent in this group of 70 patients, with 88% of the patients pain free at 6–60 months. It is hard to argue with the contention that this technique should be considered the initial treatment for trigeminal neuralgia in aged and medically disabled patients.—R.M. Crowell, M.D.

Implantation

Implantation of Human Fetal Ventral Mesencephalon to the Right Caudate Nucleus in Advanced Parkinson's Disease

Henderson BTH, Clough CG, Hughes RC, Hitchcock ER, Kenny BG (Univ of Birmingham, England)
Arch Neurol 48:822–827, 1991 28–8

Background.—Animal models of Parkinson's disease (PD) support clinical trials of implantation of human fetal DNA neurons. Fetal ventral mesencephalon was implanted in 12 patients with advanced PD, and the patients were followed up for 12 months.

Methods.—The implant tissue consisted of disaggregated ventral mesencephalic tissue from single aborted human fetuses ranging from 11 to 18 weeks of gestational age. All tissues were obtained according to existing British ethical guidelines. The tissue was implanted using stereotaxic methods and in a consistent striatal site, regardless of the asymmetry of the patients' disease. No immunosuppressive therapy was used; the patients were all receiving optimal levodopa therapy. Follow-up examinations were done every 3 months for 1 year.

Results.—Three patients showed significant and sustained improvements at 1 year. In 2 cases, the motor fluctuations were completely absent. In the group as a whole, modest improvements were noted through the first 6 months. These included better quality of "on" and "off" phase, more "on" times, and particular improvements in bradykinesia of the contralateral upper limb. The mean levodopa requirements were reduced to 64% at 6 months and to 61% at 1 year. In 9 patients, follow-up was consistent for the full year; 3 of the 9 had deterioration to below baseline ratings.

Conclusion.—Patients with advanced PD can benefit from implantation of midgestational human fetal tissue. Improvements are noted in the motor state in both "on" and "off" phases. In some cases, they are sustained and accompanied by reductions in levodopa requirements. The patient's severity of disease may be an important factor; more study is needed to identify the patient factors affecting outcome.

▶ Hitchcock and colleagues present data on 12 patients with advanced Parkinson's disease indicating that grafting of midgestational human fetal tissue (ventral mesencephalon) to the caudat nucleus can lead to improvement in neurologic performance. Further data will be needed both to identify the host factors influencing outcome and to establish the clinical indications, if there are any. It will be necessary to overcome moral concerns about this approach before such studies can proceed in this country.—R.M. Crowell, M.D.

Intraputaminal Infusion of Nerve Growth Factor to Support Adrenal Medullary Autografts in Parkinson's Disease: One-Year Follow-Up of First Clinical Trial

Olson L, Backlund E-O, Ebendal T, Freedman R, Hamberger B, Hansson P, Hoffer B, Lindblom U, Meyerson B, Strömberg I, Sydow O, Seiger Å (Karolinska Inst, Stockholm; Haukeland Hosp, Bergen, Norway; Uppsala Univ, Uppsala, Sweden; VA Med Ctr and Univ of Colorado, Denver; Danderyd Hosp, Stockholm)

Arch Neurol 48:373–381, 1991   28–9

Purpose.—In animal studies, the efficacy of chromaffin grafts has been increased by infusion of the nerve growth factor into the grafted area for a period of time after grafting. A trial of supporting grafted adrenal chromaffin tissue in the putamen of a patient with an infusion of nerve growth factor was assessed. Woman, 6, had a 19-year history of Parkinson's disease complicated by on-off phenomena and drug-induced hyperkinesia.

Methods.—The left adrenal gland was removed, and the medulla was dissected into pieces in a solution of nerve growth factor purified from mouse submandibular gland. The pieces were implanted in the left putamen and infused for 23 days with 3.3 mg total of nerve growth factor.

Results.—The patient experienced no ill effects from the procedures, and antibodies to murine nerve growth factor did not develop. The marked decrease in rigidity on the patient's right side and the decrease in hyperkinesia in the first postoperative month had diminished by the second postoperative month. Diminished improvement is common in patients with adrenal grafts without nerve growth factor support. However, this patient continued a slower phase of improvement for the next 11 months. Improvement was seen in scores from global ratings of hypokinesia and/or rigidity and amplitude of the motor-readiness potential. The scores for hyperkinesia, speed of walking, and fine motor control did not change.

Conclusion.—In this study of a single patient with Parkinson's disease, nerve growth factor was administered to the brain to support chromaffin autografts with no negative effects. The Parkinsonian symptoms gradually decreased in the patient over 11 months. The use of nerve growth factor treatment is safe in humans and may even prolong the effect of adrenal chromaffin autografts.

▶ This report gives very detailed information on a 63-year-old woman with Parkinson's disease that was treated with adrenal medullary autograft and intraputaminal infusion of the nerve growth factor. A marked initial improvement was noted, as was a slower phase of improvement extending for almost a year. The results parallel the results in rodents, which indicate an increase in survival neurite sprouting, and functional effects of grafts in the presence of nerve growth factor. Great caution and further studies will be needed to confirm these findings, but this may give new life to the program for adrenal transplantation in Parkinson's disease.—R.M. Crowell, M.D.

United Parkinson Foundation Neurotransplantation Registry on Adrenal Medullary Transplants: Presurgical, and 1- and 2-Year Follow-Up
Goetz CG, for the United Parkinson Foundation Neural Transplantation Registry (Rush Univ, Chicago)
Neurology 41:1719–1722, 1991   28–10

Background.—In 1987 and 1988, investigators involved in neurotransplantation studies developed a voluntary registry of American and Canadian patients undergoing adrenal medullary transplantation for Parkinson's disease. The data collected from the 13 participating groups at baseline and at 1 and 2 years postsurgery were summarized.

Methods.—The voluntary registry collected demographic, safety, and effectiveness data using the same scoring measures during a follow-up period of 2 years. The Baseline data on 61 patients and follow-up data on 56 patients were studied.

Findings.—A total of 18% of the patients died during the study period. Half the deaths either were related to or *might* have been related to surgery. Global improvement was seen in 32% of the remaining 45 patients at 2 years postoperatively. Significant group improvement at follow-up remained in the amount of daily "on" time and the quality of "off" function, but other measures were not significantly better than baseline values. When global improvement was based on the total sample, including those patients who died and those who were lost to follow-up in the "not improved" category, only 19% were improved 2 years after surgery. Of the survivors, 22% had persistent psychiatric morbidity that was not seen before their operation.

Conclusion.—A modest group improvement in "off" function after neurotransplantation occurred in the patients studied. However, there was a serious amount of morbidity and mortality. Although neurotransplantation may hold promise in the future, the surgical protocol (as outlined in this study) has been discontinued.

▶ This important presentation from the Neurotransplantation Registry provides important results: 2-year follow-up data on 56 patients undergoing adrenal medullary transplantation for Parkinson's disease were presented. There was a modest improvement in all "off" function after transplantation, but 18% of the patients died during the study (half of these deaths were related to surgery), and 22% had persistent, new postoperative psychiatric deficits. These results provide a serious question regarding further use of this treatment.—R.M. Crowell, M.D.

Microvascular Decompression

Microvascular Decompression for Hemifacial Spasm: Analyses of Operative Findings and Results in 310 Patients
Huang C-I, Chen I-H, Lee L-S (Veterans Gen Hosp-Taipei; Natl Yang-Ming Med College, Taipei, Taiwan)
Neurosurgery 30:53–57, 1992   28–11

Background.—In most cases, hemifacial spasm results from a vascular compression of the facial nerve at the root exit zone to the brain stem. Microvascular decompression (MVD) is universally accepted as the best available surgical procedure for the treatment of patients with HFS. A total of 310 Chinese patients with HFS were operated on at 1 center in Taipei between 1983 and 1990, and the operative findings and immediate and long-term results were reviewed.

Patients.—The patients were 167 men and 143 women aged 25–76 years. All underwent MVD. The follow-up ranged from 6 months to 8 years, with a mean of 4.3 years.

Outcomes.—A total of 88% of the patients were completely relieved of spasm within 3 days of the MVD. The remaining 12% had no immediate postoperative improvement. Of the 37 initially unresponsive patients, 5% later had complete relief immediately after a second MVD. Another 1% had delayed complete relief 6–11 months after the first MVD. The remaining 1.6% had only partial relief at 2–9 weeks after 1 MVD. One percent of the patients had late recurrence.

Conclusion.—Reoperation may be postponed for 3–4 weeks if a patient's condition does not immediately improve. A second MVD seems to be of value in some cases.

▶ This report is of interest, not only in that it supports the contention of Janetta that MVD can relieve many cases of hemifacial spasm, but also because it comes from Taiwan, the Republic of China. The authors carefully followed 310 patients—a very substantial experience, and they note that there are recurrences in some individuals and complications of the 7th or 8th cranial nerve dysfunction in others. Overall, however, the 88% complete relief of hemifacial spasm postoperatively bolsters Janetta's position substantially.—R.M. Crowell, M.D.

Hemifacial Spasm: A Review
Wilkins RH (Duke Univ, Durham, NC)
Surg Neurol 36:251–277, 1991   28–12

Background.—Many types of abnormal spontaneous facial movement have been described. Hemifacial spasm is one such abnormal movement.

Hemifacial Spasm.—Hemifacial spasm is a syndrome of spontaneous and gradual onset. Its hallmark is the intermittent twitching of the muscles of facial expression on one side of the face. It typically begins near the eye, spreading later to involve other muscles innervated by the ipsilateral facial nerve, sometimes including the platysma. Atypical hemifacial spasm begins in the buccal muscles and progresses upward over the face. In either form, tonic muscular contractions may appear. A series of twitches, increasing in frequency and intensity, is characteristically followed by a sustained spasm. The involuntary contractions of this syndrome may be triggered by voluntary facial movements, and efforts to relax the face may result in a momentary, slight diminution of spasm. The syndrome is often intensified by fatigue, stress, anxiety, or self-consciousness. A change in head and body position may alter the severity of the spasms. The spasms may persist during sleep. Individuals who have had the condition for some time may subsequently have mild ipsilateral facial weakness.

Diagnosis and Treatment.—Clinicians can diagnose hemifacial spasm by observation and clinical history. Many approaches to treatment have been attempted. The most effective is microvascular decompression of the facial nerve at the pons. However, that treatment is associated with well-recognized risks, such as ipsilateral deafness. This complication can usually be avoided through the use of intraoperative monitoring of auditory evoked potentials.

Conclusion.—Hemifacial spasm is thought to originate mainly during compression of the facial nerve at the pons, typically by an adjacent artery. To date, the most effective treatment is microvascular decompression of the facial nerve at the pons, a procedure that is associated with well-recognized risks.

▶ Dr. Wilkins's exhaustive review documents the essential features of this illness beyond a reasonable doubt. The illness may be diagnosed on characteristic features noted at the bedside. The most common cause is compression of the facial nerve at the pons, usually by an adjacent artery. In experienced hands, Janetta's procedure of microvascular decompression is highly effective, with a low rate of complications. Complications may be prevented by appropriate monitoring, particularly auditory potentials to prevent hearing loss.—R.M. Crowell, M.D.

Neurovascular Compression and Essential Hypertension: An Angiographic Study
Kleineberg B, Becker H, Gaab MR (Medizinische Hochschule Hannover, Germany)
Neuroradiology 33:2–8, 1991   28–13

Objective.—It has been proposed that arterial compression of the left root entry zone (REZ) of cranial nerves IX and X by looping arteries may play a pathogenetic role in essential hypertension. To verify this hypothesis, vertebral angiographies of hypertensive patients were reviewed retrospectively.

Methods.—Using 10 cadavers, the REZ of left cranial nerves IX and X were localized radiographically. By using a pattern of REZ topography developed from the anatomical information obtained from these cadavers, the vertebral angiographies of 99 patients with definite essential hypertension and 57 normotensive controls were evaluated using these patterns.

Findings.—For the hypertensive patients, 81% of the evaluable angiographies showed an artery in the REZ. These patients frequently demonstrated a cranial loop of the anterior medullary segment toward the REZ of the left cranial nerves IX and X. The most frequent artery in the REZ was the posterior inferior cerebellar artery, followed by the vertebral artery. In contrast, only 41.7% of normotensive patients showed an artery in the REZ. The difference between normotensive and hypertensive patients was statistically significant.

Conclusion.—These findings support the hypothesis that essential hypertension is caused by or is associated with neurovascular compression of the REZ of the left cranial nerves IX and X. These findings coincide with the results of clinical studies by Janetta, in which most hypertensive patients who underwent microvascular decompression of the REZ of the left cranial nerves IX and X showed a significant reduction in blood pressure. Prospective studies are warranted to better clarify this association.

▶ It is interesting that 81% of the angiographies done on hypertensive patients showed a loop artery capable of compressing nerves IX and X on the left. This supports Jannetta's theory of the origin of essential hypertension. On the other hand, there are some problems for the theory: What about the 19% of hypertensives without that kind of angiographic evidence of loop? What about the 41% of normotensive patients who had such a loop?—R.M. Crowell, M.D.

Magnetic Resonance Imaging of Vertebrobasilar Ectasia in Tic Convulsif: Case Report
Harsh GR IV, Wilson CB, Hieshima GB, Dillon WP (Univ of California, San Francisco)
J Neurosurg 74:999–1003, 1991   28–14

Introduction.—Magnetic resonance imaging can provide high-resolution images of posterior fossa anatomy. Imaging enhanced by gadolinium is an especially sensitive means of demonstrating tumors and vascular anomalies.

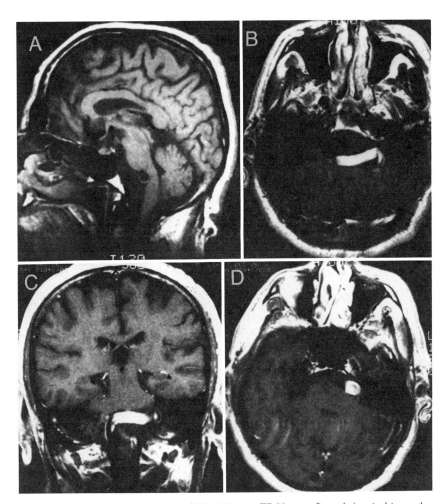

Fig 28–2.—MR images. **A,** T1-weighted (TR 600 msec, TE 20 msec, first echo) sagittal image depicting a vessel indenting and posteriorly displacing the pontomedullary junction. **B,** gadolinium-enhanced T1-weighted (TR 400 msec, TE 20 msec, first echo) axial image confirming the horizontal course of this vessel and depicting its acute turn in the left cerebellopontine angle. **C,** gadolinium-enhanced T1-weighted coronal image showing compression of the caudal pons at the left facial nerve-root exit zone. **D,** gadolinium-enhanced T1-weighted axial image demonstrating compression of the rostral pons at the left trigeminal nerve-root entry zone. (Courtesy of Harsh GR IV, Wilson CB, Hieshima GB, et al: *J Neurosurg* 74:999–1003, 1991.)

Case Report.—Man, 54, was hypertensive and had had left hemifacial spasm for 5 years and left trigeminal neuralgia for 2 months. Most of the muscles near the left eye and cheek contracted spasmodically. Lancinating pain originated above the left eye and radiated into the area of the supraorbital nerve; the trigger zone was in the orbitotemporal region. Computed tomography showed a retroclival mass, and angiography showed ectatic vertebral and basilar arteries, including a much elongated, dilated right vertebral artery. The proximal basilar artery was displaced laterally. Enhanced MRI demonstrated an acutely angulated vessel in the lateral medullary cistern, which compressed the ventrolateral brain stem on the left in the area of the trigeminal root entry zone (Fig 28-2). A massively ectatic vertebrobasilar junction was seen at suboccipital craniectomy, distorting both the brain stem and the cranial nerves. Supraselective subtotal rhizotomy of the first-division fibers was carried out, and a felt paddy was interposed between the remaining fibers and the basilar artery to displace an anterior inferior cerebellar artery loop from the root exit zone. Trigeminal neuralgia and facial spasm were absent postoperatively. Hypesthesia of the first trigeminal division persisted.

Division.—This is 1 of 13 reports of tic convulsif associated with an ectatic vertebral or basilar artery. All cases were left sided. Selective rhizotomy or microvascular decompression of the trigeminal and facial nerves have relieved symptoms in nearly all of these cases.

▶ This interesting report describes MRI evaluation of a patient with trigeminal neuralgia and hemifacial spasm caused by compression of the fifth and seventh cranial nerve root entry zones by a dilated vertebrobasilar artery. The studies provided show with very substantial anatomical detail the nature of the problem; they also suggest appropriate surgical decompression by the Jannetta approach. Both the surgical treatment and the successful outcome are described. Clinicians who face such problems should be aware of the great usefulness of MRI and MR angiography in these cases. In most instances, conventional angiography will still be required.—R.M. Crowell, M.D.

Ablation

Stereotactic Ventrolateralis Thalamotomy for Medically Refractory Tremor in Post-Levodopa Era Parkinson's Disease Patients
Fox MW, Ahlskog JE, Kelly PJ (Mayo Clinic and Found, Rochester, Minn)
J Neurosurg 75:723–730, 1991   28–15

Background.—Not all patients with Parkinson's disease respond well to medication. Surgical treatment still has a role in such cases. The early surgical results and complications in a series of 36 patients who underwent thalamotomy for control of medically refractory parkinsonian rest tremor were evaluated.

Patients and Methods.—The patients underwent ventrolateralis thalamotomy at the Mayo Clinic between 1984 and 1989. All either had been or were being treated with carbidopa/levodopa, but tremor control was unsatisfactory. Modern stereotactic techniques, including microelectrode recording, were used in all cases.

Outcomes.—Thirty-one patients, or 86%, had complete abolition of tremor. Three patients, or 5%, had significant improvement. In 2 patients, tremor recurred within 3 months of surgery. However, the rest of the patients had no recurrences during follow-ups of 14–68 months. Persistent complications occurred in 5 patients, but they were a source of disability only in 1. These complications included arm dyspraxia, dysarthria, dysphasia, and abulia.

Conclusion.—The progression of Parkinson's disease cannot be changed by thalamotomy, but disabling tremor can be abolished in 86% of patients and can be decreased significantly in another 5%. With careful patient selection, accurate preoperative documentation of neurologic deficits, precise surgical localization and lesion production, and the judicious use of postoperative antiparkinsonian medications, many patients with Parkinson's disease may be able to have more tremor-free years.

▶ In the era of widely available medical therapy for Parkinson's disease, patients are seldom referred for stereotactic thalamotomy. This publication from the Mayo Clinic shows that, for patients with disease refractory to medical treatment, thalamotomy remains a highly effective, low-risk treatment option. Both neurologists and neurosurgeons should keep this in mind when treating this common illness.—R.M. Crowell, M.D.

Cingulotomy for Refractory Obsessive-Compulsive Disorder: A Long-term Follow-up of 33 Patients
Jenike MA, Baer L, Ballantine HT, Martuza RL, Tynes S, Giriunas I, Buttolph L, Cassem NH (Massachusetts Gen Hosp, Boston)
Arch Gen Psychiatry 48:548–555, 1991   28–16

Introduction.—For the few patients with obsessive-compulsive disorder (OCD) who fail to respond to behavioral measures and/or drug treatment, cingulotomy is an option. In 1962, Ballantine et al. began a study of bilateral anterior stereotactic cingulotomy performed for very severe psychiatric illness or chronic pain.

Methods.—The results of cingulotomy done in 35 patients over a 25-year period were reviewed; all but 2 patients met the *Diagnostic and Statistical Manual of Mental Disorders, Third Edition, Revised, (DSM-III-R)* criteria for OCD. Six of the patients died, 4 of them by suicide. Of the other 27 patients with OCD, 17 returned a questionnaire and 1 patient agreed to an interview. The patient reports were corroborated by an informant in 10 instances.

Results.—Occasional seizures that were readily controlled by phenytoin were reported by 3 patients. The rate of suicide was 12%. Of the 14 patients reevaluated using the Yale-Brown Obsessive Compulsive Scale, 8 showed moderate-to-marked improvement at follow-up a mean of 5 years after initial cingulotomy. In all, improvement in 9 of 29 patients could be ascribed to surgery itself; 5 patients attributed their improvement to measures other than cingulotomy.

Conclusion.—Early prospective findings suggest that at least 25% of patients with OCD may gain significant benefit from cingulotomy after other measures have failed. Improvement may result from the operation itself, or from its interaction with postoperative behavioral or pharmacologic therapy.

▶ Since the advent of effective psychotropic agents in the 1950s, interest in psychosurgery has waned. Despite identification of the failures of psychopharmacologic therapy, and despite scientific validation of psychosurgery for selected patients, psychosurgery has retained a stigma from earlier times and is uncommon in modern American practice.

Therefore, it is particularly important to read this report on the long-term follow-up of 22 patients treated with restricted psychosurgery (steotactic cingulotomy) for refractive OCD. The first author and most of the research team is composed of psychiatrists (including the Chief of Psychiatry at Massachusetts General Hospital). The results indicate that at least 25% to 30% of the patients substantially benefit from the procedure.

These results indicate that patients with refractory OCD should be carefully considered for cingulotomy by an experienced psychosurgical team.—R.M. Crowell, M.D.

29 Nerve

Suprascapular Nerve Entrapment: A Series of 27 Cases
Callahan JD, Scully TB, Shapiro SA, Worth RM (Indiana Univ Med Ctr, Indian-apolis)
J Neurosurg 74:893–896, 1991   29–1

Background.—Entrapment of the suprascapular nerve as it passes through the suprascapular foramen can lead to chronic shoulder pain and weakness, but this condition is frequently overlooked in the differential diagnosis of shoulder pain. Twenty-seven cases of suprascapular nerve entrapment were examined.

Summary of Cases.—The medical records of 23 patients who underwent 27 surgical procedures for suprascapular nerve entrapment during a 10-year period were reviewed. The patients had a mean age of 37 years and a mean duration of symptoms of 2 years and 10 months. Twelve patients had onset of symptoms after an episode of trauma or heavy lifting. Before receiving the diagnosis of suprascapular nerve entrapment, 6 patients had undergone thoracic outlet procedures, and 3 had received anterior cervical diskectomies without relief of symptoms. Nineteen patients were seen with tenderness over the suprascapular notch, and 15 had positive cross-adduction tests. Thirteen patients evidenced muscular atrophy and motor weakness. The patients initially were treated conser-

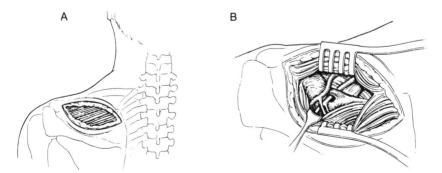

Fig 29–1.—Artist's illustrations during release of suprascapular nerve entrapment. **A,** placement of the initial skin incision and the incision splitting the trapezius muscle *(broken line)*. **B,** the suprascapular nerve is seen as it passes through the notch, and the suprascapular artery and vein are shown coursing over the transverse scapular ligament. (Courtesy of Callahan JD, Scully TB, Shapiro SA, et al: *J Neurosurg* 74:893–896, 1991.)

vatively, but all 23 ultimately underwent surgical release of the entrapped nerve (Fig 29–1).

Results.—Twenty-one patients were pain-free immediately after surgery. Two patients had minimal residual shoulder pain but sought no further treatment, whereas 17 patients remained free of pain and had complete resolution of preoperative weakness. Four patients had recurrent symptoms. Of these, 3 underwent reoperation, which revealed the nerve encased in scar tissue. All 3 patients underwent neurolysis with immediate and sustained relief of symptoms. The fourth patient was lost to follow-up. There were no incidences of wound infection or other postoperative complications.

Conclusion.—Suprascapular nerve entrapment should always be included in the differential diagnosis of chronic shoulder pain. An electromyogram should be obtained if this entrapment neuropathy is suspected, but a negative study does not exclude the diagnosis. All patients should undergo a nerve block. If conservative treatment fails, surgical release of the entrapped nerve is likely to provide complete pain relief and resolution of weakness.

▶ The patients complain of posterolateral shoulder pain. Nerve block transiently relieves pain. Section of the transverse scapular ligament is curative in a great majority of patients. Neurosurgeons should be aware of this entity and its surgical management.—R.M. Crowell, M.D.

Nerve Transfer in Brachial Plexus Traction Injuries
Samardzic M, Grujicic D, Antunovic V (University Clinical Ctr, Belgrade, Yugoslavia)
J Neurosurg 76:191–197, 1992   29–2

Introduction.—The results are usually poor with traction injuries of the brachial plexus. This is especially true in spinal nerve root avulsion, for which the only possibility of repair is nerve transfer. The results of nerve transfer were analyzed in 37 patients with traction injury of the brachial plexus.

Patients.—The patients were all followed for at least 18 months. The age range was 11–57 years, with 81% of the patients being in their twenties or thirties. Twenty-three had upper brachial plexus palsy, and 14 had complete brachial plexus palsy; avulsion injury was present in 32 patients. The patients had a total of 64 reinnervations of the musculocutaneous nerve, axillary nerve, or both, using the upper intercostal, spinal accessory, and regional nerves as donors.

Results.—A total of 70% of the procedures resulted in recovery of useful function. The best recovery rate, 84%, was seen in patients who had upper brachial plexus palsy repaired with the use of regional donor nerves, such as the medial pectoral, thoracodorsal, long thoracic, and subcapsular nerves. Significantly lower recovery rates were seen for procedures using the spinal accessory nerve (64%) and those using the upper intercostal nerve (56%).

Conclusion.—In nerve transfer for the repair of spinal nerve root avulsion in patients with brachial plexus palsy, the use of regional nerves offers a better chance of useful functional recovery than use of the intercostal or spinal accessory nerve. Recovery was most common with combined use of donors, particularly when the regional nerves were used; however, this is controversial. Recovery of even a little function is very important to these patients.

▶ This communication describes 37 patients with 64 innovation procedures for brachial plexus injury. The results show an 83.8% rate of functional recovery in regional nerve transfer (medial-pectoral, thoracodorsal, lung-thoracic, and subscapular nerves). This is superior to the functional results for intercostal transfer (55.5%), spinal accessory transfer (50%), and combined transfer. Although further experience is needed, local nerve transfer appears to offer superior results.—R.M. Crowell, M.D.

30 Miscellaneous

Postoperative Low-Dose Heparin Decreases Thromboembolic Complications in Neurosurgical Patients

Frim DM, Barker FG II, Poletti CE, Hamilton AJ (Massachusetts Gen Hosp, Boston; Univ of Arizona, Tucson)

Neurosurgery 30:830–833, 1992   30–1

Background.—Previous experience with low-dose heparin in neurosurgical patients suggests that perioperative administration can lead to wound complications secondary to bleeding, if not to hemorrhage at the operative site. Venous thrombosis is reduced by low-dose heparin in this setting.

Objective.—Heparin was evaluated in 138 consecutive adult patients undergoing major neurosurgical procedures. The control group included 473 patients who had previously had surgery on the same neurosurgical service, and who had been managed with pneumatic compression boots only.

Management.—Compression boots were used intraoperatively. Starting on the first postoperative day, the study patients received 5,000 units of heparin subcutaneously, twice a day, until they were fully ambulatory. The compression boots were discontinued 24 hours after the start of heparin therapy.

Results.—Thromboembolism occurred in 3.2% of the control group. Seven of these patients had pulmonary embolism, and 4 of them died of related complications. One control patient had bleeding at the operative site. None of the heparin-treated patients had clinical deep venous thrombosis or pulmonary embolism (table), and none had hemorrhagic complications at the operative site. One patient had catheter-related su-

Number of Thromboembolic Complications in
PCB/Heparin-Treated Patients and in Historical Controls

	Control Patients	Heparin Patients
Thromboembolic complications	15 (3.2%)	0 (0%)
Total patients	473	138

(Courtesy of Frim DM, Barker FG II, Poletti CE, et al: *Neurosurgery* 30:830–833, 1992.)

perficial thrombophlebitis in the upper extremity which progressed to deep venous thrombosis and responded to local care.

Conclusion.—Low-dose heparin administration and intraoperative pneumatic compression boots significantly lower the risk of thromboembolism in neurosurgical patients and are considered safe.

▶ Thromboembolic complications continue to plague neurosurgical patients. Although pneumatic compression boots decrease the incidence of lower extremity deep vein thrombosis, they do not affect the incidence of pulmonary embolus, the fatal complication that is of most importance. This small experience suggests that prophylaxis with pneumatic compression boots and postoperative subcutaneous heparin (5,000 units given twice daily) significantly reduces the incidence of thromboembolic complications without causing hemorrhagic complications. Further studies are needed to follow-up on this important initial observation.—R.M. Crowell, M.D.

Subject Index

A

Abulia
organic, bromocriptine and lisuride in, 94

Abuse
analgesic, with migraine, drug withdrawal in, 161
cocaine, neurovascular complications of, 40

Academics
eminent, aging of, 81

Acidosis, lactic (see Lactic acidosis)

Acoustic
imagery, occipital and temporal brain regions in, 77
neurinoma, intracanalicular, 305
neurofibromatosis as distinct from von Recklinghausen's neurofibromatosis, 307
tumors, conservative treatment, 306

Actinomycin D
for cerebral vasospasm prevention, 336

Adrenal
medulla
autograft, nerve growth factor infusion into, in Parkinson's disease, 420
transplant in Parkinson's disease, 421

Age
atrial fibrillation and cerebral infarction risk, 46

Aged
cognitive impairment, mild, 82
dementia estimated prevalence in black and white community residents, 80

Aging
of scientists and academics, eminent, 81

AIDS
CNS lymphoma in, radiotherapy of, 396
(See also HIV)

Alzheimer's disease
amyloid P immunoreactivity in neurofibrillary pathology of, 89
cognitive alterations in, 85
desferrioxamine in, intramuscular, 91
familial, chromosome 19 linkage in, 88
gene for, segregation analysis, 87
memory and attention in, 83
natural killer cell activity in, 63
proteoglycans hypothesis, 86
synapse loss in cognitive impairment, 85
tacrine in, 92

Amantadine
in ataxia, heredo-degenerative, 222

Amebic
meningoencephalitis, successful treatment, 209

Amyloid
angiopathy, cerebral, surgical risk of hemorrhage in, 353
P immunoreactivity in neurofibrillary pathology of Alzheimer's disease, 89

Amyloidosis
transthyretin, DNA in diagnosis, and mutations, 130

Amyloidotic
polyneuropathy, familial, liver transplant in, 131

Amyotrophic lateral sclerosis (see Sclerosis, amyotrophic lateral)

Analgesic
abuse with migraine, drug withdrawal in, 161

Anesthesia
general, for carotid endarterectomy, 315
local, for stereotactic suboccipital transcerebellar biopsy, 266
regional, for carotid surgery, 312

Aneurysm
carotid artery, unruptured internal, at C3 and C4, 324
cerebellar artery, clipping with rotating applier, 332
cerebral, ruptured, of posterior cranial fossa, CT of, 325
cerebral artery, from proximal segment, 331
circulation, hypothermic circulatory arrest in, 329
intracranial
multiple aneurysms, surgery of, 334
saccular, cerebral artery fenestrations, 332
unruptured, and arteriovenous malformation, 344
unruptured familial, subarachnoid hemorrhage two years after negative angiography, 323
intranidal, in cerebral arteriovenous malformation, 343
intraoperative rupture, without hypotension, 326
subarachnoid hemorrhage in, AT877 for cerebral vasospasm after, 335
surgery
clipping in, temporary, technique and results, 328
timing of, International Cooperative Study on, 326

Angiography
in carotid artery evaluation, extracranial, 105
in cerebral arteriovenous malformation, 340

Author Index

A SIMPLE, ONCE-A-YEAR DOSE!

Review the partial list of titles below. And then request your own FREE 30-day preview. When you subscribe to a Year Book, we'll also send you an automatic notice of future volumes about two months before they publish.

This system was designed for your convenience and to take up as little of your time as possible. If you do not want the Year Book, the advance notice makes it easy for you to let us know. And if you elect to receive the new Year Book, you need do nothing. We will send it on publication.

No worry. No wasted motion. And, of course, every Year Book is yours to examine FREE of charge for thirty days.

Year Book of **Anesthesia**® (22141)
Year Book of **Cardiology**® (22640)
Year Book of **Critical Care Medicine**® (22639)
Year Book of **Dermatology**® (22645)
Year Book of **Dermatologic Surgery**® (21171)
Year Book of **Diagnostic Radiology**® (22613)
Year Book of **Digestive Diseases**® (22625)
Year Book of **Drug Therapy**® (22630)
Year Book of **Emergency Medicine**® (22080)
Year Book of **Endocrinology**® (21174)
Year Book of **Family Practice**® (22124)
Year Book of **Geriatrics and Gerontology** (22611)
Year Book of **Hand Surgery**® (22618)
Year Book of **Hematology**® (22646)
Year Book of **Health Care Management**® (21177)
Year Book of **Infectious Diseases**® (22650)
Year Book of **Infertility** (22637)
Year Book of **Medicine**® (22638)
Year Book of **Neonatal-Perinatal Medicine** (22629)
Year Book of **Nephrology** (21175)
Year Book of **Neurology and Neurosurgery**® (22616)
Year Book of **Neuroradiology**® (21849)
Year Book of **Nuclear Medicine**® (22627)
Year Book of **Obstetrics and Gynecology**® (22636)
Year Book of **Occupational and Environmental Medicine** (22619)
Year Book of **Oncology** (22651)
Year Book of **Ophthalmology**® (22133)
Year Book of **Orthopedics**® (22644)
Year Book of **Otolaryngology – Head and Neck Surgery**® (22609)
Year Book of **Pathology and Clinical Pathology**® (21176)
Year Book of **Pediatrics**® (22130)
Year Book of **Plastic and Reconstructive Surgery**® (22635)
Year Book of **Psychiatry and Applied Mental Health**® (22649)
Year Book of **Pulmonary Disease**® (22624)
Year Book of **Sports Medicine**® (22111)
Year Book of **Surgery**® (22641)
Year Book of **Transplantation**® (21854)
Year Book of **Ultrasound** (21169)
Year Book of **Urology**® (22621)
Year Book of **Vascular Surgery**® (22612)

Mosby-Year Book, Inc. • 11830 Westline Industrial Drive • St. Louis, MO 63146